HIV IN WORLD CULTURES

To A C (my guardian angel)
You taught me that living with AIDS is just another box

HIV in World Cultures
Three Decades of Representations

Edited by

GUSTAVO SUBERO
University of Leicester, UK

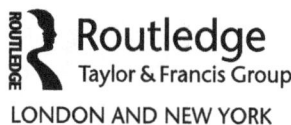

Routledge
Taylor & Francis Group

LONDON AND NEW YORK

First published 2013 by Ashgate Publishing

2 Park Square, Milton Park, Abingdon, Oxfordshire OX14 4RN
52 Vanderbilt Avenue, New York, NY 10017

Routledge is an imprint of the Taylor & Francis Group, an informa business

First issued in paperback 2020

British Library Cataloguing in Publication Data
A catalogue record for this book is available from the British Library

The Library of Congress has cataloged the printed edition as follows:
Subero, Gustavo.
 HIV in world cultures : three decades of representations / by Gustavo Subero.
   pages cm
 Includes bibliographical references and index.
 ISBN 978-1-4094-5398-7 (hardback)
 1. HIV infections--Cross-cultural studies. 2. AIDS (Disease)--Cross-cultural studies.
 3. HIV infections--Prevention--Cross-cultural studies.
 4. AIDS (Disease)--Prevention--Cross-cultural studies. 5. Patient advocacy--International cooperation. I. Title.

 RA643.8.S83 2013
 362.19697'92--dc23

                                                                          2013011984

 ISBN 978-1-4094-5398-7 (hbk)
 ISBN 978-0-367-60127-0 (pbk)

Contents

List of Figures

Notes on Contributors

Paul Attinello is Senior Lecturer at the International Centre for Music Studies at Newcastle University, UK, and has taught at the University of Hong Kong and UCLA. He has published in *Contemporary Music Review, Radical Musicology, The Journal of Musicological Research, Musik-Konzepte, Musica/Realtá*, the revised *New Grove*, and in essay collections and reference works, including *Queering the Pitch: The New Lesbian & Gay Musicology* (Routledge 2006). He is co-editor of collections on reinterpreting the Darmstadt avant-garde and on music in *Buffy the Vampire Slayer*. Current projects include a monograph on music about AIDS and a collection on contemporary composer Gerhard Stäbler.

Roland Bleiker is Professor of International Relations at the University of Queensland. His books include *Popular Dissent, Human Agency and Global Politics* (Cambridge University Press 2000), *Divided Korea: Toward a Culture of Reconciliation* (University of Minnesota Press 2005) and *Aesthetics and World Politics* (Palgrave 2009). His most recent co-edited volumes are *Security and the War on Terror* (Routledge 2007) and *Mediating Across Difference: Pacific and Asian Approaches to Security and Conflict* (University of Hawaii Press 2010). Bleiker is currently working on a project that examines how images – and the emotions they engender – shape responses to humanitarian crises.

Daniela Cápona is an actress, director and playwright. She holds a PhD in Spanish literature by the Universitat de Valencia, Spain. She has conducted research in gender studies and queer studies and their manifestations in theatre and dramatic literature, specifically in a Latin-American context. She teaches history of drama at the Universidad de Chile.

Shoshannah Ganz is Assistant Professor of English at Grenfell Campus, Memorial University, Newfoundland and Labrador, Canada. Her areas of research are in Canadian literature, religious influence on Canadian writing, travel writing, and women's writing. She has published on a number of Canadian authors including Margaret Atwood, Dionne Brand, Pamela Mordecai, Miriam Waddington, Richard B. Wright, and Elizabeth Smart, among others. She has also co-edited *The Ivory Thought: Essays on Al Purdy* (University of Ottawa Press 2008). She is currently in the final stages of editing a monograph on Canadian Literary Pilgrimage and an anthology of Canadian writing on Mexico.

John C. Hawley is Professor and Chair of the English Department at Santa Clara University. He works in postcolonial and gender studies. He is the author of *LGBTQ America Today* (Greenwood Press 2008), *Postcolonial, Queer* (SUNY Press 2001), *Encyclopedia of Postcolonial Studies* (Greenwood Publishing Group 2001), *Cross-Addressing: Resistance Literature and Cultural Borders* (SUNY Press 1996), among others.

Rut Martín Hernández has a PhD in Fine Arts and a Master's Degree in Theory and Practice of Contemporary Arts. She teaches in the Department of Painting in the Faculty of Fine Arts at the University Complutense of Madrid. Her main area of specialization is the art on HIV/AIDS. She has published extensively about this subject, and is the author of the monograph *El cuerpo enfermo. Arte y VIH/ SIDA en España* (Universidad Complutense de Madrid 2011). She has led the research projects *El cuerpo enfermo en el arte contemporáneo* and *Corporalidad e identidad en el arte contemporáneo*. Nowadays, she is part of the research project about 'Image and Philosophy' and of the research group 'Aesthetics and Philosophy of the Image'.

Johanna Hood is a Postdoctoral Research Fellow at the Australian Centre on China in the World, in the College of Asia and the Pacific at the Australian National University and a member of the north-south celebrity network. Her main research interests involve China and the social studies of medicine, health, and disease. Her current interests include medical inequality; economies of disease; health communication, racism, and representation; and public health celebrity. Her recent publications include her book *HIV/AIDS, Health and the Media in China: imagined immunity and racialized disease* (Routledge 2011); a journal article on the political and moral economy of HIV in the *International Journal of Asia Pacific Studies*, and contributions in edited volumes *Unequal China* (Routledge 2012), and *Celebrity China* (HKUP 2010). She also has forthcoming articles on gender, race and representation in China's health media to be published in *Modern China* and an overview of HIV in China in *The Routledge Handbook of Sexuality Studies in East Asia*.

Amy Kay possesses over 10 years of development experience focused in the Middle East, North and Sub-Sahara Africa. She is a global health expert and was instrumental in building the first networks of People Living with HIV (PLHIV) including Women Living with HIV in the Middle East and North Africa, and establishing the first NGOs led by and for PLHIV under USAID/Health Policy Initiative (HPI). She has also served in various capacities for the UN including as Regional Program Officer for UNDP's HIV/AIDS Regional Programme in the Arab States, as well as serving as a technical expert for a number of HIV and youth projects in Sudan and South Sudan. She is currently working for CAMRIS International as Program Manager for the USAID funded Global Health Support Initiative-II.

Felistus Kinyanjui is a socio-historian. She holds a PhD in Humanities from Rhodes University, South Africa. She teaches in the Department of History, Archaeology and Political Studies at Kenyatta University, Kenya. She is a specialist in socio-economic history, particularly in subaltern studies. Her publications are in traditional healing systems and reproductive health. Her current research interest is in the area of armed conflicts in Africa and its implication on health care provision.

Arvind Singhal is the Samuel Shirley and Edna Holt Marston Endowed Professor of Communication at the University of Texas at El Paso and also appointed as the William J. Clinton Distinguished Fellow at the Clinton School of Public Service, Little Rock, Arkansas. He teaches and conducts research in the diffusion of innovations, the positive deviance approach, organizing for social change, the entertainment-education strategy, and liberating interactional structures. He is co-author and/or editor of a number of books, including *Health Communication in the 21ˢᵗ Century* (forthcoming 2013), *Inviting Everyone: Healing Healthcare through Positive Deviance* (CreateSpace 2010); *Communication of Innovations* (SAGE 2006), *Entertainment-Education Worldwide: History, Research, and Practice* (Taylor & Francis 2004), *Combating AIDS: Communication Strategies in Action* (SAGE 2003), *The Children of Africa Confront AIDS: From Vulnerability to Possibility* (Ohio University Press 2003).

Richard Sawdon Smith is a British photographer and Head of the Arts & Media Department at London South Bank University, UK. He is Co-editor of *Langford's Basic Photography* and on the advisory editorial panel of *The Journal of Photography & Culture*. He was winner of the John Kobal / London National Portrait Gallery Portrait Award 1997 and his photographs and writing are published in a variety of books including *Spaces Between Us: Poetry, Prose and Art on HIV/AIDS* (Third World Press 2010), *Cultures of Exile: Images of Displacement* (Berghahn Books 2004), *Art & Photography* (Phaidon Press 2004) and *Male Bodies: A Photographic History of the Nude* (The University of Michigan Press 2004). His photography has been widely exhibited internationally.

Gustavo Subero is a Lecturer in Latin American and Caribbean Cultural Studies at the University of Leicester, UK. His research focuses on sexual cultures in Latin America and the Caribbean and their depiction in popular culture (especially film, literature and media). He is the author of *Queer Masculinities in Latin American Cinema: Male Bodies and Representations* (I.B. Tauris 2013). His new manuscript *HIV/AIDS in Contemporary Hispano-American and Caribbean Culture: Cuerpos suiSIDAs* will be published as part of Ashgate's New Hispanisms Series. He is currently working on a project on Horror Cinema and the Latin American Social Imaginary.

Preface

The December 2012 issue of GT (*Gay Times*) features on the front cover, and as its cover story, an article on "Australia's Olympian Ji Wallace on being out, proud and HIV positive". Although the article, perhaps quite unsurprisingly, is slightly superficial in its treatment of the life and the future of the sportsman, the photographs that accompany the article help to posit seropositivity in a rather unusual light. The front cover obviously intends to lure readers to buy the magazine by depicting Wallace in a lascivious manner: a low angle, full body picture of him lying down wearing only some beach shorts; his bulging, muscled arms slightly flexed around his head; chiselled abs and pumped chest, his very muscular body offered for the taking as he looks furtively and yet seductively at the camera. This image can be easily compared with that of Jack Mackenroth's cover photo (and also story) for PULP in October 2009, describing him as "Project Runaway favourite is Living Positive by Design", making a direct reference to Mackenroth's HIV awareness campaign. In this cover he is presented in a medium shot of his upper body, covering the full length of the cover page, dressed in a red hooded zip shirt opened up and showing his chest and chiselled torso. He also appears on the cover of reFRESH in December 2010 in which he "talks sports, fashion, design and life". This time he is shown in a full-length body shot wearing nothing but white, tight shorts and white football socks, his semi naked and perfectly muscular body once again on display.

Back in the mid-1990s, Greg Louganis' cover picture for *Out* (April 1995) was one of the first to focus on an out and seropositive athlete, whose semi naked and healthy body was directly associated with HIV in a print publication. The Louganis magazine cover is not as sexualised as the others mentioned here, yet his 'healthy' semi nakedness is, arguably, one of the first attempts to destigmatise HIV/AIDS as a death-ridden illness. David Halperin (1997), Gilad Padva (2002) and Nadia Guidotto (2006), among others, may be right to point out that the commodification of queer culture runs the risk of reducing its politics to pure consumerism; however, in the context of HIV/AIDS this may be advantageous to try and eliminate the type of negative and deadly imagery that has accompanied seropositive narratives in contemporary culture (whether gay or straight). Eroticising body images of HIV sufferers could be said to allow queer modes of consumption to count as a resistance cultural practice that has a self-transformative ethical function. In other words, by enticing the prospective reader to establish a sexual empathy with the titillating pictures of these seropositive men, the magazines are to a greater extent changing people's prejudices in relation to HIV sufferers and the illness itself. By positing these HIV positive public figures as objects of desire, the magazine subverts notions of sexual desirability – as circulated in mainstream society – by alluring the reader to regard the seropositive individual as a desirable sexual fantasy. Arguably, in this case it would be justifiable to allow queer commodification to reduce politics into a consumerist lifestyle. Featuring muscled and sexy seropositive men as queer commodities may be more effective to reach the mainstream of queer (and straight) culture than some of the work on HIV advocacy and awareness to date. As a result, queer commodification can be a useful strategy to increase the possibilities for ongoing personal and political transformation in relation to more positive HIV messages.

Heterosexual publications have also featured seropositive people to counter the stigmatisation and stereotyping suffered by such individuals in the years following the advent of the discovery of the disease. For instance, the basketball player Magic Johnson appeared on the cover of a number of prestigious US magazines in the mid-1990s after he made public his HIV status. On the cover of *People* (October 1992) *Magic's Own Story* makes headlines as the cover story. The magazine shows Johnson hugging his baby boy while his wife Cookie leans on his side and hugs him. On the side of the picture it can be read: "In a candid excerpt from his new book, he talks about: his wild years, telling Cookie he has the AIDS virus, how she helps him fight back". The photograph both reinforces the main values of middle class America (economic stability, family unity) and disavows some of the preconceptions surrounding AIDS and ethnic minorities and other populations considered 'at risk'. It is undeniable that seropositive and public celebrities "helped to put a 'human' (and heterosexual) face on AIDS" (Jones 1998: 310). This image manages to dispel fears and stereotypes in relation to black people and AIDS, and to enter the American popular imagination as a family unit whose dynamics does not threaten core values in society or the notions that sustain heteronormativity. Interestingly, Johnson received little criticism or judgement for the actions that led to his infection and was presented by the media as an AIDS survivor rather than a victim.

This is all the more obvious when analysing the trajectory of his magazine covers around the time he disclosed his seropositive status. The cover of *Newsweek* from November 1991 shows a low angle, close medium shot of a shirtless Johnson as he is ready to throw a basketball. In the middle of the cover and in big bold letters it reads 'Even me' – Magic Johnson. The implication is that even someone like him could become seropositive and be infected with the HIV virus. However, rather than alienating his fans, the ideal man encapsulated by the Johnson's star persona suffered a shift and became a symbol of heterosexual prowess as he defied the virus and its correlated stigma. Paradoxically, rather than shunning his star persona by publicly disclosing his HIV status, Johnson's image is rather eroticised in order to heighten his masculinity, even at the crucial moment of announcing his seropositive status. This image of masculine prowess continues on his next magazine cover from the February issue of Newsweek in 1996 in which he is depicted as a superhero. On this cover, a suited Johnson rips open his shirt to reveal his old Lakers' basketball shirt underneath. This photograph is clearly a pastiche of the iconic image of superman, as he reveals his superhero identity, while the magazine reads in bold red letters "It's more than magic". The issue is clearly devoted to the advances in RVT and the fact that HIV/AIDS needs no longer to be regarded as a lethal and/or terminal illness. Unsurprisingly, the other feature story on the cover of the magazine is "New hope for living longer with HIV"; a direct association between this story and Magic Johnson as its living proof is hard to miss. Historically, one can see a shift in the way the media was dealing with news about HIV/AIDS and the way they no longer portrayed the virus and its victims as people sentenced to a well-deserved death. Johnson became the archetype of the AIDS survivor as his media presence highlighted:

> medico-scientific 'breakthroughs' were seen as providing 'new hope', while others favoured 'positive thinking', 'lifestyle' factors and even people's 'naturally' strong immune systems (or constitutions) as the keys to their success. Again, little distinction was drawn between people who were gay or heterosexual in this representation, but the greatest admiration of the press was reserved for the heterosexual sporting hero Magic Johnson (Lupton 1999: 46).

This brief, and rather concise, story of the aforementioned magazine covers is a clear reflection of the way that the notion of HIV/AIDS has circulated in the social and popular imaginary since the first diagnoses appeared in the public domain. The public perception of the illness has changed over the last 30 years. The vilification and ostracism to which carriers and sufferers were once subjected has now, unfortunately, led to social mutism and indifference. The success of antiretroviral therapies has meant that the virus is no longer regarded as a deadly disease. Consequently, HIV/AIDS is no longer a current or 'hot' topic, nor is it devoted much attention in contemporary popular culture and media. Despite institutional and governmental campaigns in sexual health education and HIV prevention, little is said nowadays about HIV/AIDS in mainstream society. Nowadays, HIV/AIDS becomes current once a year around World AIDS Day (1st December), but the sort of currency it enjoyed in the 1980s and 1990s has waned to the point that it is not even a current event in the school calendar, and those populations that were once targeted as 'at risk' no longer participate actively in such programs and events. One such organisation, the AIDS Memorial Quilt, was established in 1987 by the NAMES Project Foundation. It is perhaps one of the oldest and longest running projects on AIDS awareness, and it continues to display the Quilt all over the USA and the world "to foster healing, heighten awareness, and inspire action in the age of AIDS" (www.aidsquilt.org). Although the Quilt continues to have a major presence in AIDS-related events, as well as community halls and other community venues, the impact of the Quilt as a project continues to mainly affect and touch upon the lives of those who are already affected with the virus:

The Quilt is made up of over 48,000 individual panels each measuring 3 by 6 foot. Every panel commemorates the life of someone who has died of AIDS and has usually been sewn together by family, friends and lovers of the person they wish to commemorate. It is estimated that over 14 million people have visited the Quilt at the thousands of displays worldwide and it has been the subject of books, films, scholarly papers, articles, artistic, theatrical and musical performance, and continues to play a vital role in the dissemination of individual and group stories on HIV and AIDS. However, today the Quilt needs to be understood, as suggested by Kevin Michael DeLuca, Christine Harold and Kenneth Rufo (2007), more as an archive than a monument to the AIDS crisis. In this sense, the Quilt nowadays has as its core function that of a public record, "and to make accessible a (partial, contingent) history, a history that is more than sum of the parts on its timeline" (627). In this way, the Quilt could be said to constitute an AIDS relic that attains reverence and also provides comfort to those whose lives have been directly affected by the illness. As a relic, the Quilt provides material benefit in a twofold way: to those who make the patchwork and those who observe the displays. Those who make the individual patches engage in the memorialisation, the creation of a memento mori, of a loved one lost to AIDS and the fact that, as Neil Campbell and Alasdair Kean propose, "each panel of the quilt emphasizes the individuality of the person in stark contrast to the representations that classify and universalise the sufferers" (1997: 201). For those who witness the displays, the vastness of this project is undoubtedly monumental, and it continues to be a reminder to the world of different ways in which HIV/AIDS has changed the lives of many millions across the globe, while considering the individuality of every person's experience. Mary E. O'Brien rightly points out that "The Names Project AIDS Memorial Quilt has provided for thousands of friends, partners, and other family members a treasured vehicle for grieving, remembering, and celebrating the lives of their loved ones […] Its existence will not let us forget those who have 'broken through the boundaries of death' into a different place" (1995: 76). Perhaps it would be pertinent to examine, although not the scope of this collection, the extent to which the Quilt, as a display and a ritualised experience, continues to have the same level of currency as it was originally intended to have. This is all the more poignant when one considers that, at the time of writing this, the Facebook page for the AIDS Memorial Quilt was followed by over 3,000 people – a significantly small number of followers considering that, back in 1987, during the opening display of the Quilt, it was estimated that over half a million people visited the display.

Although this book does not intend to belittle the importance and key role that the project has had in promoting the individual (and sometimes unheard) stories of those dealing with or suffering with the illness, perhaps it is necessary to turn attention to other, more current representations of HIV/AIDS around the world and the different ways in which artists, creators, activists, writers, among others, try to make sense of it, at a time when the advance in medical treatment guarantees the same life expectancy as those who do not suffer the condition. *HIV in World Cultures: 30 Years of Representations* intends to historicise and to offer an analysis of the way that HIV and seropositive subjects have been narrativised in different cultures across the globe since the advent of the 'discovery' of the disease in the 1980s. It also intends to delve into the different strategies of remembrance and/

or coping mechanisms that have been deployed by different (sub)cultural groups and individuals affected either directly or indirectly by the illness. This collection studies a variety of cultural texts and manifestations that help contextualise and historicise the trajectory that such narratives and representations have undergone over the last thirty years. This collection is by no means exhaustive, but gathers a number of representative writings on the way that HIV/AIDS is narrativised in different cultures around the world. The collection is loosely divided into geographical areas (continental experiences) in the hope that such categorisation will help the reader to map more logically the trajectories of HIV/AIDS experiences. The collection opens with works dealing with the North American region. Shoshannah Ganz's 'Canadian Literary Representations of HIV/AIDS' explores Elizabeth Hay's *The Only Snow in Havana* (1992), Tomson Highway's *Kiss of the Fur Queen* (1998) and, secondarily, Timothy Findley's *Headhunter* (1993) and Nino Ricci's *The Origin of the Species* (2008). All of these texts are set in the pre-treatment era of HIV, and the characters living with HIV all face an unknown future and generalised cultural fear and prejudice. She discusses how the narrators negotiate the 'unnamable' qualities of the HIV experience and how art is created by, and survives, disease and death. Likewise, HIV art becomes a liminal space from which to explore other cultural and historical uncertainties. The story of HIV and the resultant art will be shown to connect with other discourses of the 'unnamable' and unknown in Canadian culture, including the threats posed by the United States – a virus that could erase Canadian culture and identity – and the spread of other human-made 'diseases', and the disaster posed by plastic production and pollution, as well as the annihilation of native peoples and culture. Above all, these texts explore the ontological uncertainty of living and creating in the liminality between life with HIV and the coming deterioration resulting from the illness, and the relational, artistic, cultural, environmental, and historical discourse facilitated by memorialising through story the Canadian HIV experience in the pre-treatment era. This chapter is followed by 'Distancing the Recent Past: New Forms of Discomfort with AIDS in the U.S.' in which John C. Hawley discusses how HIV has been commonly misrepresented in the U.S. populace as a white man's disease. The history of the government's and media's lack of discussion of the topic in its early years obscured the perception of its evolution, and partly brought it into being. After years of blissful avoidance of the topic, in 1983 coverage cascaded, and with Rock Hudson's death in 1985 Americans suddenly awoke to the threat that apparently was all around them – within them, in fact. In the following decade gays themselves, in self defence against not only the disease but also the rest of society, coalesced into powerful and disruptive agents for social acceptance, full citizenship, and normalcy. With the appearance of anti-retroviral medication, this newly self-aware lobby lamented its losses in novels, films, paintings, sculpture, and in the process projected an angry and serious presence in American society. This raised the voice of gays and, arguably, other marginalised members of societies around the world. In our own time, this cohesion has been split by the queer theorists who revolt against the assimilation that an earlier, HIV-stricken generation had spent its dying days putting in place.

The argument then moves to the Latin American region with Gustavo Subero's 'Mapping Hetero/Homo-sexuality on the Caribbean, Male, HIV Body'. He is interested in exploring the implications of HIV in the popular perception of machismo and/or effeminacy as the rigid templates for male sexuality in the Caribbean, and how the illness is usually associated with a loss of masculinity (including queer masculinity). He argues that HIV is regarded as a disease that feminises the male body, through its own decay, and strips it of its culturally ascribed masculinity. He proposes that, on the one hand, although machismo is culturally regarded as an innate quality of all males in the Caribbean, it seems to operate at the interstice of hetero/homosexuality, and its loss is both feared and also a constant and real threat. On the other, HIV is regarded as a natural part of the process of sublimation of male subjects who find some form of 'enlightenment' through being positive. This chapter discusses Arnold Antonin's *Le president a-t-il le sida?* and Julian Schnabel's *Before Night Falls*, and shows how the main protagonists' positive status becomes a real threat to their purported masculinity – one that will evolve to a less caricaturised version of itself as both films progress. Finally, this chapter will argue that, in both films, HIV is used as a narrative device that transforms the characters into 'better human beings' by disavowing machismo or effeminacy as stereotypical templates for male sexuality in the Caribbean. Daniela Cápona's 'Mapping the HIV Body in Contemporary Latin American Theatre' studies a selection of plays that focus especially on the effects of HIV in the human body. This chapter addresses the diversity of representations of the HIV-affected body as it appears in plays written by both HIV positive and negative playwrights from Cuba, Venezuela, Peru, Mexico and Argentina from 1990 to 2007. This time frame will allow the articulation of a panoramic view of these representations during a period where conditions surrounding the epidemic – availability and effectiveness of treatment – varied considerably. When dealing with specific representations of the body, the impact of changes in the availability of treatment appears to be less determinant than expected, and comes second to a more prominent tendency to represent the body as the object of a fatal disaggregation of its components. She distinguishes three main ways in which the body is portrayed in its relation to the disease: a) a "fragmented body" in which limbs, fluids and symptoms are seen as isolated from the unity of the "human"; b) a "decomposing body" where the disease appears as a process that disintegrates human materiality, and c) a "venomous body" that emphasises the infectious and even lethal potential of the HIV-affected body. These representations of the somatic and its relation to HIV can also be observed in other artistic formats such as the visual arts. It suggests a certain relation between the mentioned bodily portraits in drama and some similar somatic figurations in the work of visual artists that have HIV as an important issue in their production.

The next section moves to Europe with Richard Sawdon Smith's 'Listening to Myself: Politics of AIDS Representation – a Personal Perspective'. Sawdon Smith has worked almost exclusively for the last 15 years with his own body as the subject of his photographs in various series of self-portraits exploring issues of identity and subjectivity as an HIV positive person. This chapter draws upon the inspiration and influences for this work and articulates the concerns and issues of the author's own photographic practice as an HIV positive artist. Issues of control, or the loss thereof, over one's own body is fundamental to his work, as is the desire to establish an identity by making sense of experiences of health and illness, an identity that acknowledges HIV but is not defined by it. "Listening to Myself" is a quote from the photographer Jo Spence, who came to question the control, authority and power relationship of the doctors in her treatment for cancer through a series of staged self-portraits. Sawdon Smith's practice continues these themes and ideas, although he presents his portraits as generic representations of the 'AIDS Body' that articulate concerns wider than the self. The theme of listening is picked up throughout the chapter in relation to visual representation. He argues that what one needs to do is both look at and listen because of the importance of resisting a silencing of one's voice. He investigates the phenomenon of living with a body that at times appears absent, at times alien, while resisting the categorisation of 'Other' or being classified as a representation of medical objectification. The research analyses the change in subjectivity that comes with a life threatening illness, by interrogating notions of the body defined by scientific discovery. Paul Attinello's 'Who Dies? Transformations in Derek Jarman's Last Films' focuses on the late works of British avant-garde filmmaker Derek Jarman: *The Garden* (1990), *Edward II* (1991) and *Blue* (1993), which combine musical and narrative gestures to negotiate a complex network of history, fantasy, and experience. This network is not, however, aimless or undirected; although sounds, images and stories are derived from a wide range of cultural references and sociopolitical resistances, they ultimately focus on Jarman's increasingly intense personal experience of the HIV crisis and his concomitant grief, illness, and confrontation with death. The then young Simon Fisher Turner's collage scores for all three films – created with the director's encouragement – displayed a wide range of the experimental styles and ideas typical in the late 1980s; these experiments, from minimalism to pop, punk, and electronica, parallel Jarman's play with quasi-musical structures in constructing his avant-garde narratives. Musical moods and pastiches also help to construct Jarman's insistent fusion of homophobia, violence, oppression and Thatcherite conservatism with HIV, and, after the climactic turn of *Edward II*, are themselves transformed into a purified sound world of meditative gongs for the image-less, death-driven *Blue*. Rut Martín Hernandez's 'Within the Limits of the Body: Artistic Images of HIV/AIDS in Spain and its Relation with the Cultural Industry' offers an analysis of the artistic images that have been created in Spain in order to map out this issue, through Spanish artists, works and exhibitions that deal mainly with HIV/AIDS. Taking such works and artists as a point of departure, it is possible to establish an analysis of the complexity of the epidemic in the context of the Spanish society; its mystifications, the understanding of the sick body and the strategies and mechanisms in place to confront negative effects of the illness not only on the AIDS body, but also on the social representation of the illness. The study of visibility devices and the relation between social and artistic manifestations evidences the scarce impact that such works and artists have had within the Spanish cultural industry throughout the last three decades – time in which HIV/AIDS art has not enjoyed a level of social repercussion in accordance with the social impact of the epidemic. These works very rarely receive the interest of artistic institutions – the ones who control the visibility such works may enjoy – which are more preoccupied with the changes that new technologies incorporate into the artistic language. HIV/AIDS art, when they do not constitute museum material and occupy public spaces, end up reduced to peripheral circuits. Furthermore, on the few occasions in which such works are shown, one can observe how the media repercussion is generally reduced.

The following section turns to Africa with Felistus Kinyanjui's 'The Role of Local Communities in Developing Unique and Effective Intervention Responses to the AIDS Epidemic: Experiences from Thika, Kenya'. In Kenya, HIV/AIDS has claimed many lives since 1984, when the first case was diagnosed. Initially, scientific and medical initiatives were launched and lauded as the best way to deal with the pandemic. However, due to the continued rise in new infections, an alternative approach towards dealing with the scourge was sought in the social realm. The need to employ a holistic approach, anchored in the dynamics of societies and their social structures, was perceived to be more feasible. In line with this, locally-developed health messages and channels of communication were devised across Kenya, akin to what was happening elsewhere in Africa. This chapter explores some of these unique social intervention mechanisms in the Thika district of Kenya, an area that has suffered a high toll of sero-prevalence. Local troupes, drama, poems, song and dance are used to develop sex messages, couch them and educate locals of all ages and gender on safe sexual behaviour. Troupes have managed to overcome socio-cultural barriers that silence communities on sexual matters. They reach those infected and those affected, and offer a message of caution to those not infected. To some extent these unique interventions have partly contributed to shatter myths surrounding the causes and effects of the disease; greatly helped reduce stigma and encouraged those infected on how to love positively. The study shows that sexual issues, once held as an abomination, are today shared in public domain. Using drama – deeply embedded in the peoples' customs – life situations are used to make people resonate with the reality of the virus, without eliciting a sense of disrespect and shame. The locally-constructed messages and this local mode of communication have broken silences on sexuality and empowered women to negotiate for safer penetrative sex. Arvind Singhal's 'Deconstructing and Reconstructing Cultural Representations to Strengthen HIV/AIDS Interventions in Africa' continues the study of the region. He argues that the dominant bio-medical approaches construct HIV/AIDS as a life-threatening disease to be feared, resulting from promiscuous and deviant behaviours of the 'others'. Hence most HIV/AIDS interventions have been anti-sex, anti-pleasure, and fear-inducing. While 'sexuality' involves pleasure, bio-medical approaches have rarely constructed sex as play, as adventure, as fun, as fantasy, as giving, as sharing. Devoid of such cultural considerations, many HIV/AIDS programs are largely ineffective. This chapter analyses the role of cultural values in HIV prevention programs to halt the spread of the epidemic. The limitations of the dominant bio-medical approaches to HIV prevention are highlighted, and the role of culturally-based, participatory, and community-driven strategies for HIV/AIDS prevention analysed. By drawing upon examples from this continent, he argues that, for HIV/AIDS programs to be effective, the cultural values, beliefs, and practices of the targeted community need to be thoroughly understood. Only then can communication strategies accentuate the positive undercurrents of a culture, reducing (or completely overcoming) the effects of opposing forces. Roland Bleiker and Amy Kay's 'Representing HIV/AIDS in Africa: Pluralist Photography and Local Empowerment' explores the nature and political consequences of representing HIV/AIDS in Africa, where the disease has taken its greatest toll. They examine how different methods of photography embody different ideologies through which they give meaning to political phenomena. They distinguish three photographic methods of representing HIV/AIDS: naturalist, humanist, and pluralist. Naturalist approaches portray photographs as neutral and value free. Humanist photography, by contrast, hinges on the assumption that images of suffering can invoke compassion in viewers, and that this compassion can become a catalyst for positive change. By examining a widely circulated iconic photograph of a Ugandan woman and her child affected by AIDS-related illnesses, they show that such representations can nevertheless feed into stereotypical portrayals of African people as nameless and passive victims, removed from the everyday realities of the Western world. They contrast these practices with pluralist photography. To do so, they examine a project in Addis Ababa, which used a methodology that placed cameras into the hands of children affected by HIV/AIDS, giving them the opportunity to actively represent what it means to live with the disease. The result is a form of dialog that opens up spaces for individuals and communities to work more effectively in overcoming problematic stigmas and finding ways of stemming the spread of the disease.

Finally Johanna Hood closes the collection with 'AIDS Phobia (*aizibing kongjuzheng*) and the People who Panic about AIDS (*kong'ai zu*): The Consequences of HIV Representations in China'. She argues that China's media, broadly defined, has had a tremendous impact on popular perceptions of HIV/AIDS. Television, radio, newspapers, photojournalism, public health campaigns and service announcements are the main source of information on HIV for over 90 per cent of urban China's population. Among the same group however, fear of the virus and discrimination of HIV-positive people is rife, while 'AIDS panic' has become a newly recognized psychiatric disorder. In this chapter she investigates urban China's media representations of HIV/AIDS to explain this fear and discrimination. She first examines the trends in media narratives on HIV in the early 2000s, notably the widespread coverage of the detection of HIV in particular places and people, namely those in rural China. She also discusses these representations in light of the well-developed academic literature on attitudes and fear toward HIV-positive Chinese, and on the impact China's media has in health communication of HIV/AIDS. The images and language used in these stories conveyed levels of suffering which were unimaginable for most urban readers. In the absence of widespread public health campaigns, the deathscapes portrayed in such stories forged associations between HIV and suffering, blood-selling, and rural areas and everyday experiences. These connections had disastrous consequences on popular explanatory models of HIV: HIV is now a highly stigmatised and widely feared disease; HIV sufferers have alarming rates of depression and suicide, and most urbanites believe themselves to be immune to the virus, as it is frequently shown to only exist in marginalised communities.

References

Campbell, N. and Kean, A. 1997. *American Culture: An Introduction to American Culture*. London and New York: Routledge.

Danto, A.C. 1981. *The Transformation of the Commonplace: A Philosophy of Art*. New Jersey: Harvard University Press.

DeLuca, K.M., Harold, C and Rudo, K. 2007. Q.U.I.L.T.: A Patchwork of Reflections. *Rhetoric & Public Affairs*. Vol. 10 (4), Winter: 626-649.

Gay Times. 2012. December 12, Issue 413.

Guidotto, N. 2006. Cashing in on Queers: From Liberation to Commodification. *Canadian Online Journal of Queer Studies in Education*. Vol. 2 (1). http://jqstudies.library.utoronto.ca/index.php/jqstudies/article/view/3286/1414. Last accessed December 2012.

Halperin, D. 1997. *Saint = Foucault: Towards a Gay Hagiography*. Oxford: Oxford University Press.

Jones, R.H. 1998. Two Faces of AIDS in Hong Kong: Culture and the Construction of the 'AIDS celebrity'. *Discourse & Society*. Vol. 9 (3): 309-338.

Lupton, D. 1999. Archetypes of Infection: People with HIV/AIDS in the Australian Press in the mid 1990s. *Sociology of Health & Illness*. Vol. 21 (1): 37-52.

Newsweek. 1991. November 18.

Newsweek. 1996. February 12.

Nochlin, L. 2006. *Bathers, Bodies, Beauty: The Visceral Eye*. New Jersey: Harvard University Press.

O.Brien, M.E. 1995. *The AIDS Challenge: Breaking Through the Boundaries*. Connecticut: Greenwood Publishing Group.

OUT Magazine. 1995. April.

Padva, G. 2002. Heavenly Monsters: The Politics of the Male Body in the Naked Issue of Attitude Magazine. *International Journal of Sexuality and Gender Studies*. Vol. 7 (4): 281-292.

People Weekly Magazine. 1992. October 19.

PULP Magazine. 2009. October 2. Vol. 12 (3).

reFRESH. 2010. December. Issue 58.

The AIDS Memorial Quilt and The NAMES Project Foundation. http://www.aidsquilt.org/about. Last accessed December 2012.

Chapter 1

Canadian Literary Representations of HIV/AIDS

Shoshannah Ganz

While this study is an attempt to look at the Canadian literary representations of AIDS, the starting point for this discussion will be a more generalized discussion of AIDS art and the representational politics of AIDS literature and art. According to James Miller "[p]redictably, most AIDS fiction functions like the usual kinds of AIDS art – as instruction, memorial, or commodity" (1992: 266). However, other theorists focusing on the metaphorical usage of disease in art, such as Brian Patton – building on the work of Susan Sontag's *Illness as Metaphor* (1978) and *AIDS and its Metaphors* (1989) – argue that the predominant metaphor for HIV/AIDS is military: the immune system is seen to be at war (274-275). The artists, writers, and particularly activists in the AIDS crisis have, likewise, seen their work to be engaged in a fight – one whose object is more than instruction or memorial, although both are certainly a part of the work. An unnamed AIDS activist at the 2010 Mexico City Human Rights Commission AIDS conference put it simply as "at the beginning we were just fighting for the right to bury our dead" (December 2010). It is not surprising then, that the films of the 1990s, collectively called New Queer Cinema, are characterized by what Michele Aaron describes as "defiance" (2004: 3) – works that are "unapologetic about their characters' faults" and "defy the sanctity of the past" (4). And while Peggy Phelan sees "interrogation of causality" – what is the cause of homosexuality and AIDS? – as the central question of works such as *Silverlake Life* (1997: 159), Gabriele Griffin's *Representations of HIV and AIDS: Visibility Blue/s* (2000) focuses on "why HIV/ AIDS, a visually under-determined illness, surfaced in visually over-determined media (film, theatre, photography, poster campaigns, art)" (17). In fact, campaign and art projects like the one started by three Canadian artists in New York, who took the Acquired Immune Deficiency Syndrome acronym AIDS and rearranged and proliferated this logo to resemble the similar LOVE logo (*Imagevirus* 2010: 1), seem to be forcing everyone to both see AIDS and identify the disease with the most elevated of human emotions and one that, while invisible, can infect everyone. According to Gregg Bordowitz "[t]urning LOVE into AIDS seems to draw some kind of causal connection between a powerful human emotion and a deadly disease" – this symbol exploded and proliferated – like the virus itself to combat the "reinvigorated deep-seated homophobia" (2010: 1-2).

The Canadian literary scene did not explode with proliferating representations of AIDS like the AIDS logo of the previous discussion. In fact, to date there are very few Canadian novels that deal to any great extent with people living with or dying from HIV/AIDS, and it is this very lack of proliferation of Canadian AIDS literature that constitutes one of the secondary questions of this chapter. The answer reaches almost certainly beyond the scope of a literary study and into the realm of cautious cultural speculation. The primary intent of this study is to explore four novels: Elizabeth Hay's *The Only Snow in Havana* (1992), Tomson Highway's *Kiss of the Fur Queen* (1998) and, to a lesser extent, Timothy Findley's *Headhunter* (1993) and Nino Ricci's *The Origin of the Species* (2008). All of these texts are set in the pre-treatment era of HIV/AIDS – the 1980s – and the characters living with HIV/AIDS therefore all face an unknown future with certain death and generalized cultural fear and prejudice. In both Hay and Highway's contemporary Canadian texts, the first-person narrator becomes witness to the life and death of a close friend or relative who has contracted HIV/AIDS. This chapter discusses how the narrator negotiates the 'unnamable', 'unknowable', and 'unseen' characteristics and qualities of AIDS, and how visual art is created by the character with AIDS in the text and survives both the disease and the death of the AIDS artist. Likewise, AIDS art becomes a liminal space from which to explore other cultural and historical uncertainties. The story of HIV/AIDS and the resultant art will be shown to connect with other discourses of the 'unnamable' and unknown in Canadian culture, including the threats posed by the United States – regarded as a virus that could erase Canadian culture and identity; the spread of other human-made 'diseases'; the disaster posed by plastic production and pollution, as well as the annihilation of native peoples and culture. Above all, these texts explore the ontological uncertainty of living and creating in the liminality between life with HIV and the coming deterioration resulting from AIDS, and the relational, artistic, cultural, environmental and historical discourse facilitated by memorializing through story the Canadian HIV/AIDS experience in the pre-treatment era.

Elizabeth Hay's *The Only Snow in Havana* is described on the back cover as "[b]lending memoir, biography, travel writing and history". As such, and as characteristic of all four genres, there is an assumption that the writing is the record of something that has happened in real time to an historical person. The blending of these genres underscores the fluidity of these genres, the text and writing, and also underscores what I will eventually describe as the fluidity of the art of disease and, particularly in this case, AIDS art.

The Only Snow in Havana opens in both contradiction and fluidity. Hay writes: "North elides into south" (3) and "Two avocados ripened on top of the fridge, two cold sores blossomed on my lips" (3). The Northern narrator of the text meets the Southern traveler to Mexico, and, signaled by the word "elides", slides from the frozen North into the melting South. The change of states is important to this image. Likewise, the southern fruit/vegetable of the avocado – itself in an uncertain state – ripens on the fridge, a place of preservation of a particular state, but the avocado is outside of and on top of this mechanical stasis. The "cold sores blossomed" is significant in its immediate signal of viral unpredictability but unexpected in the pairing of disease and contamination – and specifically, sexual disease – with the rebirth and beauty implied in blossoming. These seemingly strange juxtapositions signal immediately the author's intention of exploring the 'state inbetween', or the liminal nature of viral disease, and the possibility of beauty and art "blossoming" from virus. It is interesting to note that Hay pairs herself and the first person narrator with a sexual virus and art; she claims the cold sores to be "blossoming" on "my lips" (3). Further, the following and third paragraph of the text explores identity and the fluidity of identity. It seems both intentional and significant that the discussion of the author/narrator's identity directly follows the claiming of personal virus and the resulting beauty of the "cold sores blossom[ing] on my lips" (3).

The majority of *The Only Snow in Havana* meditates on the uncertainties of the self and Canadian identity, sometimes in relation to the people of the culturally-defining land mass that separates Canada from Mexico (that is, The United States of America). Leonard Cohen's *Beautiful Losers* (1966) in a similarly oblique manner reflects on the victimization of Canada by the United States. Peter Wilkin, building on Linda Hutcheon's claim that "Leonard Cohen's *Beautiful Losers* allegorizes Canada's historical-political situation", extrapolates that "Anglophones and francophones, according to this logic, are both victims and oppressors, while the Indians are simply victims and the Americans are simply oppressors" (1966: 1). The oppression by America is one that threatens to annihilate Canadian culture through the unilateral obliteration of cultural differences. In the final scene of the text, the narrator I, who has morphed into F, is swallowed and consumed by an American film star, thus completely engulfing every version of Canadian identity that the narrator has studied, meditated on and eventually become. Responding to the consuming culture of the United States, perhaps itself a metaphor for ravaging disease and HIV/AIDS, is one of the ongoing narrative strands of the Elizabeth Hay text. The story deals with the American takeover and destruction of culture and acts to destabilize the history and cultures of both Mexico and Canada, yet the response is very different on the part of the two countries. For Canadians the response appears to be a loss of self and a forgetting of history (just as it is represented in the Leonard Cohen novel); perhaps a mirror for the Canadian cultural response to AIDS, a forgetting of the history of AIDS in Canada and an erasure of the stories of Canadians with AIDS through a gaping hole in the majority of Canadian fiction. While the military metaphor for AIDS seems justifiably resonant in the American context, Canadian identity is keyed to its role as a 'peace keeper' and thus the arguably predominant metaphors employed for HIV/AIDS lose their resonance in the Canadian context. The relative lack of exploration of AIDS in the Canadian cultural landscape seems to at least suggest the lack of military metaphoric resonance and possibly a problem with representation within the symbolic framework of Canada. What would be the metaphor for 'peace keeping' with AIDS? Surely the closest representation of this relationship is the one that is produced in these texts: the friend or relative caring for and loving the person with AIDS and watching rather helplessly as the person suffers and eventually dies. As the Leonard Cohen example suggests, Canada's history provides many examples of victimization and erasure. Speculations on cultural productions of meaning aside, both Hay and Highway's texts clearly link HIV/AIDS and northern Canada.

Hay's text discusses Northern explorers, inhabitants and history as part of an attempt to define or name Canadian cultural identity as unique and different from the threat of the American cultural virus produced by the consumer and consuming markets of the United States. But the North is also a metaphor for the HIV/AIDS virus, and eventually the North becomes connected almost seamlessly with the section entitled *"David"*, and the exploration of AIDS and art. The letter that begins this chapter is contained within a "barely readable envelope" (92) and the card inside has nothing on it. In the paragraphs that follow there is an intertwined discussion of various forms of physical deterioration and its mirror image in the art, but it is not until the second break in the text and following five pages of discussion of an unnamed disease that AIDS is named for the first time. Historically, Canadian writers have discussed diseases with negative metaphoric resonances by similarly not naming the disease. Most famously perhaps, Nellie McClung's early twentieth century Pearl Watson trilogy fails to name the disease of tuberculosis in chapter after chapter of discussions with doctors of symptoms and cures. While all of the symptomology points to tuberculosis, the taboo of naming is not transgressed. Hay seems to follow this historical precedent of silence around a disease with similarly negative metaphoric resonances. A blank card acting as the opening image to the 'biography' of David seems significant. In Canadian literary AIDS discourse the writer rarely names the virus, and it is only by varying degrees of unnameability – here the blankness – that signals the unspeakable disease. For David's family members, David, the artist with AIDS, is already in the past tense: there is no possibility of future rebirth or beauty. When David is talking to the narrator on the phone he says that he is "worried about [his] friends. They all think I'm dead. But I'm not dead" (93). His mother tells the narrator that David "was so brilliant" and that this former state of brilliance makes the present all the more unbearable: "[t]hat's what's so hard. To see him now" (93). His mother in fact mirrors his movements and follows David, creating with him a dance of insomnia driven by the disease and in turn creating a new art in the present. When David cannot sleep "… he wanders around and changes everything in the house, writes on things, paints on them, cuts them up and pastes them to things" (93). While David has continued to create from his past art new patterns and images that reflect upon his new state of disease and decline, he is also very aware of the limit to his future creations. David gives the narrator "buttons, embroidery thread, pieces of scrap Christmas paper in a box already full of things he had saved for us. He threw in a handful of change. 'Do something with them'" (94). David here is gathering together the odds and ends of his life – the little and seemingly insignificant objects he had saved in all probability to make art – but here he is rather thrusting the future potentiality of these objects to become art away from himself and his decline, towards the narrator, who has become in many ways both a receptacle and a mouthpiece for his memory. The section "David" is both a work of art, a narration of David's art, and also a memorial to the artist's life. The narrator looks at the pictures on David's wall of them in Mexico, "bathing our feet in the stream at Palenque, buying tortillas, climbing a ruin" (93). In the two pages that follow, the narrator collects together images, objects, people, places and conversations from her travels in Mexico with David. She concludes these bright memories with a very Mexican juxtaposition of death and life, and in the process transforms David's death through a creative rebirthing. The narrator first concludes with "For over a year" during their travels together "David had [...] deep and vicious boils that wouldn't go away" (96). And in the final paragraph of this section "One afternoon while he slept outside in a hammock, Alec and I made love in the tent and conceived our daughter. I've always thought of David as her guardian angel. Death? As a guardian angel?" (96). Hay here gives no commentary on what or why she has made this connection. She leaves both as questions and unanswered questions, but it seems in her treatment of her relationship with David that she notes everywhere the death and rebirth of his art as something else following the advent of his disease.

While much of the narrative recounts the narrators' time with David in Mexico during a particular time in his illness, there is from the very beginning of this section a deep and abiding connection between David and the North. The connection is so profound that it is tempting to suggest that the North is an extended metaphor for creating art from the seeming deathscape of AIDS. The second paragraph is the first link between David's current viral demise and the North. The narrator describes a photograph that "hangs above my desk. One of a series shot in Yellowknife of weeds in water, weeds in snow. This one is weeds in snow. The stems stick up like fine, precise calligraphy: stick legs, his legs, now" (92). Weeds like virus and later the infection in David's leg "went crazy" (92). And the weeds, the sticks, become David's legs, withered by the spread of the viral infection. In Atwood, Highway, and Hay – all winners of the highest Canadian honour for fiction, the Governor General's Award – HIV/AIDS is linked by character to the North. This is a seemingly strange juxtaposition at first glance, in all cases. Why the North? In the case of Hay, the exploration of the North begins with the spread and contamination of white diseases to the first Esquimaux inhabitants and the ever-multiplying crazy slaughter of the life-sustaining animals of the North. Hay goes into the archives and searches for the writings and marginal mentions of the Esquimaux in the grand narratives of the great Canadian explorers of the North. Like the Esquimaux and the slight writings and art created out of the struggle for life in the severest of climates, David's art and the art that emerges from the infected artist is marginalized in our culture. There is the fear of contamination and the belief that David expresses that he has been forgotten and that others think he is already dead. There is also the connection of his state to madness, a connection also noted in Findley's portrait of an artist with AIDS, which further condemns the AIDS artist to the margins or even to invisibility. Like the disease, which for most of this memoir is not even named, the work of artists with AIDS lacks a public space, for with a public space there must be the acknowledgement of the beauty and life that also springs from the site of infection. And perhaps above all, as the narrator notes in her fears about bringing her daughter to see David, and her condemnation of herself for her unfounded but nonetheless acknowledged fear, there is a societal desire to look away from AIDS and to forget about the generative qualities of the virus and its possible manifestation in the proliferation of art from the diseased artist. Like the North, marginalized by geography, access, fear and the seeming deadness or nothingness of snow and ice, the AIDS artist is marginalized and secluded within the walled rooms and corridors to which we offer up our sick. Canadian literature has a long history of striving for survival and even taming of nature. The North is perhaps one of the last places where this has not occurred, and, like the North, AIDS represents the unknown and untamed threats to human survival. The very lack of writing about AIDS in Canadian literature supports a theory of marginalization as a result of fear and terror. Even those writers who do speak about AIDS often leave the disease unnamed. While study after study will look at various aspects of the disease from clinical and medical models, the cultural impact of the art and literature that strives to represent the 'unrepresentable' has not been the subject of a single study in Northern Literature or even more broadly Canadian Literature.

Hay names the AIDS virus for the first time in relation to David's uncertainty about the diagnosis and in relation to the art he was making at the time of this liminal state – between the unknown and the condemned. Hay remembers that:

> [i]n the months when David suspected he had AIDS but before he knew for sure, he made a series of drawings using black ivory pigment made from burned bones. He set up a tent in his studio, laid pieces of paper inside, used a bellows to blow in the pigment, and allowed it to settle on the paper. He drew on the dust with his fingers. He said he wanted the drawings to resemble the marks left in snow on a tranquil day. (97)

In the early and liminal stages before the diagnosis, he is working in the pigments of the North and using "pigment made from burned bones" (97). But by the end of his illness, ravaged by disease, his mother says that he demolishes everything. And this taking apart or destroying of order and establishing of chaos is the very fear that AIDS represents. There is no cure. There is no barrier against death. There is only the madness and chaos of the unknown. And when the artist genuinely represents this, it induces terror in even those persons closest to the artist, who have witnessed the AIDS journey and the art created and destroyed as a response to the physical attack of disease and threat of death that has been launched on the human body.

Timothy Findley's *Headhunter* (1993), while not a text under primary consideration in this paper, provides an interesting starting point for a discussion of subjects associated with the discussion of AIDS in Tomson Highway's *Kiss of the Fur Queen*. Findley is preoccupied in much of his writing with humanity's ability to turn away from the suffering of fellow human beings and animals. A number of Findley's works, including probably most famously *The Butterfly Plague*, explore the slaughter of the Jews in the holocaust, the turning away from the physically and mentally ill and homosexuals, as well as the wanton destruction of animals. Like the plague of evil and butterflies in *The Butterfly Plague*, in *Headhunter* Findley employs the language of plague to describe a bird-related disease that has become deadly to humans, named sturnusemia. It seems possible that the plague is related to environmental destruction, human evil or some other unnamed and unknowable force that is culling humanity. And the narrator notes that "though no other explanation had been forthcoming, and even in spite of the mounting death toll, the population at large gave every indication of ignoring the threat of sturnusemia" (10). The narrator goes on to say that this reaction is far from unique and that "[i]n an earlier decade, the majority had turned away from the evidence of AIDS" (10) linking in this invocation of AIDS the human reaction of turning away and the sheer unknowability of the current and past plagues. What is further interesting in *Headhunter* and with *Kiss of the Fur Queen* are the other unmentionable and unnamable subjects – in both cases the sexual abuse and betrayal of young boys and the acquiescence and even permission granted by figures of authority. For a time, characters in both texts circle around the questions of diagnosing the sickness, in part because of the amazing art being created – in Timothy Findley and Julian Slade's large and daring masterpieces and in Tomson Highway and Gabriel Okimasis' challenging experimental dance and theatre – and the impossibility of pairing this art and performance with the physical and mental decline of the AIDS artist. However, through the symptomology most commonly employed in describing the visible and invisible marks of AIDS – pneumonia; lesions that will not heal; repeated and prolonged illness; emaciation and weakness – it becomes apparent that the artist/actor/dancer is dying of AIDS.

In *Headhunter* we are introduced to the artist Julian Slade at the opening of what will be his last exhibition when he is already in the final stages of his illness. The audience at the opening can see immediately that something is wrong with Slade, to the extent that a member of the audience and central figure of *Headhunter*, Kurtz, "immediately saw that Slade was ill. His body, always thin, was now emaciated. Sturnusemia? AIDS? It was impossible to tell without a closer view, but clearly – all too clearly – Julian Slade was dying" (95). Kurtz purchases one of Slades' paintings to hang in the Parkin Institute, noting that "[h]e had decided that Slade had explored mental illness as avidly from the inside and with the same scientific skill as Sommerville and Shelley had explored it from the outside. He had decided that *The Golden Chamber of the White Dogs* transcended art to become a scientific statement. *For a desperate disease – a desperate cure*[1]" (171). The "desperate disease" is not named by Kurtz and the diseases of the text seem to multiply with every chapter, however the painting of the AIDS artist looks at mental illness and AIDS from the inside with such acuteness that Doctor Kurtz pronounces it science, and the art itself becomes

---

1   Italics in original.

linked to a "desperate cure". When Kurtz discusses Slades' painting with another client she tells him that Slade is dying. Kurtz questions whether he is dying of AIDS and his patient answers that he is dying of "[e]verything. AIDS. Life. Schizophrenia. Not a great combination" (265). But Kurtz responds that "[i]t produced great art" (265) bringing together life, AIDS, and mental illness, and acknowledging that this combination produces great and terrifying art. In the final diagnosis of Findley, it is not the individual that has become sick but that "[c] ivilization – sickened – had itself become a plague" (388). And while *Headhunter* does tell a devastating story of humanity's further descent into evil, madness and disease, the story is not without hope; that hope is in bringing the unnamable to light and displaying AIDS, life, mental illness and the sexual abuse of children in the great works of terrifying and convicting art. AIDS art then, according at least to Findley, has a function beyond the recording or scientific exploration of the disease. Interestingly, the question of causality when it comes to AIDS is thrown back at society – it is not the fault of the individual but civilization itself that has the disease, life itself. The other causality that is brought to the fore seems to be sexual exploitation in general. While not the cause of AIDS, the sexual abuse of children is linked by both Findley and Highway to the sickness of the individual and the culture that breeds these diseases – mental and physical. The AIDS virus then, becomes merely another manifestation of the overall sickness of society, and the cure or hope is in the healing of society by the bringing to light of all the underlying abuses of human rights.

Tomson Highway's *Kiss of the Fur Queen* begins in Northern Manitoba, the home of the Okimasis brothers. The brothers are ripped from their home, their language and their culture and placed in a residential school where both boys are renamed and then repeatedly abused by the Catholic priests. A great deal of the novel is a working out of this abuse and the struggle of the boys becoming artists in a culture that discriminates against them, and in a language which is foreign to them. It is not until part six and the final section of *Kiss of the Fur Queen*, "*Presto con fuoco*", when the brothers have already succeeded as artists – one as a musician and the other as a dancer – that there are the first hints of the unnamable disease. Gabriel questions "[w]hat's this? The blemish on his neck still there? After two weeks?" (275) and the narrator goes on to note that "Gabriel had had the flu twice this year, so this might be the third, but was anyone immune at this time of year?" (275). While the late nights of sex with strangers for money and/or pleasure have featured somewhat prominently in the narrative, the undercurrent has always been the on-going psychological stress and nightmares from the boyhood sexual abuse at the hands of the priests. This telltale "blemish on his neck" is the first mention of any AIDS related symptoms. From this moment onwards, the narrative decline of Gabriel is rapid. For Gabriel, his dancing career had reached its pinnacle in this last performance for his brother's play. Even before the final performances he is physically failing, becoming more and more tired, sick and dependent on medicine. When Gabriel goes to the doctor there is yet no discussion of the disease but only that "[t]he poker-faced technician removed the needle and pressed a bandage over Gabriel's bared forearm" (281). Gabriel then proceeds to ignore the "rack of pamphlets on various diseases" and then goes "[b]ehind the clinic" with "the leather man" and finally emerges from the alleyway "with a new fifty-dollar bill" (282). In these oblique and partial lines Highway informs of blood tests, pamphlets on diseases and male prostitution. Taken together with the aforementioned "blemish on his neck" there is almost conclusive hints towards the disease Gabriel may have contracted. But importantly there is no positive proof at this point in the text and the next mention is Gabriel wondering "of all the days on Earth, how could I have chosen this day to go back to the clinic for the results?" (284). But the "results" are not given and again there is only the question by another actor of "[w]hat's the matter, babe?" (284). The narrative continues with exhaustion, sweat, pills, "rare pneumonia" (292) and the discussions with the doctor again include all the signs of the disease, but never the naming.

However, the complication in naming for the Cree brothers appears to be one with language, "[h]ow do you say AIDS in Cree, huh? Tell me, what's the word for HIV?" (296). AIDS is rather represented by Gabriel as Weetigo feasting on human flesh. The image of the devouring tongue of Weetigo is paired in Gabriel's repeated question with regards to the priests' molesting of the Cree boys. Gabriel pleas, "Haven't you feasted on enough human flesh?" (299). Later, the cannibal spirit takes on the face of one of the molesting fathers (299-300) devouring his boyhood body and then again his AIDS ravaged body.

While there are only a handful of Canadian novels that deal with HIV/AIDS, it seems important to underline that the Canadian novels that have been written do attempt to answer some of the central questions that theorists of literature and art exploring HIV/AIDS have suggested are central to the study of AIDS art and literature. Elizabeth Hay and Nino Ricci both take on the issues of homophobia and fear of contamination, and the problems of representation: how do you name or show something that does not exist except as a group of possibly related symptoms? Elizabeth Hay, Timothy Findley and Tomson Highway all broaden the question of causality beyond the simplicity of sexual relations and orientation to question the ways in which HIV/AIDS intersects with other forms of victimization, disease and societal sickness. Alongside the study of the sickening of the human body through HIV/AIDS, as shown briefly in Findley's *Headhunter*, HIV/AIDS seems to figure in minor ways in other discourses of disaster (environmental or otherwise) and plague. Most recently, Governor General Award Winning author Nino Ricci in his 2008 *The Origin of the Species* engages the protagonist in an emotionally intense relationship with a woman who is dying from MS and a man who is entering the final stages of AIDS. The woman suffering from MS, in explaining her disease, compares it unflinchingly to the AIDS virus. And Alex, in his association with a student suffering from AIDS, is forced to confront his own homophobia and fear of AIDS, and in his process of interaction with both of these immune system sufferers he wrestles with the questions of evolution and negative human participation in the survival and destruction of the species. The attack of the immune system on the body or its failure is part of this discussion, and both

MS and AIDS figure then as metaphors for climate change; the survival of the species; destruction of life, and in the end are simply aspects of the devastating and never-ending – though clearly coming to an end – battle for life of the species. Nino Ricci manages to bring the Canadian AIDS discourse into a more global discussion impart through the employment of the military metaphor, with the battle for life extending beyond the individual to the species and planet.

References

Aaron, M. Ed. *New Queer Cinema: A Critical Reader*. New Jersey: Rutgers UP.

Bordowitz, G. 2010. *General Idea: Imagevirus*. London: Afterall Books.

Findley, T. 1993. *Headhunter*. Toronto: HarperCollins Ltd.

Gilman, S.L. 1988. *Disease and Representation: Images of Illness from Madness to AIDS*. Ithaca: Cornell UP.

Goldstein, D.E. 2004. *Once Upon a Virus: AIDS Legends and Vernacular Risk Perception*. Logan Utah: Utah State UP.

Green, J. and Miller, D. 1986. *AIDS: The Story of a Disease*. Toronto: Grafton Books.

Griffin, G. *Representations of HIV and AIDS: Visibility Blue/s*. Manchester: Manchester UP.

Hay, E. 1992. *The Only Snow in Havana*. Toronto: Cormorant Books.

Highway, T. 1998. *Kiss of the Fur Queen*. Toronto: Anchor Canada.

Kuppers, P. 2007. *The Scar of Visibility: Medical Performances and Contemporary Art*. Minneapolis: University of Minnesota Press.

Leibowitch, J. 1985. *A Strange Virus of Unknown Origin*. Trans. Richard Howard. New York: Ballantine Books.

McGovern, T. 1997. *Bearing witness (to AIDS)*. New York: A.R.T. Press, 1999.

Miller, James. AIDS in the Novel: Getting it Straight, in *Fluid Exchanges: Artists and Critics in the AIDS Crisis*, edited by J. Miller. Toronto: University of Toronto Press, 257-271.

Morris III, C.E. 2011. *Remembering the AIDS Quilt*. East Lansing: Michigan State UP.

O'Connor, M.F. 1996. *Treating the Psychological Consequences of HIV*. San Francisco: Jossey-Bass Publishers.

Palmer, S. 1997. *AIDS*. Toronto: University of Toronto Press.

Patton, B. 1992. Cell Wars: Military Metaphors and the Crisis of Authority, in *Fluid Exchanges: Artists and Critics in the AIDS Crisis*, edited by J. Miller. Toronto: University of Toronto Press, 272-286.

Phelan, P. 1997. *Mourning Sex: Performing Public Memories*. New York: Routledge.

Piel, J. 1985. *The Science of AIDS: Readings from Scientific American Magazine*. New York: W.H. Freeman and Company.

Reed, Christopher. 2011. *Art and Homosexuality*. Oxford: Oxford University Press.

Ricci, N. 2008. *The Origin of the Species*. Toronto: Anchor Canada.

Sontag. S. 1977. *Illness as Metaphor and AIDS and Its Metaphors*. Toronto: Doubleday.

Watney, S. 2000. *Imagine Hope: AIDS and Gay Identity*. New York: Routledge.

White, E. 2001. *Loss within Loss: Artists in the Age of AIDS*. Wisconsin: University of Wisconsin Press.

Chapter 2

Distancing the Recent Past: New Forms of Discomfort with AIDS in the U.S.

John C. Hawley

In his introduction to this collection, Gustavo Subero makes reference to the AIDS Quilt, a reference made especially significant since the year 2012 marked its 25th anniversary. The whole quilt had been last displayed in 1996; in the summer of 2012, 8,000 panels were rotated each day in the National Mall in Washington, DC. The quilt, composed of thousands of 3' x 6' panels (intentionally the size of a human grave), currently consists of over 48,000 panels honoring more than 94,000 individuals who have died of AIDS. In the early days of the quilt, in the 1980s and 1990s, the quilt grew at a rate of 11,000 panels a year; these days there are about 500 panels added each year. The Executive Director of the NAMES Project Foundation overseeing the quilt, Julie Rhoad, nowadays has sections displayed in various locales around the country, and tailors the choice of panels to fit particular communities (for example, those commemorating Jewish individuals might be gathered and displayed in a synagogue, and so on), and Rhoad is determined that Americans "never leave a population uncared for" (UlabyJune 27, 2012). She recently noted that the newest panels are returning to the custom of commemorating individuals only by first name; these most recent additions, she says, are often for African American victims of AIDS. Though some, like bell hooks, argue that "black homophobia" is a myth resulting from the mistake of stereotyping African Americans as speaking with one voice (hooks), Rhoad asserts that this lack of a surname for some recent quilt panels is suggestive of the stigma that still remains in that community against those with the disease, and repeating the stigma that attached to all early victims in the 1980s, and that was similarly symbolized by the lack of surnames in the earliest panels. Thus, one might think that the very idea of a quilt would be a perfect metaphor for the community of AIDS sufferers, yet for a number of reasons that is not actually the case. If they were laid out side by side, the quilt's thousands of panels would stretch for more than 50 miles, though those commemorating African Americans who have died of the syndrome would make up only one half of one mile of those 50.

This suggests in a pictorial way one of several imbalances in the description, reporting, and imagining of the epidemic that have shaped the understanding of HIV and AIDS in the United States. According to the Center for Disease Control and Prevention, in 2009, African Americans comprised 14 per cent of the US population but accounted for 44 per cent of all new HIV infections ("the estimated

rate of new HIV infection for black men was more than six and a half times as
high as that of white men, and two and a half times as high as that of Latino
men or black women" [http://www.cdc.gov/hiv/topics/aa/]), yet the most common
perception among the US populace is that HIV is a white man's disease. This is
a direct result of the skewed representation of the syndrome and its associated
illnesses in the United States. Jacqueline Foertsch, for example, laments that we
have seen "so far, mostly white, middle-class AIDS novels, plays and poetry"
(1999: 57). If it ever was a white man's disease, these most recent statistics suggest
that things are changing in the United States. How that is happening is partially the
subject of this chapter.

The Great Recoil: Subalterns, Aliens, Monsters, the Damned

For those who were sexually active at the time and are still alive, the growing
fear of the early 80s in the United States is impossible to forget. Those who
frequented the gay bath houses awoke one morning to a small article that belied its
prophetic importance: this was the *New York Times*'s memorable first article on the
syndrome, written by their science columnist, Lawrence Altman. Published on 3
July 1981, and entitled "Rare Cancer Seen in 41 Homosexuals", his brief column-
length entry was somewhat hidden on page 20, as if the event being described was
a curiosity that some might take note of as roughly comparable to an outbreak
of influenza in Thailand. But gays, at any rate, sat up and took notice, and began
the worrying that would all-too-soon be confirmed for them on a growing and
terrifying scale.

    Even those most concerned did not know where to turn for more information
about what was happening. *Newsweek*'s cover story of 18 April 1983, "was
optimistically subtitled 'The Search for a Cure,' even though most of the experts
working on the disease were still not certain what caused it, much less how to go
about looking for a cure" (Kinsella 1989: 94). The article corrected earlier mistakes
about how it was transmitted, and gave a thorough description of the various
groups who had been contracting the syndrome. Nonetheless, misinformation, or
a general lack of information, continued to confuse Americans. "Sex in the Age
of AIDS" was *Newsweek*'s cover on 14 March 1988, and it confidently spread
incorrect information on the ease with which the virus was being transmitted (for
example, on toilet seats). At this time of unreliable information it is not surprising
that the rest of the country tried its hardest to completely ignore the new health
problem, principally compartmentalizing the threat as mercifully ghettoized within
a group in society that was, well, the less said about them, the better.

    This would eventually change, but it would take some screaming from those
most affected. As has often been the case, the art community was focused on this
issue well before the rest of society: by 1992, "500 professional artists in the
United States put AIDS at the center of their work":

> Suggestions of a homosexual 'sensibility' attuned to Aesthetic sensitivity, camp whimsy, or subtle codes were supplanted by images of homosexuals as forceful political advocates using collectively produced and mass-distributed imagery to advocate on their own behalf. (Reed 2011, 208)

Randy Shilts, the best early chronicler of the progression of the syndrome and American society's head-in-the-sand resistance to acknowledging the growing threat, notes that it took the sudden eruption of gayness itself, like a ripping off of clown masks at some domestic birthday celebration, to awaken the country to what had been going on in their very midst for some years. "By October 2, 1985," writes Shilts:

> the morning Rock Hudson died, the word was familiar to almost every household in the Western world. AIDS. . . . Indeed, on the day the world learned that Rock Hudson was stricken, some 12.000 Americans were already dead or dying of AIDS and hundreds of thousands more were infected with the virus that caused the disease. But few had paid any attention to this; nobody, it seemed, had cared about them. (1987: xxi)

But they cared about Rock Hudson, less so, perhaps, after his sexuality became more widely known, but he was, nonetheless, not the "typical" gay: he was not mincing; he *looked* like a real man. If *he* was one of them, then how were we supposed to steer clear of that kind of person? Suddenly, after thousands had died miserable deaths, Americans *en masse* felt not compassion, but threat.

James Kinsella and Randy Shilts have argued that non-homosexual Americans had been lulled into a false sense of immunity by such prestigious institutions as the *New York Times,* not by what it had written about the syndrome, but rather by the fact that it had not reacted to it *at all.* And as the newspaper of record, if they did not think it worth getting upset about, then it appeared that life could continue as always for the normal citizen. As Kinsella records, "'At first AIDS was a gay story,' said a senior [*New York*] *Times* editor, describing the news evolution of the epidemic at the *Times*: 'And then it became a scientific story. And finally, it was a story about government.' Only in that last phase did AIDS become an important ongoing story that reports throughout the newspaper were covering. Finally, the epidemic had become a *Times* story" (1989: 85). That was the Spring of 1984. By contrast, the *Times* had run 13 articles on the Philadelphia outbreak of Legionnaire's disease in *one week*, and three of them were on the front page, but "the first two years of the AIDS crisis prompted no front-page story in the *Times* on the epidemic" (1989: 66). Larry Kramer, a founder in 1982 of the Gay Men's Health Crisis and later founder of the more militant ACT UP, wrote his play *The Normal Heart* (1985) to protest this lack of attention; the popular play "chronicles the unwillingness of government officials and much of the gay community to take AIDS seriously" (McCabe: 17).

On May 25, 1983, the Assistant Secretary for Health and Human Services announced that AIDS was now a major health concern in the United States, prompting the *New York Times* to publish its first front-page story on the syndrome. Indeed, "in the summer and fall of 1983, American media's coverage of the epidemic leaped almost 600 percent over the previous six-month period" (Kinsella: 73), prompted by the false news that the disease could be transmitted through casual contact. In that first decade in the epidemic, there were three peaks in AIDS reportage:

> In 1983, fear of widespread and rampant infection was triggered by rumors that AIDS could be spread by simple household contact. In 1985, actor Rock Hudson's death spurred a wave of interest because it appeared as though the disease was affecting even all-American types. And in early 1987, the discussion around containing the threat with widespread testing for the AIDS virus caused another explosion in news coverage. (Kinsella: 4)

Yet the public was surely getting mixed messages in the remarkable silence on the issue that continued in the highest reaches of the government. By 1986, "in public, the president had uttered the word 'AIDS' only once" (Kinsella: 3).

Less responsible journalists used the miasma to stir up trouble, typified by the *New York Post*, which ran a front page on 12 October 1987, stating: "'AIDS Monster': Cops: He may have given deadly virus to dozens of L[ong] I[sland] child victims" (Kinsella: 153). As the muffled hysteria spread, stoked by coverage such as the *Post*'s, Susan Sontag published a follow-up to her acclaimed study of the misrepresentation of cancer in American society, *Illness as Metaphor* (1978), in which she had criticized the "blame the victim" approach to coverage of that ongoing health scare. Ten years later, she saw in AIDS and its representation in the American press a new manifestation of what she had attacked in her earlier book, a manifestation that was all the more insidious because it broadcast a more compelling moral message of condemnation against those suffering from AIDS. As she writes:

> The unsafe behavior that produces AIDS is judged to be more than just weakness. It is indulgence, delinquency—addictions to chemicals that are illegal and to sex regarded as deviant. [...] AIDS is understood as a disease not only of sexual excess but of perversity. [...] Getting the disease through a sexual practice is thought to be more willful, therefore deserves more blame [...] From the beginning, the construction of the illness had depended on notions that separated one group of people from another—the sick from the well, people with ARC from people with AIDS, them and us—while implying the imminent dissolution of these distinctions. (26, 31)

This is, perhaps, at least not surprising coming from certain quarters in the early imagination of those who had contracted the virus. But it continued, and in

1997 Tim Lawrence concludes that, in portrayals of those with AIDS, what is underscored in much of the representation until, perhaps, the end of the twentieth century, is that:

> debilitated, sick, and almost dead, people with AIDS are desperate in the face of their inevitable death. Such representations play into deep and reactionary cultural narratives. AIDS has become a convenient symbol for moral majoritarians who want to hammer home their sense of contemporary moral decay: the virus is a retribution for past and current sins, a deserved and necessary ending caused by the 'sexual revolution.' The disease has come to stand for the danger of sex outside the heterosexual family – in particular of gay sex, with the distinction between gay men and AIDS regularly erased, replaced by the equation Homosexuality = AIDS = Death. Doom, powerlessness, and hopelessness are central themes: there is little chance of the diseased person having a productive life; the overdetermined body images of the person with AIDS are evidence of inner depravity. (Lawrence 1997: 243; see, also, E. Albert)

As Sontag had observed, "The most terrifying illnesses are those perceived not just as lethal but as dehumanizing, literally so [...]. the signs of a progressive mutation, decomposition" (1988: 38, 41). Much like the "thingification" by the French colonizers that Aime Cesaire had condemned as the precondition for the enslavement of those in the Caribbean, those determined to distance themselves from gay men in the 80s and 90s in the United States had first to underscore that this was something that gay men had brought upon themselves, something that gave evidence of, and also brought about, their dehumanization: AIDS sufferers were to be condemned and ostracized, rather than welcomed into the broader civil society. Many gay activists objected to the unrelenting visual portrayal of those with HIV and AIDS as passive emaciated victims, horrifying corpses that hadn't yet died.[1]

Suddenly, of course, gays were "appearing" all over the United States, and some in the most surprising places. Sontag notes that "to get AIDS is precisely to be revealed, in the majority of cases so far, as a member of a certain 'risk group', a community of pariahs. The illness flushes out an identity that might have remained hidden from neighbors, job-mates, family, friends" (25). This continued to change the "face" of the homosexual in the United States, and thereby throughout the

---

1 See Simon Watney's "Read my lips: AIDS, art & activism" in his *Imagine Hope* (2000: 89-105). Christopher Reed records that:

> At a 1988 MoMA exhibition of Nicholas Nixon's (b. 1947) photographs of people with AIDS, activists from the group ACT UP (AIDS Coalition to Unleash Power) sat in the gallery with photographs of energetic people captioned as 'living with'—not dying of—AIDS. The activists talked to viewers about their criticism of the art on display and handed out fliers that concluded with the demand 'STOP LOOKING AT US; START LISTENING TO US.' (2011, 209)

world: "we're here, we're queer, get used to it" eventually, though not in the beginning, became a watchword of defiance from these former pariahs. As with any shunned group, such massive rejection by the larger segment of society prompted a counter-offensive: a self-identification with the ghetto, now seen as a source of political power. To be revealed, willy-nilly, "confirms an identity and, among the risk group in the United States most severely affected in the beginning, homosexual men, has been a creator of community as well as an experience that isolates the ill and exposes them to harassment and persecution" (Sontag 1988: 25). There had already been, of course, the comparatively long-established ghettoes – the Castro region in San Francisco; Greenwich Village in New York; Boystown in Chicago, and so on – but people were getting AIDS in Iowa, in Alabama, in Colorado … what in hell was going on?

In the face of apparent indifference on the part of government and the majority of Americans, gays in the major cities began to mobilize in self-defense. At the ACT UP rally in Albany, New York, on May 7, 1988, Vito Russo sent out a call to arms for the gay community to pull together. "I'm here to speak out today as a PWA," he told his audience, "who is not dying *from*—but for the last three years quite successfully living *with*—AIDS" (Russo 1990: 408). Unlike wartime, when a common enemy united a people in a shared experience, this "war" has divided Americans, Russo warns. Unlike us, he reminds the crowd, the "real people in this country", those who are not "fags and junkies," (408) do not have to spend days and months trying to acquire experimental drugs for exorbitant prices:

> And they don't sit in television studios surrounded by technicians who wear rubber gloves and refuse to put a body mike on them because it isn't happening to them so they don't give a shit … They don't spend their waking hours going from one hospital to another, watching the people they love die slowly of neglect and bigotry … They haven't been to two funerals a week for the last three, four, or five years. (409)

Thus, Russo explicitly urges those who are actually enduring the onslaught to band together and fight for governmental recognition of their health needs. "And after we kick the shit out of this disease," he concludes, "I intend to be alive to kick the shit out of this system so that this will never happen again" (410).

This was an underscoring of the power, the agency, that AIDS-sufferers could still manifest in taking at least some control – as a community if not as individuals – in the face of what, at the time, was an unstoppable and horrible fate. Such independence from the heterosexual community in the United States was a double-edged sword: on the one hand, as with the black power movement, frightening the mainstream Americans who were already avoiding gays; on the other hand, actually getting some results from the elected officials in some parts of the country. Russo's and Kramer's anger in ACT UP did, indeed, offer a counter-narrative to that repeatedly inscribed by pictures of those with late-stage disease. Gaunt gay men with Kaposi sarcoma, mere skin and bones, had been flashed across magazines and television newscasts, but powerful men with the virus, whether gay or straight, had not yet become the kind of symbol that Magic Johnson became in 1991. As Tim Lawrence observes, writing only slightly after the success of the protease cocktail of medications began to be seen:

> they are rarely portrayed as being active, fit to work, and able to have safe sex. As such, the subjectivity of the person with AIDS disappears, while the body with AIDS remains visible. Furthermore, the focus on the individual means that the public dimension of the crisis, especially the failure of governments to provide adequate money for medical research and information campaigns, has seldom been articulated. Individualization becomes a strategy of depoliticization. (Lawrence 1997: 243)

At the same time, while the syndrome itself was becoming better understood, there remained "the persistent representation of the person with AIDS as white, gay, middle class, and promiscuous" (244). This was the situation in 1994 when Timothy Murphy, reflecting on the ethics proper for what appeared to be a status quo for some considerable time into the future, writes that:

> Barring an unexpected breakthrough in research for a treatment or vaccine, HIV disease will be a permanent part of the catalog of human suffering. AIDS will certainly not be defeated by 'get tough' measures whose attraction will diminish with passing years, rising costs, and the foreseeable inability of dramatic headlines to energize a public inured to the epidemic. It thus becomes important that the energy of anti-AIDS measures be sustained, that it cross generations. (1994: 185)

Near the end of the twentieth century, Murphy suggests, the gay man is seeking "freedom to be HIV-positive, freedom from atavistic moral conceits that AIDS is a mark of difference signaling death, ruin, and social decay" (1994: 187).

A Growing Keen: Compassion, Loss, Nostalgia

In the meantime, thousands of gay men were dying. Russo's anger is clear, but even more obvious is the growing sense of irretrievable loss that was spreading throughout the gay community, which, thereby, was becoming even more obviously that: a community set apart from the larger group that was not as clearly traumatized. As evidenced in the AIDS quilt, many companions and friends sought ways to memorialize their loved ones.[2] Many novels, many memoirs, sought to keep alive the essence of the young men who had died prematurely. Many writers who had celebrated their new sexual freedom in the 70s and 80s, and who had

---

2   See Simon Watney's "Acts of Memory" in his *Imagine Hope* (2000: 163-168).

watched friends suddenly die, looked with melancholy at what had been lost. Felice Picano's 1995 novel, *Like People in History*, follows its characters through three decades, concluding with a determination to live, despite the losses:

> I stood in the freezing darkness and desolation, and that radiator chugged and rattled and spouted, and its whistle hissed out steam so noisily and with such intensity of purpose that I slowly – amazing myself – became certain it really *did* have a purpose: to carry on as long as it had the power to do so, and while it remained active, to do what it did best – even if that meant attempting to warm up the entire immense, vitrescent, frigid, indifferent night. (512)

A great number of gay readers appreciate the novel's fictionalized history of the crucial decades from 1960 to 1990 when so many milestones changed American perceptions of gay and lesbian life in the United States, an era of personal liberation and intense support within the gay community that many look back upon with nostalgia.[3]

Paul Monette's loving tribute to his lover, *Borrowed Time: An AIDS Memoir* (1988), records the small turns taken in the last months and days in a loved one's life, almost shouting to the world that this person mattered, despite his relative anonymity and comparative youth. Monette identifies the apparent randomness with which the virus struck members of the gay community in the early days, as if it were playing with individuals who tried to take precautions against an enemy that was not well understood. He and his lover were very careful in their sex lives, starting in 1982, yet Roger was diagnosed as positive in 1985. Monette's frightened observation records the realization by many that they had begun taking precautions a bit too late:

> A lot of us were already ticking and didn't even know. The magic circle my generation is trying to stay within the borders of is only as real as the random past. Perhaps the young can live in the magic circle, but only if those of us who are ticking will tell our story. Otherwise it goes on being *us* and *them* forever, built like a wall higher and higher, till you no longer think to wonder if you are walling it out or in. (5-6)

We see in Monette's metaphor a prescient sense of the split within the gay community between those who were positive, and those who remained free of the virus, suggesting, perhaps, a split in generations as well: the young, with more warning, now careful to avoid the older and contaminated in their midst, and thereby nurturing a deceptive sense of invulnerability.

---

3   One blogger records that "it has helped me dust off the glitter on the faded red sequined hot pants of my own gay identity." Daniel G. at http://www.goodreads.com/book/show/449189.Like_People_In_History.

Monette records the sense of helpless ignorance that haunted those with the earliest diagnoses:

> "It's not till you first hear it attached to someone you love," he writes, that you realize how little you know about it. My mind went utterly blank. The carefully constructed wall collapsed as if a 7.5 quake had rumbled under it. At that point I didn't even know the difference between KS and the opportunistic infections. I kept picturing that swollen gland in his groin, thinking: What's *that* got to do with AIDS? And a parallel track in my mind began careening with another thought: the swollen glands in my own groin, always dismissed by my straight doctor as herpes-related and "not a significant sign." (7-8)

Many pages later, he's awakened by a phone call informing him of Roger's death, and his memoir ends much as did Picano's novel, and as do so many of the novels and memoirs of the late 80s and mid-90s: "I swam back to bed for the end of the night, trying to stay under the Dalmane. Putting off as long as I could the desolate waking to life alone – this calamity that is all mine, that will not end till I do" (342); Monette died of AIDS-related complications in 1995. This fear of being alone for the rest of one's life, this lesson of the dangers of surrendering to loving another gay man in the age of an epidemic that appears to be strangely targeted on the same community that you have tried hard to build, this yearning for a happier time of innocence, runs through all these accounts.

Poets also sought to capture in words some semblance of the AIDS experience and the appalling toll it was taking in the gay community. Thom Gunn was preeminent in this group, especially in his 1992 collection, *The Man with Night Sweats* (1992), in which he "assembles an elegiac response to AIDS reminiscent of the AIDS Memorial Quilt, a 'patched body' that represents both grief and hope, and stands as a successful form of nonseparatist political action" (McNeil 2012: 36). Playwrights and eventually screenwriters also produced works to commemorate the loss, and most honored among this group was Tony Kushner's *Angels in America* (1993). This Pulitzer-winning pair of plays accomplishes several important feats: it encourages its audience to accept the presence of the epidemic in their midst as long-term, and it incorporates AIDS-sufferers into full citizenship as Americans. In this second goal, Kushner's play distinguishes itself from Larry Kramer's *The Normal Heart* (1985), which Terry McCabe describes as "the last great play that posited gay life as a subculture within, but separate from, American life" (17). Kushner's play not only sees the gay subculture as having been increasingly incorporated into mainstream American society, but also makes bold to see its suffering as emblematic of American citizenship in the late twentieth century. Claudia Barnett argues that Kushner's plays suggest that:

> AIDS is not only death but a precondition for life, as Prior [the central character] learns on his prophetic journey. He *sees* because he has AIDS; he survives because he sees; and, in the end, he shares his vision with humanity [...] This

middle space [of comparative hope] is [...] modern drama's positive pole of Purgatory, a space of possibilities [contrasting with] the negative extreme of Samuel Beckett's drama. (Barnett 2010: 472)

This is a mundane version of the divine *afflatus*, one supposes. For Barnett, "Kushner's Purgatory [...] [is] a murky space of promise and loss – a journey to Heaven and back, a walk on damp leaves, a body ridden with disease – from which some emerge blessed [...] [and] the blessing is Purgatory" (473). It is as good a metaphor for the condition of HIV-sufferers as any, perhaps: living somewhere between heaven and hell, a metaphor that allows one to avoid complete despair. "Purgatory," Barnett writes, paraphrasing Stephen Greenblatt, "is a story that allows the dead to live on and be remembered" (2010: 492).

Indeed, "Since *Angels* [*in America*], playwrights no longer write gay-people-as-victims scripts" (McCabe 2003: 17). Nonetheless, if there were those like Kushner attempting to clear a space for some possible hope for the future, one emotion that also informed all these memoirs – the novels, plays and poems written by those of the earlier generation – was a recognition and simmering resentment that the ghettoized world of camaraderie and sexual experimentation was quickly transmogrifying into something hollow, bland and pedestrian, if not reactionary. Edmund White (2001), in his introduction to a collection of brief memoirs of artists recently dead from AIDS-related diseases and written by other artists who were their friends, typifies the nostalgia:

> Most of these memoirs [...] are about a specific time, one that Benjamin Taylor calls 'the sunlit late seventies' [...] I suppose we should never forget that the one social milieu that was open to the homosexual in the period before Stonewall was the bohemian – and this acceptance defined much of subsequent gay artistic history. The whole idea of making art – of setting up shop in workaday America and declaring oneself an artist – was as unthinkable to most Americans of the epoch as was sexual dissidence. (4)

This world died out with AIDS. In the late eighties, magazines liked to publish full spreads of photos picturing all the talent wiped out by the disease, but what these photos didn't suggest was that a way of life had been destroyed. The experimentalism, the erotic sophistication, the prejudice against materialism, the elusive humor, the ambition to measure up to international and timeless standards, above all, the belief that art should be serious and difficult – all this rich, ambiguous mixture of values and ideas evaporated (9).

Understandably, the great majority of these memoirs are written by men. One effect of the route that the epidemic was taking in its manifestation principally in men, though, was the increasing leadership roles that lesbians were assuming in maintaining the overall gay/lesbian community. This was noted with gratitude by gay men, yet some critics, in looking back over these years, lament that literature by men still does not honestly reflect these demographic leadership changes, and instead "gay authors' continued efforts to downplay or ignore women's important roles as supporters, healers, activists, and fellow-sufferers dissolve the radical potential of the AIDS text into the misogynist tradition that typifies the heterosexualized Western canon" (Foertsch 1999: 57).

The memoirs multiply as the years advance, and often at various removes from the individuals being commemorated; written by observers less emotionally connected to the dead, or by heterosexual caregivers whose medical specialization necessitated a constant and repeated contact with AIDS-related deaths. Abraham Verghese is one of these doctors, someone who found himself in 1985 – early in his career – working in a small town in eastern Tennessee and unexpectedly overseeing Johnson City's first case of AIDS. The response among his co-workers is, by now, a familiar one that has generally dissipated:

> Word spread like wildfire through the hospital. All those involved in his care in the ER and ICU agonized over their exposure. The intern remembered his palms pressed against the clammy breast as he performed closed-chest massage. Claire remembered starting the intravenous line and having blood trickle out and touch her ungloved skin. The respiratory therapist recalled the fine spray that landed on his face as he suctioned the tracheal tube. The emergency room physician recalled the sweat and the wet underwear his fingers encountered as he sought out the femoral artery. Even those who had not touched the young man—the pharmacist, the orderlies, the transport personnel—were alarmed. (1994: 10)

Not surprisingly, "the hometown boy was now regarded as an alien, the father an object of pity" (11). The death of the young man was not the end of the hospital's panicked dilemma, since the contagion was still a novelty, even four or five years into the epidemic. Thus, the question of quarantine becomes an issue, exemplifying the insults against which Vito Russo railed:

> The respirator was unhooked and rolled back to the respiratory therapy department. A heated debate ensured as to what to do with it. There were, of course, published and simple recommendations for disinfecting it. But that was not the point. The machine that had sustained the young man had come to symbolize AIDS in Johnson City. Some favored burying the respirator, deep-sixing it in the swampy land at the back of the hospital. Others were for incinerating it. As a compromise, the machine was opened up, its innards gutted and most replaceable parts changed. It was then gas disinfected several times. Even so, it was a long time before it was put back into circulation. (12)

This complex emotional response to AIDS suddenly manifesting itself in one's own familiar surroundings, away, one had thought, from the gay ghettoes that one could happily avoid and never discuss, typified the early years of the epidemic. In towns tucked away in rural America Christian charity warred with atavistic self-preservation. Gays had always seemed alien and wrong-headed; now there was reason to more openly say so.

Rebirth: Inscrutable Territory, and Amnesia

In more recent times, a sense of stark loss among those with HIV and their communities has been replaced by an ironic sense of humor, as if life itself has now become somewhat less serious, less meaningful, because one is never again fully alive and happy. Consider, for example, Alistair McCartney's *The End of the World Book* (2008), which is written as an apparently casual set of definitions, as in the following:

> **Porn, Pre-Condom**. Just like you, I love watching pre-condom porn. My favorite film is probably *He Seems to be Reaching for Something*, directed by Praxiteles, the greatest Greek gay porn director of the 300s BC. In this film, some of the Gods (today we call them cholos) wander around, cruising through the maze of antiquity, while others just stand around, waiting to be picked up, with one hip thrust out into space in the pose that was dubbed the S-curve of Praxiteles, the *S* standing for sex. All of them have a look of dreamy, ice-creamy contemplation on their faces; life's good in the sex-curve. They all appear very relaxed, probably because they are Gods, not to mention the fact that AIDS is such an impossibly long way away. (197)

The wry joking accompanies a callow hankering for some earlier time of freedom and experimentation that McCartney, born in 1971, has heard about from an older generation of gays.

Such humor, tentative and detached though it may be, will nonetheless strike some older readers whose friends or lovers have died terrible deaths, as premature, to say the least. As we have noted, the 1980s and well into the 90s had been an era in which the medical community had grown almost as fearful of the syndrome as had the general public. In comparing the epidemic with earlier diseases that seemed unavoidable – and therefore became oddly attractive – Sontag describes the "syphilis-envy" of 1920s Romania, in which artists would embrace the disease as supposedly bringing with it, just before madness, a great burst of creative intensity. "But with AIDS," she writes, "– though dementia is also a common, late symptom – no compensatory mythology has arisen, or seems likely to arise. AIDS, like cancer, does not allow romanticizing or sentimentalizing, perhaps because its association with death is too powerful" (1988: 23-24).

Palliative care seemed the only option for doctors, regardless of the sophistication of their hospital setting. "In the absence of a magic potion to cure AIDS," writes Verghese, "my job was to minister to the patient's soul, his psyche, pay attention to his family and his social situation [...] My training had not really prepared me to be this kind of doctor" (1994: 271-272). It was becoming abundantly clear that all workplaces, and not just hospitals, would need to put in place policies and procedures that had been well-thought-through, as advised by Earl C. Pike, the AIDS and Training Coordinator for the Chemical Dependency Program Division of the Minnesota Department of Human Services: "I have come to recognize," he writes in 1993:

> how critical the organization's role is, and will be, in fighting this epidemic— both in terms of treating clients and employees with HIV or AIDS well, and in terms of providing education and support for behavior change to reduce the transmission of HIV [...] Although debate continues in some arenas, the vast body of knowledge, and the mass of policy that has derived from it, is constant. Administrators need not avoid policy development for fear that 'things will change. (1993: xiii-xiv)

Pike's words clearly indicate that, by 1993, there was a growing understanding that the epidemic was here to stay, and was likely to get worse. The need to institutionalize protocols for dealing with AIDS patients accompanied a growing understanding that, with an escalating epidemic, caregivers themselves were experiencing severe psychological problems of despair and burn-out, and physical exhaustion. Reflecting in 1995 on his work with Shanti, a worldwide organization of volunteer caregivers working with the dying, its founder, Charles Garfield, writes that "I think it's clear by now that acknowledgment and support are vital for those people who work and sometimes live in the vortex of trauma and loss that are part of the AIDS pandemic" (283).

This approach also suggests that the human suffering that had become so evident throughout the United States had slowly worked as a solvent on the hardened prejudices of American society. Somewhat surprisingly – but only after years of terror-mongering in some quarters – American society was growing more understanding of, if not respectful of, gay men in its midst. As Gregory Herek argues in 1997, "AIDS could have created a major backlash of prejudice and hostility against gay men and lesbians, but it did not" (212), and the gay community had a hand in this. He asserts:

> The [gay and lesbian] community recognized early on that AIDS could be used to eradicate the hard-won victories of the 1970s, and it organized quickly to prevent such an outcome. Gay people were supported in this effort by largely sympathetic public health and medical establishments that incorporated civil rights safeguards into their traditional responses to communicable disease [...] Although members of the political right attempted repeatedly to use AIDS as a justification for repressive measures, they failed because the public became convinced that such measures were unnecessary and ineffective. (213)

As it gradually became clear how many Americans were dying from AIDS, and as authorities extrapolated from this figure to estimate the appalling number of those infected with HIV who did not yet themselves know, changes slowly came to American attitudes towards those in their midst who had no future, except that of a horrible death. As noted above, "by creating new visibility for gay people, their relationships, and communities, the epidemic may have hastened the emergence of new public identities and roles for gay men and lesbians" (Herek 1997: 212-213). And six years after he saw his first patient, Dr. Abraham Verghese recognized the changes. "I think if [that first AIDS patient's] voyage were to happen today," he writes in *My Own Country* (1994), "he might find a community in Johnson City better equipped to deal with him, to accept him. I have faith in the town and its people. I remember the acts of human kindness that illumine our world" (429). This optimism, whether supported by any facts or not, can be comforting in an age of hopelessness in the face of the syndrome, which was still the case in 1994 when Verghese published his book. This changed, beginning around 1995, when the representation of sero-positivity as an inevitable death sentence seemed miraculously to fight its way towards the more hopeful representation of HIV infection as a manageable, though chronic, set of health problems that could be managed with a very careful regimen of very expensive medications. The epidemic, though by no means over, was now becoming treatable. This regularization of the prognosis for the virus evolved further in October 2012, when a home test kit became available over-the-counter, very similar to a home pregnancy test. Such a test would likely never have been produced if there were not also some hope that a positive test result would not lead to a spike in suicides. As one writer notes, "in the past, some advocates have opposed home testing on various grounds: that finding out one is infected is so stressful that it should be done only in the presence of a counselor, that the uncertainty around the test would be stressful, and that getting a false negative could encourage someone to have unprotected sex. But since the disease is no longer an inevitable death sentence and it is clear from the epidemic's continuing spread that Americans are having unprotected sex anyway, those objections began to pale" (McNeil: 2).

The medical advances were a belated echo of the legal corrections that had been steadily transforming the role of gays in American society. In 1986, for example, the Supreme Court upheld, in *Bowers v. Hardwick*, laws against sodomy (and 66% of Americans felt that homosexual relations between consenting adults should be illegal). Just 17 years later, in *Lawrence v. Texas* (2003), the court overturned that ruling (and 60% of Americans felt that homosexual relations between consenting adults should be legal). "What made the difference between the 1986 and 2003 rulings," writes Terry McCabe, "was not some new legal theory, but society's growing acknowledgment of gay rights as civil rights, plain and simple" (McCabe: 17).

From an economic point of view, many companies came to recognize this newly-visible community of gay (HIV positive) men as a potential niche market, and this had the welcome side effect of validating the group as representatives of a much larger, and arguably culturally influential "tribe." Sherry Wolf writes that:

> The gay advertising drought of the eighties, resulting from the explosion of AIDS
> and a spate of gay militancy that advertisers shunned, gave way in the nineties
> to a dramatic rise in national brands targeting the market. One spokeswoman
> for Miller beer explained her company's ubiquitous ad campaigns in gay
> neighborhoods and bars matter-of-factly: "We market to gays and lesbians for
> business reasons because we want to sell our product to consumers. It doesn't
> get more complicated than that". (Wolf 2009: 153)

Admittedly, the stated motivation is not very complicated; in fact, it is perfectly
normal, and that is perhaps the point. Gays and lesbians in the 90s had become a
legitimate, visible, vocal, and courted market in the United States. They had not
been, heretofore.

The emerging, if sometimes begrudging, acceptance of homosexuality in
American society wrought unexpected changes in attitude among this "target"
population of new customers. The evolution of an effective "cocktail" of pills
coincided with an odd combination of, on the one hand, what Edmund White
describes as "a new queer Puritanism – the appearance of many gays who want
to marry, to adopt, to blend in, and to become virtually suburban" (2001: 9) and,
on the other hand, the rise of "barebacking", anal copulation without the use of a
condom.

The changing consciousness is well-encapsulated in two entries in Alistair
McCarthy's novel: first, *Extinction*:

> Sometimes when I look in the mirror on the medicine cabinet in our bathroom, I
> am reminded of the time my mother took me to the Museum of Natural History.
> We saw a tiny fossil of a small, strange, winged creature. The pattern of its
> wings was so delicate. It was as if the ancient bird was hurtling toward us, flying
> through the slate-gray rock. As I looked, my face pressed up to the glass case,
> some joy in me snapped.

> Thought took us to the brink of extinction, but on further reflection, we have
> decided to come back. (78)

Second, *Masque of the Red Death*. In the entry with this title, McCarthy compares
Poe's story to a porn movie well-known in the gay community, *The Other Side
of Aspen*, in which gay skiers welcome a masked stranger to their lodge, without
fear, which is the opposite of what Poe's characters do; Poe's characters more
understandably flee death:

> However, whereas the guests in Poe's story are horrified by this ghoulish masked
> stranger, who is Death himself, and attempt to turn away – an attempt that of
> course in the end proves to be futile – the guests in *The Other Side*, perhaps
> knowing that there is no longer any point in hiding and that any attempt to do so

would be ineffectual, welcome the masked stranger, who is Death himself, into
the fray. (158)

This is an interesting commentary on the 1983 movie, produced in the years when
death did seem to be seriously stalking the gay community, and last, desperate
orgies at a snow lodge might have special appeal. What McCarthy might have
considered, however, are the subsequent films in that series. *The Other Side* part
VI, for example, was released in 2011, and the participants are visibly careful
to use condoms. One 20-year veteran pornography director, Chi Chi LaRue, has
decided never to film bareback scenes, and includes a warning against such activity
in each of his films. Many other directors have clearly come to other conclusions,
and are trumpeting the erotic potential of unprotected anal intercourse. The point
McCarthy makes about the carpe diem atmosphere in which the first film in the
series was made, in any case, makes great sense. What does not make as much
sense, is the quickly expanding market in "bareback" pornography in the gay
community and, of more concern for those tracking increasing rates of STD and
HIV transmission, the apparently increasingly popular engagement by younger
gay men in barebacking itself.[4] This is accompanied by a truly bizarre activity
known as bug-chasing, in which an individual actively seeks out HIV-positive
men who are willing to bareback and pass the virus along; this is called "gift-
giving" (Cooper 2003). Such activity seems very much to support the notion of
amnesia that we will discuss in what follows.

    Queer theorists nowadays, as well as some older gay men, criticize a growing
comfort among gays with settling in as normal American citizens: "There is a
transition under way," writes one, "in how queer subjects are relating to nation-
states, particularly the United States, from being figures of death (that is, the AIDS
epidemic) to becoming tied to ideas of life and productivity (that is, gay marriage
and families)" (Puar 2007: xii). Some, principally from the Stonewall generation,
lament what is being lost in the process of incorporation and domestication.
"In the arts an edginess, a quirkiness, even a violence has given way to stylistic
blandness," writes Edmund White:

> Gay fiction has now become a wading pool for minor talents to dabble in; the
> novels often sound transcribed from the film scripts they long to become: novel
> as novelization. Publishers, who recognize that few gay novels can be expected
> to sell more than twenty thousand (or even ten thousand) copies, are now
> content to throw dull genre fiction out into the world and let it sink – or paddle
> – unaided. Gay bookshops are closing down (from seventy-five two years ago
> to fifty now [2001]), and most of the serious gay literary publications (with the
> exception of the *James White Review* and the *Gay and Lesbian Review*) have

---

    4 A clear and concise introduction to this rapidly changing topic is offered on the
'bareback' entry on Wikipedia: http://en.wikipedia.org/wiki/Bareback_%28sex%29/
Accessed 12 July 2012.

stopped publishing. A tackiness, a sort of steroid-injected sex-shop conformism, has replaced the old transgressiveness of gay art (2001: 10).[5]

With the greater visibility of gays in American society, there seems to be a whiff of "you can't go home again" in White's lament that in contemporary fiction, film, and television "what isn't being shown are gay men in a gay world, people as fully expressed socially as sexually" (10). And, one must admit, the old gay enclaves have now become remarkably similar to heterosexual communities, extremely commercialized places that are not very transgressive, at all (if one overlooks the proliferation of pornography shops, which, arguably, do not fill the social role that bookstores once did). White and his brethren lament the loss of gays as countercultural, as anti-institutional. One might think of the comparative seriousness of the Mormon church in *Angels in America* versus its silliness in *Book of Mormon* (Trey Parker, Robert Lopez, Matt Stone, 2011), where the message, while surely informed with heavy-handed criticism of the church's hypocrisy, seems to be encouraging the audience at every turn to shout: "let's have some fun, the crisis has passed." To give the playwrights their due, there is a compelling song early in the musical that reminds the audience that the virus is decimating large percentages of the African population.

Increasingly, some critics are objecting to what they describe as a comforting amnesia, an unseemly putting-behind-us of the epidemic, as if it were over, as if there were not many thousands of Americans (let along those in the rest of the world) living with HIV. Richard Canning laments the erasure of this reality from the popular arts by a younger generation of gays that just wants to get the party started. "Again and again," he writes, "popular narratives have returned us to the convenient, ubiquitous storyline of coming to terms with one's marginal sexuality and 'coming out'" (2011: 26). In other words, to the world of adolescence:

> The wider world of HIV infection, which continues at epidemic levels and is decimating host populations, must expect no look-in, barring the rare, exceptional art house vehicle [...] Surely there is something massively forgetful about our contemporary moment and its fostering of all manner of GLBT identities in, as it were, a historical bubble—one that avoids the years 1981 to 1997, and which pretends that the world post-1997 is HIV-free. (27)

---

5 Viewed from a broader perspective, though, Christopher Reed argues that:
   By the turn of the millennium – a century after Wilde made the aesthetically sensitive, persecuted homosexual a paradigm for the modern artist and a quarter century after Warhol made camp a paradigm for postmodernism – the connotations of 'gay art' equally included the 'in-your-face' anger, political engagement, and sexual explicitness associated with ACT UP, Mapplethorpe, and Wojnarowicz (2011, 228).

His point is that the "drug-cocktail-dependent person [...] no longer experiences – if s/he ever did – the visceral, salutary uplift of restorative good health, but instead plows on in the imperfect, always uncertain here and now" (26), but this is rarely represented in novels, poems, or films in the United States in the twenty-first century. This gives the impression that, as gays increasingly assimilate, their motto has become: the less said, the better, as far as the bad old days of AIDS are concerned.

This concern underscores the problem that historians of the gay liberation movement have with some queer theorists, whom they accuse of papering over the messiness of the early decades, including the horrors of AIDS, as a tactic for moving on. What is objected to is "the gesture of disavowing a gay past in order to procure a queer rigor." (Castiglia and Reed 2012: 5). This was especially true in the first wave of queer theory, which Christopher Castiglia and Christopher Reed suggest "arose at a particular moment for reasons other than greater intellectual acuity and [...] at least one of those reasons was the general unremembering that took hold in the aftershock of the first years of AIDS" (5). The community was traumatized, and reacting as a trauma victim would to the assault from an unstoppable epidemic. "It was that context that not only demanded a 'queer subject,' solitary and outside history, but that also detached itself from its intellectual roots in ways that made 'gay theory' seem an anachronistic oxymoron" (5).

The second wave of queer theorists, they contend, is more "historically grounded, socially engaged, multiethnic, and sensitive to the spatial and temporal operations of sexuality" (4), and thus has helped mitigate what the two critics call "coercive unremembering and queer countermemory" (4), but they nonetheless want to reaffirm, in the face of some queer theorists, that "sexuality *should* matter: it should be the thrilling, dangerous, unpredictable, imaginative force it once was and no doubt still is, although more often quietly and out of public sight" (9), thus, the new puritanism that White sees dominating today's gay community.

Much like Edmund White, Castiglia and Reed lament what has been lost since the unifying struggles against a deadly disease:

> The collective trauma of AIDS was a fact of life. Just when we most needed models of culture that would allow us to mourn our losses and strengthen ourselves to resist the conservatism that made those losses seem inevitable, just when our pleasures and the cultural spaces for enjoying them were most precarious, we began a process of temporal isolation, distancing ourselves from the supposedly excessive generational past in exchange for promises of 'acceptance' in mainstream institutions. The signs of these losses are everywhere: in the monopoly of 'gay marriage' in place of debates about sexual world-making; in the assimilation of sexual minorities and the subsequent abandonment of supposedly restrictive gay 'ghettos'; in the insistent invisibility of AIDS or sexual liberation in popular media; in the dearth of radical, public, and collective challenges to mainstream institutions. (9)

However wounded such authors may legitimately feel themselves to be, though, this brief survey cannot conclude without a return to the observation made in its opening: there is at least one community in the United States in which AIDS has not been brought under control. For a complex set of reasons that would go beyond the scope of this essay, the various African American communities are still underrepresented in fiction, film, and gay community newspapers. Marlon Riggs's 1989 film, *Tongues Untied*, Keith Boykin's *Beyond the Down Low* (2004), and Cathy Cohen's *The Boundaries of Blackness* (1999) demonstrate the complexities of silencing and shame within black communities on this issue, but also indicate the racism within gay white America that perpetuates the marginalization of this group of gay men. The same could be said, though less uniformly, about the representation of Hispanic men infected with HIV. The amnesia that is growing among a younger white generation of gay men, the "de-generation" that Castiglia and Reed lament, literally pales in comparison to the inadequate representation of AIDS among America's racial minorities.

References

Albert, E. 1986. Illness and deviance: the response of the press to AIDS, in *Social Dimensions of AIDS*, edited by D. Feldman and T. Johnson. Westport, Connecticut: Praeger.

Anonymous. 1999. HIV/AIDS: crisis among young black and latino gay men and other men who have sex with men (MSM). National Alliance of State and Territorial AIDS Directors (NASTAD) Youth Issue Brief #1. http://www.nastad.org/Docs/highlight/2009130_Youth%20Issue%20Brief%20No%201.pdf. Accessed 13 July 2012.

Barnett, C. 2010. AIDS = purgatory: Prior Walter's prophecy and *Angels in America. Modern Drama* 53.4. 471-94.

Boykin, K. 2004. *Beyond the Down Low: Sex, Lies and Denial in Black America.* New York: Carroll and Graf.

Bruni, F. 2012. Love among the spuds. New York Times online. 10 July. http://www.nytimes.com/2012/07/10/opinion/bruni-love-among-the-spuds.html?_r=1&hp&pagewanted=print. Accessed 10 July.

Canning, R. 2011. The epidemic that barely was. *Gay and Lesbian Review Worldwide*, 18.2, 25-27.

Castiglia, C. and Reed, C. 2012. *If Memory Serves: Gay Men, AIDS, and the Promise of the Queer Past.* Minneapolis: University of Minnesota Press.

Centers for Disease Control and Prevention. HIV among African Americans. http://www.cdc.gov/hiv/topics/aa/. Accessed 7 July 2012.

Cohen, C. 1999. *The Boundaries of Blackness: AIDS and the Breakdown of Black Politics.* Chicago: University of Chicago Press.

Cooper, A. 2003. Interview with Louis Hogarth. YouTube 6 June 2003. http://www.youtube.com/watch?v=Bo_n0IPsC7g. Accessed 8 July 2012.

Coppola, V. 1983. The AIDS epidemic: the search for a cure. *Newsweek* 18 April. http://www.whatisaids.com/newsweekarticle.htm. Accessed 4 July 2012.

Foertsch, J. 1999. Angels in an epidemic: woman as 'negatives' in recent AIDS literature. *South Central Review*, 16.1, 57-72.

Garfield, C. 1995. *Sometimes My Heart Goes Numb: Love and Caregiving in a Time of AIDS.* San Francisco: Jossey-Bass Publishers.

Gross, L. and Woods, J. eds. 1999. *The Columbia Reader on Lesbians and Gay Men in Media, Society, and Politics.* New York: Columbia University Press.

Herek, G. 1997. The HIV epidemic and public attitudes toward lesbians and gay men, in *In Changing Times: Gay Men and Lesbians Encounter HIV/AIDS,* edited by J. Levine. Chicago and London: The University of Chicago Press, 191-218.

Hoffman, T. 2000. Representing AIDS: Thom Gunn and the modalities of verse. *South Atlantic Review*, 65.2, 13-39.

hooks, bell. Homophobia in black communities. *ONTD Political* June 6, 2010. http://ontd-political.livejournal.com/6369860.html. Accessed 11 August 2012.

Kinsella, J. 1989. *Covering the Plague: AIDS and the American Media.* New Brunswick and London: Rutgers University Press.

Lawrence, T. 1997. AIDS, the problem of representation, and plurality in Derek Jarman's *Blue. Social Text*, 52/53, 241-264.

Levine, M., Nardi, P. and Gagnon, J. eds. 1997. *In Changing Times: Gay Men and Lesbians Encounter HIV/AIDS.* Chicago and London: The University of Chicago Press.

McCabe, T. 2003. Angels in our midst. *The Chronicle of Higher Education* 5 December. 17.

McCartney, A. 2008. *The End of the World Book.* Madison, WI: Terrace Books/ University of Wisconsin Press.

McNeil, D. 2012. Quick at-home H.I.V. test wins federal approval. *New York Times* online, 3 July. http://www.nytimes.com/2012/07/04/health/oraquick-at-home-hiv-test-wins-fda-approval.html?_r=1&hp. Accessed 3 July 2012.

Monette, P. 1988. *Borrowed Time: An AIDS Memoir.* New York: Harcourt Brace Jovanovich, Publishers.

Murphy, T. 1994. *Ethics in an Epidemic: AIDS, Morality, and Culture.* Berkeley: University of California Press.

Picano, F. 1995. *Like People in History.* New York: Viking.

Piggford, G. 2000. "In time of plague": AIDS and its signification in Hervé Guibert, Tony Kushner, and Thom Gunn. *Cultural Critique*, 44, 169-196.

Pike, E. 1993. *We Are All Living with AIDS: How You Can Set Policies and Guidelines for the Workplace.* Minneapolis: Deaconess Press.

Puar, J. 2007. *Terrorist Assemblages: Homonationalism in Queer Times.* Durham: Duke University Press.

Reed, C. 2011. *Art and Homosexuality: A History of Ideas.* New York: Oxford.

Riggs, M., dir. 1989. *Tongues Untied: Black Men Loving Black Men.* Frameline distributors.

Rotello, G. 1997. Creating a new gay culture: balancing fidelity and freedom. *Nation* 21 April. 11-16.

Russo, V. 1990. A test of who we are as a people: ACT UP rally, Albany, New York, May 7, 1988, in *Democracy: Discussions in Contemporary Culture*, edited by B. Wallis. Seattle: Bay Press. 299-302. Rpt. in Gross, L. and J. Woods, eds. 1999. *The Columbia Reader on Lesbians and Gay Men in Media, Society, and Politics*. New York: Columbia University Press. 408-410.

Shilts, R. 1987. *And the Band Played On: Politics, People, and the AIDS Epidemic*. New York: St. Martin's Press.

Signorile, M. 1997. *Life Outside: The Signorile Report on Gay Men: Drugs, Muscles, and the Passages of Life*. New York: HarperCollins.

Sontag, S. 1988. *AIDS and its Metaphors*. New York: Farrar, Straus and Giroux.

Ulaby, N. 2012. Pieces of AIDS quilt blanket nation's capital. National Public Radio 27 June 2012. http://www.wnyc.org/npr_articles/2012/jun/27/pieces-of-aids-quilt-blanket-nations-capital/ accessed 28 June 2012.

Vargas, H. and Inniss, H. LGBT health is about life and death. *Advocate.com* http://www.advocate.com/commentary/2012/06/20/reminder-lgbt-health-about-life-and-death?goback=.gde_4061263_member_126798420 accessed 28 June 2012.

Verghese, A. 1994. *My Own Country: A Doctor's Story*. New York: Random House.

Watney, S. 2000. *Imagine Hope: AIDS and Gay Identity*. London and New York: Routledge.

White, E., ed. 2001. *Loss Within Loss: Artists in the Age of AIDS*. Madison: University of Wisconsin Press.

Wolf, Sherry. 2009. *Sexuality and Socialism: History, Politics, and Theory of LGBT Liberation*. Chicago: Haymarket Books.

Chapter 3
Mapping Hetero/Homo-sexuality on the Caribbean, Male, HIV Body

Gustavo E. Subero

HIV/AIDS is recognised as an increasingly major problem in the Caribbean. According to the AVERT (International HIV and AIDS charity), the Caribbean is the second largest region in the world to be affected by the illness. The size of the region, as well as the diversity of cultures, beliefs and socio-political systems that co-exist in this area, make it difficult to plan strategies that are effective through the entire region to prevent and combat further transmissions. Unlike other regions in the world affected by this problem, the Caribbean (in much of a similar fashion to the African region) has traditionally suffered from a self-imposed silence in relation to the reality of its HIV problematic. Overall, the main route of HIV transmission in the Caribbean is heterosexual sex. Transmission usually occurs via commercial sex and/or sex tourism or by gender-orientated, culturally-fostered ignorance, as seropositive men pass the syndrome to their girlfriends or wives through sex. Sex between men (whether gay or men who sleep with men) also plays a major role in the way the syndrome is transmitted amongst the population. According to the Caribbean Task Force on HIV/AIDS, it is estimated that HIV is the leading cause of death amongst the 15–44 year age group. Furthermore, it is claimed that cultural and behavioural patterns such as early initiation of sexual acts, as well as taboos related to sex and sexuality; gender inequalities; lack of confidentiality; stigmatisation and economic need, are some of the factors that most greatly influence vulnerability to HIV and AIDS in the Caribbean.

The system whereby sexual culture(s) operate in the Caribbean plays a key role in the high incidence of HIV transmission amongst the population. Research by the World Bank reports that "to prove their *machismo*, many men in Caribbean countries […] engage in high-risk behaviours such as having early and frequent sex with multiple women. Such behaviours amplify both their own vulnerability and their partners' vulnerability to HIV infection" (2001: 25). This can be explained by the fact that macho men are expected to be knowledgeable about sex, however – and paradoxically – they are socially and culturally discouraged to obtain information and/or access services for safer sex.[1] On the other hand, women become reliant on men's sexual knowledge and experience whilst they are also expected to be compliant and not challenge men's sexual demands, even when they suspect or know that their partners are infected. Another influential factor in the transmission of HIV is the early initiation of sexual activity amongst young people (especially boys). Macho attitudes and beliefs, peer influence, as well as influence by parents and older relatives, music such as Reggaeton and Dance Hall (characterised by the objectification of women and sexually explicit and violent lyrics) are some of the factors that strongly encourage children and adolescents into early sexual practices. For instance, in an adolescent health survey carried out by PAHO in 1998, it showed that of those youths who declared themselves to be sexually active, more than 40 per cent stated that their first sexual encounter had been at the age of 10, whilst an additional 20 per cent had started at age 11 or 12. Similarly, "adolescent girls and some boys may accept unprotected sexual relations with older men in order to access resources. These practices are supported by the cultural norm that men should provide financially for their sexual partners" (Bombereau and Allen, 2008). By the same token, the World Bank report adds "some men and women, and even children, in the Caribbean are forced by economic and political conditions to leave their families to find work or to become sex workers in order to survive" (2005: 26). It could be easily predicted that, in such cases, safe-sex information is scarcely provided or available to such individuals. Similarly, the lack of control over sex work in the region, in conjunction with the cost of condoms and other safe-sex protection, makes both clients and sex workers high-risk groups. Kamala Kempadoo also asserts, "it appears that the demand on the part of men not to use condoms is still high, and the pressure on women to work unsafely is still a major factor" (1996: 77). Such individuals also tend to move from one city or island to another, thus they become mobile carriers of HIV infection wherever they go. The economic environment and associated gender disparities that are evident in the region continue to provide men (heterosexual) with the ownership of desire in matters of sex and, as a result, young people and women are often exposed to or become the victims of physical abuse that puts them at risk of HIV. At the same time, the lack of a clear national or regional strategy that may reduce HIV infection amongst the population, as Gaelle Bombereau and Charles Allen argue "may undermine public health goals by encouraging new infections. Criminalisation of homosexuality and sex workers, lack of strong policies regarding sexual abuse, and differential access to care and treatment options put various sub-populations at risk for HIV" (2008).

---

1   The Report of National Knowledge, Attitudes, Behaviour & Practice Survey (2000) indicates that a high level of knowledge about ways to prevent HIV coexists with various myths about HIV. The public awareness campaigns launched by the government with the theme "AIDS kills" have left a lasting impression on the general population who believe that HIV diagnosis equates to an imminent death.

Besides the social and political factors that contribute to the proliferation of HIV cases in the Caribbean, the system through which sexual cultures operate in the region plays a key role in the way that people face or engage in their own sexual practices. Unfortunately, certain elements within the Caribbean's popular culture further reinforce male hegemony in sexual matters and, as a result, only serve to maintain male supremacy in the popular imaginary. Perhaps one of the most influential forms of artistic expression that contributes to maintain the status quo of gender and sex relations in the region is music, especially Dance Hall and Reggaeton. Although both music/dance genres have very specific elements that distinguish them from one another, they both also share overt sexual lyrics (in which women are depicted as sexual objects and gay men are vilified, whilst heterosexual, male listeners are encouraged to subjugate them) and a particular form of dance that practically emulates sexual intercourse. As Donna P. Hope rightly argues, "masculine identity is negotiated via a route that wrests power (sexual and otherwise) from the feminine other, resulting in the upliftment of an intensely heterosexual, polygamous and ultimately powerful form of male identity" (2007: 377). The language employed in the lyrics of the songs becomes one of the main tools to exercise and maintain male dominance.[2] Direct references to female genitalia, sexual positions/instances during sex and (homo)sexual identity are described by using words such a punaany (vagina) or battyboy (gay men), which also function as devices that make abject aspects of sexuality and/or gender that are regarded (and even feared) as feminine in such macho cultures.[3] The constant use of such language then filters into mainstream society, to the extent that the words become part of everyday usage (and even come to replace the original in the popular usage). Alongside this, the style of dancing that accompanies such musical genres also reinforces a hierarchical system based on gender identity, in which men are articulated as superior. As Alfredo Nieves Moreno points out, "this superiority is articulated from the very perreo, in which a woman swings her hips to the rhythm of the music while the male partner, standing right behind her, rocks slowly" (2009: 255). This form of pseudo-intercourse, although it challenges traditional views on sexual practices (by disavowing the missionary position as the only "accepted" or "decent" position in sex in accordance to religious beliefs), it still subjugates women by placing them as passive objects of

---

2   Errol Miller (1991) argues that the Caribbean is experiencing the marginalisation of the black male, as they are increasingly absent from the high position within the family, the classroom and the labour force. This research, however, takes side with Keisha Lindsay (2002) who proposes that the presence of more women in such strata within Caribbean society does not necessarily imply a correlation between female empowerment and the family structure or even the wider society.

3   Carolyn Cooper (2000) rightly argues that some female artists, such as DJ Lady Saw, challenge culturally-rooted paradigms in relation to women's appropriate behavior, however her behavior is usually frowned upon and therefore receives a form of censorship for being too "slack".

desire. Male domination continues to be paramount in the construction of gender identity in the region, a type of domination that "enhances the figure of the man and situates him in a position of constant symbolic authority" (idem). This could be taken even further by suggesting that the dances which accompany Dancehall and Reggaeton are, as Jan Fairley points out, both "symbolically masturbatory dance" and "apes troilism and pornographic 'spit roasting,' that is, a woman serving one man sexually while another man is having sex with her" (2009: 286). With such images of sex and sexuality circulating in the mainstream of culture and fuelling the popular imagination (and libido) of the population, it is not surprising that challenging sexual paradigms in relation to gender relations and safe sexual practices is a very difficult task for both policy makers and sexual health workers.

It is from this point of departure that this chapter is interested in exploring the implications of HIV in the popular perception of *machismo* and/or *mariconería* as a template for male sexuality in the Caribbean, and how the illness is usually associated with a loss of masculinity (including queer masculinity). It will argue that HIV is regarded as a disease that feminises the male body, through its own decay, and strips it of its culturally ascribed masculinity. The chapter evidences that, on the one hand, although machismo is culturally regarded as an innate quality of all males in the Caribbean, it seems to operate at the interstice of hetero/ homosexuality, and its loss is both feared and also a constant and real threat. On the other hand, HIV is regarded as a natural part of the process of sublimation of male subjects who find some form of "enlightenment" through being positive. To this end, this chapter will mainly focus on Arnold Antonin's *Le president a-t-il le sida?* and Julian Schnabel's *Before night falls,* and show how the main protagonists' positive status becomes a real threat to their purported masculinity – one that will evolve to a less caricaturised version of itself as both films progress. The first part of the chapter will provide a close analysis of Antonin's film and evidence that, despite the didacticism with which the film was made (one that has sought to stress the intrinsic message that both protected sex is primordial in order to prevent further HIV contagion and that medical attention is key to control the illness), the storyline has relied heavily on the protagonist's body and love interest to stress his masculinity and guarantee its permanence, since HIV is depicted and narrativised as a latent threat that culminates in the loss of masculinity. For heterosexual men, becoming seropositive becomes a shameful experience and makes their bodies abject in relation to sexual cultures within their own societies. Shame and stigma remain paramount in the construction of positive identity for heterosexual males and the way such bodies are constructed within the popular imaginary. The second part of the chapter will provide a close analysis of the trajectory that Schnabel's protagonist's body undergoes in order to narrativise HIV as a form of gay martyrdom. Schnabel decides to obviate aspects of the narrative (as described in Arenas' posthumous autobiography on which the film is based) that would call into question the "sanctity" of the depiction of the character and his own suffering, both as a gay man persecuted in a homophobic regime of power and as a seropositive man living in poverty in the USA. Finally, this chapter will argue that, in both films, HIV is used as a narrative device that transforms the characters into 'better human beings' by disavowing machismo or mariconería as stereotypical templates for male sexuality in the Caribbean.

Changing men and masculinity in *Le president a-t-il le Sida?*

Haiti is one of the poorest countries in the Caribbean; it has faced several hardships in the form of a cruel dictatorship, political violence, widespread abject poverty and, more recently, a devastating earthquake that left the country in political and economic turmoil. However, despite all the problems faced by this country, filmmaking seems to still thrive as a popular form of mass consumption and as a much-needed form of relief from the harsh reality faced by Haitians. Although the vast majority of the population cannot afford portable DVD players and the distribution of films is very limited, portable cinemas have been set up around the island and "often packed to the brim the screenings offer new hope and a form of escape from the nightmare that exists" (Kanema www.mubi.com). Arnold Antonin, a documentarist and film director, emerged from a new generation of Haitian filmmakers in the 1970s and has seen cinema as an instrument to educate the masses and a as weapon against the dictatorial regime. Antonin's work is mainly constituted by institutional or educational films, and since his return to Haiti from exile in 1986 he has worked closely with the Centre Pétion-Bolivar. However, in 2006 Antonin made the feature film *Le president a-t-il le Sida?*, a film that tells the story of Dao (Jimmy Jean-Louis), a famous singer who leads a wild life fuelled with promiscuous sex and drugs, and who becomes HIV positive as a result. The film follows his experience with Voodoo and Evangelical priests as they try to rid him of the illness until he eventually accepts medical treatment for HIV. During this time, Nina (Jessica Geneus), who is his first real love, tries desperately to help him accept his positive status. In the end, accepting his HIV condition and undergoing medical treatment are the only option in order to lead a healthy and normal life.

From the very beginning of the film it is clear that Antonin's goal is to provide a form of agency to the HIV positive individual whilst also criticising (and trying to challenge) macho attitudes and sexism on the island. As has been previously suggested, Caribbean masculinity, in a very similar fashion to the rest of Latin America, relies heavily on the performance of gender and masculinity. The film, however, does not seem to challenge the way that masculinity is constituted or internalised amongst Caribbean males, but the way that masculinity is practised or exercised. This idea follows Kamala Kenpadoo when he argues that Caribbean masculinity must be understood in terms of sexual praxis. He points out:

> the focus on praxis rather than identity is for two main reasons: a) sexuality does not form a primary basis for social identification in the Caribbean, consequently sexual behaviours, activities and relations have become the central focus for

analyses of sexuality in the region; and b) the specification of sexual identity groups often elides the very varied sexual arrangements in the region, and can work to hinder broader understandings of how Caribbean peoples relate sexually. (2009: 2)

This is all the more evident in the opening scenes of the film in which a contrast between Jean (played also by Jean-Louis) and Dao, and their assumed masculinities, is established. The film opens with Jean and Myrlene (Chantal Pierre-Louis) in bed after a failed attempt at sex. Jean is shown covered up to his waist (revealing his muscular and chiselled torso) whilst Myrlene is fully covered by the bed sheet. She justifies the failed sex encounter by blaming Jean for not offering her either economic security or marital stability (which seems to be the two criteria for the fulfilment of a successful relationship). As Jean stands up to get dressed, she takes the opportunity to point out that if Jean were to cut his dreadlocks (the only thing that visibly differentiates the two characters played by Pierre-Louis) and look more like Dao, she would be more willing to lose her virginity with him. It is clear that the sexual transaction here is dominated by fantasies of fame and power and by the desire to attain economic mobility. This kind of message, however, seems to be in direct opposition to the notions of masculinity that circulate in the popular imaginary, since women are expected to be passive recipients of male desire. Although it could be argued that this scene empowers female identity, it also demonstrates that many sexual transactions on the island are based on the possibility or prospect of economic mobility and therefore put people more at risk of engaging in practices without fully protecting themselves.

The scene then cuts to Dao's mansion as spectators see him rushing into his bathroom and being sick in the toilet. Although he is only wearing his underwear, his body is already depicted as a sick body and is somewhat de-eroticised by the external manifestation of his illness. Once he has finished being sick, Dao goes to check himself in the bathroom mirror and he says to himself "Dao, you're the best musician in the country, the most handsome, the president" and after sniffing some cocaine he adds "You're not ill. Nothing can happen to you". This scene already sets the tone for the film to regard illness as a metaphor, following Sontag's (1965) famous theorisation, and to associate the protagonist's illness with a deviant lifestyle. By using his body as a vehicle to negate the reality of his seropositive condition, Dao also demonstrates an awareness of what Charles Horton Cooley (1992) and Kathy Charmaz and Dana Rosenfeld (2006) call the "looking glass self", in which the individual constructs his identity via the corporeality of the body, or as Charmaz and Rosenfeld argue "looking at the relationships between the body, self and identity" (2006: 36). However, the protagonist also makes the audience aware of his own mortality and the fact that neither his skills as a musician nor his good looks and virility can overcome his HIV condition. This demonstrates that Dao is more concerned with the way the illness will affect his depiction of his star/ masculine persona than any concerns with the problems that may be associated with the illness he is suffering. This scene cuts to Dao, found in bed with three naked women by Georges (his manager). After getting rid of the three women, Georges (Manfred Marcelin) expresses surprise at not finding residual or unused condoms in the room. Dao proceeds to take him to a secret room at the top of his mansion where he has created a Voodoo altar and tells the manager that he does not need condoms because he is protected by magic. Antonin's didactic approach to the subject matter is evident in this scene (and many others in the film) as Georges says "Nothing supernatural will protect you against AIDS, only self-protection". However, Dao's macho attitude and mentality chimes with David Plummer and Joel Simpson who claim "Caribbean masculinities are defined by taking risks; and [...] masculine reputations are made through demonstrating sexual prowess" (2007). Dao's masculinity is constructed on his body, a body that is both desired by women and reified by their behaviour towards it, and envied by men who wish to attain his degree of masculinity (and seek to compensate this lack by means of imitation, as in the case of Jean). It could be argued that Dao's masculinity is constructed through body transactions, as his body becomes a form of currency that provides inner value to him, as a man, and can be also used as a form of exchange (in this case, to obtain sex at will). In *Le president*, the self-figuration of Dao as the filmic epitome of a black Caribbean male identity, relies heavily on the way his body is read (both sexually and culturally) by the people around him. He depends on his body to continue the status quo of his socio-sexual identity and, as Fran Fanon suggests in his analysis of black (negro) identity, "represents the sexual instinct (in its raw state). The Negro is the incarnation of a genital potency beyond all moralities and prohibitions [...] the Negro [acts] as the keeper of the impalpable gate that opens into the realm of orgies, of bacchanals, of delirious sexual sensations" (1993: 177).

However, Dao's masculine identity is threatened by his decaying body, as he runs the risk of becoming de-masculinised and, by default, feminised by the illness. Interestingly, this de-masculinisation in the film does not rely on external factors (or symptoms) that may show his positive status, but by the mere suspicion of having the illness and, therefore, questioning the bearer's masculinity. For instance, the first time that Nina and Dao meet on a date, Nina is warned by a group of women, whose advances Dao has rejected, that she should be careful not to contract HIV from him (although they do not know that he is seropositive) because "men like him swing both ways". This scene, thus, operates in two ways; on the one hand, it evidences that HIV continues to be considered, in the popular imaginary, as an illness that only affects gay men or men who have sex with men. On the other, and more importantly, it highlights the importance of female complicity to maintain male power by means of proclaiming and stressing their partner's maleness. As Linden Lewis asserts, "masculinity also has much to do with men's relationships to women. There is a sense in which men in society collectively define masculinity for themselves, but they are always cognizant of the influence of women in their definition" (2003: 95). This complicity is, therefore, paramount in the construction and maintenance of black masculinity as it means that the male subject will be able to reaffirm his maleness through the recounting of his experiences of sexual prowess. It is understandable, therefore, that later on in the film Nina is kicked out of Dao's mansion when she asks him to wear a condom in order for them to have sex. Asking him to use a condom only serves to dig into the protagonist's insecurity and his own fears in relation to the symptoms he has been showing since the beginning of the film. It is also obvious that, for Dao, Nina has betrayed him by challenging his maleness. As he stands semi naked in front of his lover, his words are testimony of his hurt macho pride as he yells at her "I'm the best, the biggest. Do you think I'm sick?" In this instance, he uses his muscular body, as he gestures to himself, to reassure her that he does not need to wear a condom because he is a 'real man'.

Dao tries to use his body to avoid stigma and to prove that there is nothing wrong with him. He realises that the body is a social symbol and that his (Caribbean) masculinity, like most hyper-masculine identities, is read on the surface of the body. This clearly follows Erving Goffman (1963), who argues that stigma is most clearly visible on the subject's body when such a body is recognised as a social construction and allows for the recognition of an intrinsic difference. This difference is based on a specific characteristic that only serves to devalue its bearer. However, whether Antonin's intention to use Jean-Louis's body to de-stigmatise the HIV positive individual is successful must be called into question. The director certainly presents Dao as a sex symbol from the very beginning of the film whilst constructing and reifying his masculinity through his muscular body. For instance, when his mother (Huguette Saint Fleur) takes him to see the Voodoo priest in order to exorcise the bad spirits that afflict her son, the film wastes no time in offering Dao as the object of the erotic filmic gaze. Although at this stage in the narrative Dao is supposedly quite sick, there is nothing on his external appearance that shows a degradation or deterioration of his body; in fact, only his acting tries to convey the 'severity' of his illness. It is undeniable that HIV encapsulates all three of Goffman's categories of stigma: abominations of the body, blemishes of individual character and tribal stigmas (1963), and yet none of these aspects are discernible on the protagonist's body. Dao's seemingly decaying body is shown shirtless as the Voodoo ritual begins. He is then tied up to a post and the camera proceeds to pan very slowly in close shot from his bulging biceps to his chiselled abs. This then cuts to a close-up of his face looking down, with part of the rope around his neck and a very small amount of blood trickling down his lip and nose. The way this image is presented does very little to invoke the stigma that HIV individuals suffer; instead it follows a tradition of masochistic eroticisation in which the male protagonist must temporarily suffer at the hands of the villain(s), whilst his torture is presented as a fetish (Holmlund, 1993; Brown, 2002) and the viewer is temporarily positioned as voyeur. Even when Nina eventually rescues him from the priest's house, the only visual element that tries to narrativise (or diegetically portray) the deterioration of his body is dust from the floor of the shank in which he was being kept captive. Paradoxically, the overt eroticisation of his body arguably disavows the criticism that the film tries to provide against engaging in popular or religious practices[4] and beliefs as a way to combat the illness. However, as the film progresses, the audience will witness a gradual de-eroticisation of the protagonist's body, as the narrative moves closer to the moment when he is officially diagnosed with his seropositive condition.

It could be argued that, in this film, the protagonist's stigma derives from the silence surrounding the speculations about his HIV condition rather than the stigma that arises from bodily marks. As Régine Michelle Jean-Charles comments in relation to the film, "that the title [of the film] is framed as a question, which the narrative confirms in the affirmative, comments on the perception of AIDS in a larger cultural context. This is not, as the title suggests, about whether he [Dao] has AIDS but rather about whether he will publicly acknowledge his disease" (2011: 67). The stigma surrounding the protagonist's body begins, as previously mentioned, in the scene in which the three women warn Nina about Dao's potential positive status. This silent stigma continues when Dao is asked at a radio interview whether the rumours that his health is precarious are true. Interestingly, Dao's double-entendre reply clearly shows the importance of the *teledjol* (system of information based on rumours and speculation) within Haitian society. He answers the radio presenter with a "*Je suis malade avec mon publique*", which can be taken as either "I'm sick of my public" or "My public is sick with me". The first answer (provided as the sole option in the English subtitles) would simply convey Dao's annoyance at the fact that his star persona and his masculinity are called into question by speculating about his health. However, the second interpretation is all the more interesting, as this permits to revert stigmatisation and to make Dao's public (or those who were questioning his health) abject. This answer simply dehumanises Dao's followers by making them the subjects of an illness of which he is the sole cause. This idea is further illustrated by a comment he makes earlier on in the film when, just before the start of a concert, he tells an interviewer "people are looking for a cure to Dao's music". The metaphor of illness famously discussed by Susan Sontag (2001), in which the sufferer of an illness (especially those which procure visible marks on the patient) is dehumanised, is reverted onto the assumedly healthy music fans. This action reifies that, as Jonathan Vaknin argues in relation to abjection, "the boundary between subject and object fades, and the meaning constructed by this dichotomy breaks down" (2010: 4). By positing Dao's audience as sick patients, he reverts the subject position that operates in the abjection of the self when the subject (the sufferer in this case) recognises that he and his body no longer belong to the realm of the normative. The fact that Dao's music is so 'contagious' and that people are not able to help but succumb to his music allows the singer to posit himself, if only temporarily within the diegesis of the film, to a position of supremacy and to revert stigmatization. The "collective disgust" that Vaknin (2010: 5) points out, following the analysis of Manuel Ramos

---

4   Edward Crocker Green (2003) points out that more established church organisations have been involved in awareness and prevention programmes, however non-institutionalised congregations continue to construct HIV/AIDS as a demonic act.

Otero's *Invitación al polvo* (1991), becomes now an individual disgust as Dao can be the one who looks down on his public for showing the evident signs of their musical malady.

Nonetheless, the narrative will soon re-posit Dao as an AIDS-constructed body, whilst reframing his identity as a positive subject at the expense of the loss of his sex appeal (and with it part of his black masculinity). Firstly, the narrative returns to Jean and Myrlene's sub-plot. After losing a bet to some of his friends, Jean is forced to get rid of his dreadlocks and shave his head, revealing his 'uncanny similarity' to the film's protagonist. He is then talked into setting Myrlene up by passing as the real Dao in order to finally take her virginity (the cultural signifier of his masculinity that was denied to him at the beginning of the film). After the two have finally had sex, and as they enjoy their post-coital glow whilst watching some television, the camera switches to a live television interview with the real Dao. Although the rest of the scene primarily focuses on Jean's deception, it would be more interesting to turn attention to the contrast between Dao and Jean and what they come to represent. In the television interview, Dao is once again asked about his health, and he successfully manages to dispel any doubts about its precarious condition. However, at this point in the narrative it is very clear to the audience that Dao is positive, and the film further stresses AIDS stigma by contrasting his body to that of Jean's. Jean seems to be, now, the bearer of the ownership of desire and the object of the filmic gaze, an object position that the protagonist will not recover again throughout the film. Jean is shown almost naked, his muscular body in full view of the audience and his body acting as a constant reminder of what Dao is slowly losing. The presence of Jean in the film only serves to further stress the fact that "AIDS stigma is both a personal phenomenon, reflecting a potential threat to physical well-being (i.e., to one's identity as a healthy person), and as a social phenomenon, reflecting a threat to core social values involving sexual behavior, morality, and religion" (Devine et al. 1999: 1213). Although the film's ultimate intention is to challenge social and cultural misconceptions associated with HIV and those who suffer it, it cannot be denied that aspects of AIDS stigma are still present in it.

HIV reflects a potential threat to the protagonist's physical well-being, as portrayed in the bathroom scene that was previously analysed, or in a later scene in which, feverish and drenched in sweat, he goes back to his home altar only to cry for help; "Oh, my goddesses! Don't let your lover down! Come to my rescue!" before passing out. Dao's illness poses a threat to the Caribbean system of social values because his masculinity, and the system of imaginary masculinity that circulates amongst his audience based on his star persona, is called into question and is destabilised. The stigma associated with being HIV positive is challenged by the film; the physical changes that Dao undergoes by the end of the film shows that certain aspects of AIDS stigma remain unchanged in the popular imaginary, especially those related to the physicality of the HIV male body. Although Dao is eventually vindicated as a positive subject within the film, his body is still made abject by the way it is portrayed on screen. As Michelle Jean-Charles clearly indicates, Dao's body is at first "consciously inserted into a sexual economy that marks the hypersexual, heterosexual, and hypermasculine body as a site of desire" (2010: 69). However, by the end of the film, he is stripped of his hypersexual and hypermasculine attributes (he will retain his heterosexuality by keeping Nina as his girlfriend), as evidenced in the last concert in which he appears onstage fully dressed (in contrast to his first onstage appearance in which he was shirtless). By covering his body, the film continues to Other him – within Caribbean sexual discourses- and reveals an intrinsic fear towards the corporeality of the HIV body. Despite the fact that the film makes it clear that HIV is nowadays a treatable and controllable disease, the denial of his sex appeal produces, as Julien S. Murphy argues in relation to AIDS, reproductive technology and ethics:

> a severe dismemberment of the social body. Not only might we see the body of someone else with AIDS as out of control and near death [...] we begin to fear the entire social body as being out of control and rampant with disease and death. The fear of AIDS becomes manifest in public panic over the fear of the body – the ground of our own mortality. (1995: 15)

Although Dao's body is not 'out of control' or 'near death' or even ravaged by the disease, his masculinity is. His positive condition has, ultimately, affected his purported black masculinity, since this is defined by "equating successful masculinity with physical and emotional strength and social dominance" (Plummer and Simpson, 2007). Although the film clearly suggests that Dao will be able to live a long life (following viral treatment that he can only afford since his position as a singer allows him to do so), he will no longer be regarded as the erotic, desirable and sex symbol figure that the film constructed him as from the beginning. Despite the fact that Dao continued to be accepted as an 'equal' by Georges, band members and the general public, his HIV condition renders him desexualised, perhaps in an attempt by the film director to avoid alienating the film's prospective Caribbean audience. This is all the more evident when Antonin declares that "*l'un des messages du film [...] est que le sida ne se traite pas par des procédés magiques. Une idée largement répandue dans les milieux vaudou et* évangélique. *L*ᵼ*autre aspect du film est la violence faite aux femmes dans notre sociét*" (Juste, 2006).⁵ If the film is primarily concerned with raising awareness about the importance of obtaining clinical treatment for HIV, as well as to denounce gender violence on the island, then it seems strange that there are so many instances of male corporeality that would otherwise remain unproblematized by the protagonist's HIV body.

---

5   One of the messages of the film [...] is that HIV cannot be treated by magic procedures. This is a notion that has been largely promoted by voodoo and evangelical sites. The other aspect of the film relates to the violence women face in our society.

Mapping the (d)evolution of the queer AIDS body in *Before night falls*

It is undeniable that at the core of Schnabel's film there is a desire to demonise Fidel Castro's regime as a highly homophobic State whose persecution of homosexuals could be almost compared with that of gays during the Holocaust. Certainly, the Marxist ideology that was to shape the revolutionary consciousness in Cuba privileged the idea of the heterosexual man as the sole subject of socio-political change. The notion of *hombre nuevo* (new man) rids itself of any abstract conceptualisation of men (rather than mankind) and searches for an historical and social vision of men – a notion that is concretely humanistic – and one in which men are creators and a result of the society in which they live. The *hombre nuevo* is a man who would give his life for the revolutionary cause, a man who is capable of transforming his immediate reality and who can value himself as an object and subject of the process of development. As Juan Manuel del Aguila suggests, the *hombre nuevo* is "a selfless, committed, highly motivated citizen willing to immerse himself totally in shaping a new order without [...] bourgeois prejudices" (1984: 88-89). In Cuba's socialist society this kind of mentality has undoubtedly served to deeply root a *machista* view of the world, and to decrease to some extent the possibility of sexual equality, especially in relation to male homosexuality. During the 1960s and 1970s, the creation of the UMAP Camps (camps created to reform subversive elements of society) and the famous Mariel Exodus to the United States (a mass movement of Cubans who were allowed to go into exile in the USA, as the Cuban government regarded such individuals as anti-revolutionary), were but a few examples of the sexual discrimination to which gay individuals were subjected during the first three decades of the socialist regime. With these measures, the Government hoped to eliminate the remaining subversive people left in Cuba (many of whom were homosexual). Back on the island, the Church, the army and many other social and political institutions became outlets of institutionalised homophobia (Lumsden, 1993). Homosexuality operated clandestinely for a few decades, and yet the work of many artists (writers, filmmakers, actors, amongst others) remains testimony to an emerging and thriving gay subculture. As argued elsewhere, the clandestine nature of queer practices and the spaces in which such practices operate "is the result of necessity; on the one hand, to offer a locus for gay socialisation, and on the other, to separate two different strata of life: socially acceptable versus what is considered socially unacceptable" (Subero, 2008: 272).

However, it is important to note that, until the mid-1990s, to proclaim openly to have a gay identity was considered anti-revolutionary. The coming out – that "point in time when there is self-recognition by the individual of his identity as a homosexual and the first major exploration of the homosexual community" (Gagnon and Simon, 1967: 181) – was limited to closest friends and other gay men. Most "out" artists and figures of prominence were either sent to the UMAP camps or sent into exile. Schnabel's *Before night falls*, partly based on Reinaldo Arenas' posthumous autobiography of the same name, compiles the events that led to Arenas' suicide in New York in December 1990. The film follows Arenas' (Javier Bardem) life, with a major emphasis on his intellectual life and his homosexuality; from Havana's underground world (inhabited by those excluded by the system) to the difficulties of going into exile, and his eventual suicide after becoming terminally ill with AIDS. The film seems to operate as a queer hagiography of the writer (a point to which the discussion will return in the conclusion) whilst placing great emphasis on the writer's body and the different social, cultural and sexual nuances evoked throughout his life. From the very beginning, the film seems preoccupied with the construction of the protagonist's body and takes the viewer through a corporeal journey in which social, political, ideological and sexual issues are mapped on Bardem's depiction of Arenas' body. A journey in which the body becomes increasingly desexualised as Arena approaches the point of exile from Castro's Cuba. Arenas' naked and semi-naked body becomes an arena of contestation of the mechanism whereby heteropatriarchy regulates sex and sexuality in the Caribbean. Unlike Dao in the previous film, the instances of nakedness in this film do not invite the viewer to take an active subject position within the heteronormative realm. For instance, the first sexually charged image in the film disavows the naturalness of heterosexuality by presenting a teenage Arenas (Vito Maria Schnabel) who, upon visiting a brothel in Huelga with his friend Carlos (Diego Luna), is taken by a *mulata* prostitute to lose his virginity. The camera, positioned from behind the prostitute in a high angle and medium shot, permits to see the naked Arenas (his lower body covered by the head of the prostitute as she performs fellatio on him) displeased by the ministrations he is receiving. In spite of the slightly shocking image of such a young boy being sexually active, the film does not try to conceal the boy's real sexual desires. Thus his homosexuality is further stressed by this scene, cutting to Arenas' imagined image of Carlos as he looks lasciviously and seductively at the protagonist.

Arenas' body will remain, throughout the film, at the very centre of the narrative discourse and at the core of the construction of (queer) masculinity. The film offers three distinctive phases to the corporeal construction of the character: a) the early years in Havana characterised by the eroticisation of the protagonist's body, b) the years of the political persecution characterised by a degradation and subjugation of his body, and c) the AIDS years characterised by the physical changes on the body produced by the illness. The film makes clear use of activist aesthetics (Kruger, 1996; Davidson, 2003) as a way to deal with the adversities that the protagonist faces during it. His body becomes the main theme of such aesthetics, as it is through the protagonist's body that struggle, resistance and liberation is experienced and conveyed. The notion of activist aesthetics must be taken further from the simple didacticism with which the aforementioned theorists envisaged writing as a mechanism that "expresses doubt and/or the realization that sustainable political reform of HIV/AIDS-related issues [or any issues] involves the questioning and dismantling of deeply entrenched cultural prejudices about identity and contagion" (Davidson, 2003: 55). Thus in *Night*, the director's activist aesthetics are preoccupied with not only the way that Arenas' HIV condition is externalised, but also with using the protagonist's body for a clear anti-Castro campaign. Arenas' body becomes the channel through which illness as a metaphor can be visually acknowledged. However, illness must be understood as a social construction and in its broadest sense. In this way, it is proposed here that Arenas' subversive literature, his homosexuality, his dissidence, his capitalist ideas and his AIDS condition are the narrative illnesses the film tries so hard to denunciate. The connection between the ideological and the physical is constantly present within the narrative, as his body always seems to suffer major physical changes in direct relation to his life experiences. This is all the more poignant as Schnabel decides to revisit certain themes within the story to offer a sharp contrast between the "healthy" Arenas (athletic; in good health; pro-revolutionary) and the "unhealthy" Arenas (dissident; suffering malnutrition; physically abused in prison; HIV positive).

The first half of the film constructs Arena's body as the recipient and object of the stereotypical Caribbean fantasy of (queer) male masculinity.[6] One of the first scenes of the adult Arenas already depicts the symbolic importance of his body as a site of sexual, social and political contestation. In the common showers of the university, he checks his naked reflection – shown in a long shot – in a mirror. He keeps tensing and relaxing his buttocks and seems very pleased with his own physicality; a pleasure that is only interrupted when other men enter the changing room. The filmic gaze in this part of the film seems to be unashamedly gay as Arenas is constructed as the object of desire. His Cuban identity is both "Othered" and exoticised. When he first meets Pepe (Andrea Di Stefano) he makes it clear that he is different from other men in Havana because "I'm a guajiro from oriente", the film suggesting that Arenas is a different and exotic man even for those who are originally from the island. This part of the film is also characterised by many instances of semi and full nakedness in which male bodies (both gay and straight) are eroticised. Arenas, his lover Pepe and his friends are seen in many scenes at the beach wearing their swimming trunks and showing their bodies. Their semi-nakedness accentuated by their sweat and a camera that wastes no time in capturing them glistening in full health under the Caribbean sun. Conversely, as Arenas becomes a dissident, his body begins a transformation that is intrinsically linked to the narrative building up his body as counter-hegemonic. From the scenes in the Parque Lenin, where he had been living in hiding and in which he has lost a lot of weight, to the scenes in the prison where his body has been the object of degradation and abuse, the film uses his body to show a trajectory that could only culminate with his seropositive condition.

After overcoming many obstacles, he finally makes it to US shores. Once there, spectators are quickly taken from the one scene in which he and his lover Lazaro (Olivier Martinez) enjoy their first snow in NYC on the top of a friend's

---

6   At this point it is important to point out that the accuracy of Arenas' posthumous autobiography should be considered carefully and, perhaps, challenged. Many instances in the book seem to be overt exaggerations (claiming, for instance, he had sex with more than 1000 men throughout his life) or just mere artistic liberties.

car, to Arenas suffering from a fever due to his HIV condition. Interestingly, the narrative never makes a direct reference to AIDS or tries to provide a name to the protagonist's condition; instead Schnabel draws from spectators' previous filmic and media references to the condition as observed in mainstream media and film. For instance – and unsurprisingly – the Arenas of this latest part of the film draws many similarities with Tom Hank's depiction of Andrew Beckett in *Philadelphia* (Jonathan Demme, 1994). His face, arms and hands are marked by lesions that resemble those produced by Kaposi's Sarcoma (KS) which, as Vaknin reminds his reader, "these lesions, then, become signifiers of the patients' status as not only being HIV-positive, but also as having AIDS, and thus being fated to suffer an imminent death" (2010: 5). By doing so, the film purposely produces a response from the audience that makes Arenas abject by dehumanising him physically and stripping him of his human subjectivity. By this point in the narrative the character is also stripped of his queer agency – evidenced by his physical dehumanisation – whilst the audience (imagined as purportedly heterosexual since the film was not released as a queer but a mainstream, that is, hetero-normative, film) can now recuperate their own hetero-hegemonic agency by inciting their disgust at the confrontation with Arenas' impending death. Furthermore, the main themes that were once used to stress the character's queer identity are now reutilised to further serve as themes that make him abject due to his positive condition. For example, in a late scene in his New York flat, Arenas checks himself out in a mirror whilst washing up. Through a close shot of his reflection in the mirror it is easy to discern his physical deterioration, as he looks extremely pale, much thinner and with the visible marks of his KS lesions. This scene appears in stark contrast to the earlier one previously discussed, in which he checks himself out in the communal changing rooms at the university. His abject position is further stressed by the fact that, as he seems lost in thought whilst looking at his decayed body, he accidentally breaks a glass he has been washing and blood pours out of his cut. As Lazaro comes to the help, Arenas simply rejects him by shouting not to touch him or get near him. Arenas' blood becomes the greatest signifier of AIDS as metaphor since it serves as the visual reminder of one of the main causes of infection (blood contagion), and any doubts within the narrative about his real condition are dissipated by this scene.

By the same token, other previous scenes are revisited in this latter part of the film but are foreshadowed by more AIDS metaphors. In one such scene, Arenas and Lazaro are eating together – a dinner consisting of boiled eggs and broccoli – however it is obvious that Arenas is struggling to eat and he finally decides to give up on the food and leave it all to Lazaro. This scene reminds the audience of an earlier one in which Arenas is eating the same food, but this time completely shirtless and under the Caribbean sun, his body glistening with sweat and looking very healthy. It is not surprising that all of the later scenes before his death are also characterised by a lack of clear lighting; greys and shadows seem to abound, as if preparing the audience for a bleak finale. However, the most metaphoric of all images in the film occurs once Arenas is discharged from hospital, where he had been taken after Lazaro found him unconscious in his flat. Arenas leaves hospital in a wheelchair, with his belongings on his lap and with a very small flowerpot in his hands (the source of which is never provided diegetically). Once he arrives back at the building where he lives, he starts climbing the stairs back to his flat and begins to show signs of being unwell and dizzy, and eventually ends up falling down the stairs. As he recovers, he realises that the flowerpot has smashed on the floor and the plant and soil are spread all over the stairs. He takes a handful of soil in his hand, squeezes it and then eats it, the camera capturing this symbolic moment in great detail through a low angle close shot. This image remits the audience to the beginning of the film in which Schnabel depicts Arenas' birth as coming directly from the earth. As Edward R. Landa slightly points out in relation to the film, "the tale has come full circle – from Oriente Province to Manhattan, from birth to death – and the soil is the visual link" (2009: 91).

However, the protagonist's AIDS body should be regarded as a tool of dissent, for it becomes the ultimate weapon to fight against the communist regime in his native Cuba, unlike Jodi Parys (2004), who regards the AIDS body as a weapon that is manipulated in order to enact revenge, and in which the individual uses HIV "to try to retaliate for the permanent biological and ultimately, physical and psychological, alterations that will be caused by the progression of the HIV virus" (2). *Night* cannot be regarded as Parys's revenge narrative because the protagonist does not make it his ultimate decision to take matters under his own control and use his sexuality and/or altered body in search of retribution. Instead, it is proposed that the film offers a counter-revenge narrative in which HIV is still regarded as a punishment; yet this punishment only serves to further enhance the political readings of the text as a counter-hegemonic text. In this context, Arenas' body should not be regarded as a body with AIDS, but instead as a body 'infected by' AIDS. His HIV positive condition is not regarded as the direct effect of his own actions, but the consequence of someone else's (in this case, as he blatantly puts it at the end of his memoir, Fidel Castro's). If the audience is to take sides with Arenas and blame the Cuban dictator for the protagonist's demise, then the notion of the suffering of the wounded storyteller, as theorized by Arthur Frank (1997), must be reworked in a different light. Frank argues that:

> suffering has two sides. One side [...] expresses the threat of disintegration. The chaos narrative is overwhelmed by this threat; disintegration has become the teller's encompassing reality. The other side, [...] seeks a new integration of body-self. The quest narrative recognizes that the old intactness must be stripped away to prepare for something new. Quest stories reflect a confidence in what is waiting to emerge from suffering. (1997: 171)

However, what is proposed here is that Arenas' AIDS narrative combines both types of suffering into one because his body must undergo a process of disintegration in order to emerge from his own suffering as a different kind of narrative figure. His death is not only symbolic but also necessary to construct him as the heroic figure, the martyr that the film so openly claims he should be taken as. Whereas in the book Arenas constructs himself as *"excluido, exilado, homosexual, perverso, erótico, anárquico, cachondo, alegre, capaz de gozar, criticar, y disfrutar, persona con sida que se suicida"* (Angvik, 1995: 31), in the film, Schnabel constructs the late Arena as a Christ-like figure whose suffering is symbolic of the suffering of the Cuban nation.

Arenas' death is, therefore, fashioned in the film as the ultimate sacrifice rather than as the imminent consequence of living with HIV/AIDS. The last sequence in the film, in which he stages his own suicide by taking some unknown tablets and watering them down with whiskey, prepares the audience to see his body being offered sacrificially. By staging his death, Arenas guarantees that his decayed body, and ultimately his corpse, are both regarded as the living proof (sic) of his struggle for intellectual freedom.[7] The physical decomposition that the character conveys through his inability to feed himself, the staging of his death without Lazaro's help (who keeps feeding him pills and whiskey), and the handheld camera that follows Arenas to the sofa on which he will eventually die, all become part of the grotesque. His body is offered as a grotesque since, as Brad Epps argues, it "is invoked as the design of a self whose life is shadowed by death and whose presence is exceeded (preceded and superseded) by an absence, a lack" (1995: 39). By the end of the film, the audience is drawn into a space of perverse fetishism in which Arenas' death becomes the source of scopophilic pleasure, for it provides visual significance and an end to his quest for liberation. Although his body is not highly stigmatised as counter-hegemonic and remains in the safe confines of an acceptable hetero-normativity (even if this is done at the expense of any queer readings of the film), its otherness establishes a safe separation between the audience and the protagonist in which the audience can relate to the suffering of the character but only as long as he is regarded as a sacrificial figure. His dying body becomes a stylised effect of the grotesque and attains political meaning, because every moment in which his body visibly suffers the ravages of HIV, the audience is asked to associate his body suffering with the struggle of many Cubans who are living under communist oppression. This HIV metaphor comes to an abrupt end by Schnabel's artistic liberty as he shows how Lazaro, who is witnessing Arenas' staged suicide, decides to asphyxiate him with a plastic bag whilst the former is resting on the sofa. Besides providing tension in the film, in what would have been an otherwise drawn-out scene of Arenas' death, it permits to bring to an end the grotesque by disavowing death as spectacle. The last image of Arenas' dead body, one in which the camera lingers for a few seconds before cutting to snapshots of Arena at different times in the narrative (when his body was healthy), shows the rhetoric of death as both a repudiated act and a site of perverse fascination. However, this very brief recount in flashback of the protagonist's story

---

7   It is important to point out that the film downplays Arenas' struggle as a gay man, and his sexual orientation becomes secondary to his struggle as a writer and subversive intellectual.

serves to ensure that the distance between the imagined audience, and its subject position as purportedly heterosexual, and the character are re-established in a way that all possible associations between Arenas, as an imagined subject position, and the audience are disavowed.

HIV as a sublime experience

The manner in which the two texts analysed here deal with HIV corporeality(ies) could not be more different. On the one hand, there is Dao, a bearer of a hypermasculine body whose HIV condition provides 'enlightenment' by undergoing a journey through the different cultural paradigms that become an obstacle to efficiently deal with the illness in Haiti: machismo, and religion. On the other, there is Arenas, a figure whose HIV condition becomes the ultimate manifestation of his condition as a dissident and exiled subject from the oppression of Castro's Cuba. However, what these two figures share in common, within the HIV filmic narrative of the texts in which they are portrayed, is the fact that, for both characters, HIV operates as a sublime experience. HIV becomes a liminal sublime experience because the way that both directors depict it on screen makes HIV look like an experience integral to human existence (even when its own presence usually fosters feelings in relation to the very loss of human existence). In both films, HIV provides agency to the central characters as their social, sexual, political, intellectual and cultural (amongst others) personas are defined through their positive status. Although this chapter does not intend to either demonise or discriminate against seropositive individuals, it is necessary to deconstruct the way the narrative in both texts uses HIV/AIDS as a pathway to the sublime by the main characters. It cannot be denied that becoming positive is not a life-changing experience, however, these texts seem to suggest that acquiring the virus is the only way in which certain cultural and political paradigms can be contested in the Caribbean. By confronting their own mortality, these characters can finally offer a critical insight into issues that would otherwise be justified or overlooked within the cultural and social politics of their own societies.

The sublime must be made a tangible experience if spectators are to become aware that their 'heroes' have finally experienced transformation and change. Filmic narrative conventions in the form of heroes and anti-heroes are utilised to further convey the HIV body as sublime. In *Le president*, the character of Larieux (Ricardo Lefevre) is portrayed as the embodiment of all the masculine vices that are found in the construction of Caribbean masculinity. He is a womaniser (and interestingly the audience is asked to make a distinction between Dao and Larieux's objectification of women, and regard the former's as a phase rather than an embedded socio-cultural identity), he uses physical violence against women and also uses his economic status to exercise power over women. In *Night*, the anti-hero is a historical figure whose name, and the regime he represents, plays heavily on the mind of the audience, and invokes an immediate and usually loaded reaction: Fidel Castro. Both figures are necessary for the sublime experience of the film protagonists because, otherwise, AIDS would become the enemy and this, in turn, would truncate the possibility of using HIV as a form of the sublime. The protagonists, therefore, follow the notion of the modern hero, as theorised by Catherin Mavrikakis who argues "the modern hero is destined to return to the grand narrative, where death is the ultimate transformation. As in all tragedies, the hero is by definition condemned to death. Consequently, the narrative also bears the markings of death" (1998: 130). Even though the two protagonists meet different endings to their HIV experiences – Dao starts medical treatment for his HIV and is expected to live a 'normal' life whilst Arenas commits suicide/is killed by the end of the film – they both foreshadow death as the ultimate human experience. The changes the characters undergo throughout the films, and which these directors provide as those the audience must internalise (for these are intrinsically didactic films), can only be experienced by their closeness to death in the form of their HIV condition. As Lap-Chuen Tsang, following Burke (1803), explains, "the sublime [is] as some kind of intense delight acquired upon our escape from the privations of the human condition, like utmost danger, or suffering and death" (1998: xv). The fact that both films are aimed at an imaginary heterosexual audience, and that they both portray HIV without as many of the negative stereotypes as were characteristic of such narratives in the 1980s and 1990s is praiseworthy. However, the narratives seem to fail to convey the notion that changes in society and in established socio-cultural patterns can be achieved without radical experiences such as becoming positive.

In short, this chapter has demonstrated how the HIV body has been used to challenge socio-cultural paradigms that govern and regulate male sexual cultures in the Caribbean. *Le president* shows the dismantling of Caribbean masculinity, through a rather didactic text, in which the mechanism whereby masculinity operates in Haiti is disavowed once the film's protagonist discovers that he is HIV positive. However, in spite of an attempt by the director to show the ravages caused on the body by the lack of medical attention to the HIV body, the protagonist's own body remains throughout the film unchanged and is, in fact, highly eroticised until the protagonist's positive diagnose is finally revealed. It is only at this point in the narrative that his body becomes a vehicle to promote equality (his masculinity no longer needing to be proved by the objectification and subordination of women) and acceptance (of HIV positive individuals as fully functional subjects), however this is done at the expense of his ownership of desire as his body is then de-eroticised. Although the film is effective in its portrayal of the importance of medical attention for HIV patients in order for them to live a long and healthy life, the film disregards, to the point of belittling, the importance of the body in the construction of masculinity amongst Caribbean males. Similarly, in *Night*, Arenas' body is at the intersection of sexuality, gender and intellectual militancy as the film devotes a third of the running time to show bodies that may challenge heteronormative paradigms within Caribbean sexual cultures. However, the film seems so preoccupied in providing a sort of gay hagiography of the historical character that, as with the previous film, it offers this at the expense of the character's ownership of desire. By the time in the narrative that spectators see Arenas dying of AIDS, his body has been completely desexualised and offered as the undeserving victim of a terminal illness that symbolises his fight against Castro's regime. For Arenas, being seropositive becomes his last quest to prove his sainthood. The marks on his face and body produced by the SK become the ultimate form of stigmata (emphasised through many close and close-up shots), as this constructs him as a saintly figure whose body represents both the struggle for freedom (from Castro's repressive regime) and as a gay man. By the same token, his seropositive condition becomes the instrument through which to experience sublimation, a characteristic also shared with the previous character, and that allows him/them to experience radical changes in their socio-sexual persona that ultimately made them become better human beings. In other words, becoming HIV positive allows them to re-evaluate, challenge and positively transform the male sexual paradigms that circulate in the popular imaginary of the Caribbean.

Filmography

Le president a-t-il le Sida? (dir. Artaud Antonin 2006).
Philadelphia (dir. Jonathan Demme 1993).
Before night falls (dir. Julian Schnabel 2000).

Bibliography

Angvik, B. 1995. *Bio-grafías y tanato-grafías: estrategias teóricas en torno a la presencia del sida en la literatura contemporánea*. Actas XII.Centyro Virtual Cervantes: 26-37.
—— 1998. Textual Constellations: AIDS and the Love of Writing in the Postmodern Era. *Journal of Latin American Cultural Studies*. Vol. 7 (2): 165-183.
AVERT: AVERTing HIV and AIDS. International HIV & AIDS charity. www. avert.org
Bombereau, G. and Allen, C.F. 2008. *Social and cultural factors driving the HIV epidemic in the Caribbean*. St. Augustine, Trinidad and Tobago: Caribbean Health Research Council.
Brown, J.A. 2002. The tortures of Mel Gibson: Masochism and the sexy male body. *Men and Masculinities*. Vol. 5 (2): 123-143.
Burke, E. 1803. *The works of the Right Honourable Edmund Burke. Vol. 1*. London: F. and C. Rivington, St. Paul's Church-Yard and J. Hatchard, Picadilly.
Caribbean Task Force on HIV/AIDS. Caribbean Community Secretariat (CARICOM). www.caricom.org.

Cooper, C. 2000. *Lady Saw Cuts Loose: Female Fertility Rituals in Jamaican Dancehall Culture.* [online] Available at http://www.jouvay.com/interviews/carolyncooper.htm [accessed 02 May 2012].

Crocker Green, E. 2003. *Rethinking AIDS Prevention: Learning from Successes in Developing Countries.* Santa Barbara: Greenwood Publishing.

Davidson, D. 2003. Difficult Writings: AIDS and the Activist Aesthetics in Reinaldo Arenas' Before Night Falls. *Atenea.* Vol, XXIII (2): 53-72.

del Aguila, J.M. 1984. *Cuba: Dilemmas of a Revolution, 3rd edn.* Westview Press: San Francisco and Oxford.

Devine, P., Plant, E.A. and Harrison, K. 1999. The problem of "us" versus "them" and AIDS stigma. *American Behavioral Scientist.* Vol. 42 (7): 1212-1228.

Epps, B. 1995. Grotesque identities: Writing, death and the space of the subject (Between Michel de Montaigne and Reinaldo Arenas). *The Journal of the Midwest Modern Language Association.* Vol. 28 (1): 38-55.

Fairley, J. 2009. How to make love with your clothes on, in *Reggaeton*, edited by R. Rivera, W. Marshall and D. Pacini Hernandez. Durham: Duke University Press, 280-296.

Fanon, F. and Markmann, C.L. 1993. *Black Skins, White Masks.* London: Pluto Press.

Frank, A. 1997. *The Wounded Storyteller: Body, Illness and Ethics.* Illinois: University of Chicago Press.

Goffman, E. 1963. *Stigma: Notes on the Management of Spoiled Identity.* London: Simon & Schuster.

Holmlund, C. 1993. Masculinity as multiple masquerade: The "mature" Stallone and the Stallone clone, in *Screening the Male: Exploring Masculinities in Hollywood Cinema*, edited by S. Cohan and I. Rae Hark. London and New York: Routledge.

Hope, D.P. 2007. "Love Punaany Bad" Negotiating misogynistic masculinity in Dancehall culture, in *Caribbean culture: Soundings on Kamay Brathwaite*, edited by A. Paul. Kingston: University of the West Indies Press, 367-380.

Juste, J. 2006. *"Le président a-t-il le Sida"? Le Nouvelliste.* [online] Available at http://www.lenouvelliste.com/article4.php?PubID=1&ArticleID=28080 [accessed 28 April 2012].

Kempadoo, K. 1996. Prostitution, marginality and empowerment: Caribbean women in the sex trade. *Beyond Law.* Vol. 5 (14): 69-84.

——— 2009. Caribbean Sexuality: Mapping the field. *Caribbean Review of Gender Studies: A Journal of Caribbean Perspectives on Gender and Feminism.* Issue 3: 1-23. [online] Available at http://sta.uwi.edu/crgs/november2009/journals/Kempadoo.pdf [accessed 02 May 2012].

Kruger, S. 1996. *AIDS Narratives: Gender and Sexuality, Fiction and Science.* New York: Garland Publishing.

Landa, E.R. 2009. In a supporting role: Soil and the cinema, in *Soil and Culture*, edited by E.R. Landa and C. Feller. New York: Springer Publishing, 83-107.

Linden, L. 2003. Caribbean masculinity: Unpacking the narrative, in *The Culture of Gender and Sexuality in the Caribbean*, edited by L. Linden. Gainesville: University Press of Florida, 94-128.

Lindsay, K. 2002. Is the Caribbean male an endangered species?, in *Gendered Realities: Essays in Caribbean Feminist Thought*, edited by P. Mohammed. Kingston: University of the West Indies Press, 56-82.

Lumsden, I. 1993. *Machos Maricones & Gays: Cuba and Homosexuality*. Philadelphia: Temple University Press.

Mavrikakis, C. 1998. To end the glorification of suffering, in *History and Memory: Suffering and Art*, edited by H. Schweizer. London: Bucknell University, 124-132.

Michelle Jean-Charles, R. 2011. The Sway of Stigma: The Politics and Poetics of AIDS Representation in Le président a-t-il le SIDA? and Spirit of Haiti. *Small Axe*. Issue 36: 62-79.

Miller, E. 1986. *The Marginalization of the Black male: Insights from the Development of the Teaching Profession*. Mona, Jamaica: Institute of Social and Economic Research, University of the West Indies Press.

MUBI Europe. Unheard Voices: Cinema of Haiti. http://mubi.com/lists/unheard-voices-cinema-of-haiti.

Murphy, J.S. 1995. *The Constructed Body: AIDS, Reproductive Technology, and Ethics*. New York: SUNY Press.

Nieves Moreno, A. 2009. A man lives here: Reggaeton's hypermasculine resident, in *Reggaeton*, edited by R. Rivera, W. Marshall and D. Pacini Hernandez. Durham: Duke University Press, 252-279.

PAHO, Unicef. 2008. *Secondary Education: The Funnel Effect*. Bridgetown, Barbados: Pan American Health Organization. Office of Caribbean Program education.

Parys, J. 2004. *AIDS and revenge: The body as Silent Weapon*. Paper presented at the Latin American Studies Association. Las Vegas, Nevada.

Plummer, D. and Simpson, J. 2007. *HIV and Caribbean Masculinities*. [online] Available at http://www.old.msmgf.org/documents/CA_home_masculinities.pdf [accessed 02 May 2012].

Simon, W. and. Gagnon, J.H. 1967. Homosexuality: The formulation of a sociological perspective. *Journal of Health and Social Behavior*. Vol. 8 (3): 177-185.

Sontag, S. 2001. *Illness as metaphor; and, AIDS and its metaphor*. US: Picador.

Subero, G. 2009. The Silent scream of the Locas in Mariposas en el andamio. *Bulletin of Latin American Research*. Vol. 28 (2): 266-283.

Tsang, L. 1998. *The Sublime: Groundwork Towards and Theory*. New York: University of Rochester Press.

Vaknin, J. 2010. Metáfora contagiosa: AIDS and metaphor in the Hispanic Caribbean. *Penn McNair Research Journal*. Vol. 2 (1): 1-14.

World Bank. 2001. *HIV/AIDS in the Caribbean: Issues and options. Volume 52*. New York: World Bank Publications.

Chapter 4

Mapping the HIV Body in Contemporary Latin American Theatre

Daniela Cápona[1]

In 1989, *Unidentified Human Remains and the True Nature of Love* by the playwright Brad Fraser, opened in Calgary (Canada). The play depicted a group of young people struggling with their romantic lives while a serial killer haunted the streets of Edmonton, killing women and leaving in his wake unidentified human remains. At first glance, it would seem that the play does not address HIV, however, a more careful analysis would reveal that AIDS, as a social phenomenon, runs throughout the entire plot.[2] The simultaneity between the search for affection and the murders creates a parallel between love and the human remains scattered around the city by the killer, an analogy that is corroborated by the title itself. The association of these two elements suggests a new and particular bond, one that goes beyond Fraser's work, as it seems to be a prevalent element in the theatre in the times of AIDS. The resulting metaphor is suggestive; love is linked not only to death, but to bodily fragmentation. As such, the metaphor seems to recover, from a different perspective, the link between love, violence and fate established by romanticism. Fraser's play serves as a point of departure to approach a particular phenomenon that we can observe in the contemporary Latin American plays that we will be examining here: the change in the forms of representations of the body that is a product of a modification of the corporeal experiences generated by the AIDS crisis. These plays present, among other characteristics, a tendency towards bodily fragmentation and the resulting emergence of a dehumanized soma whose incompleteness prohibits its total identification with the self.

When tackling the process of identification of the self with the bodily image, it is necessary to refer to Lacan's specular image theory (2004) as it addresses the moment when the infant recognizes his image in the mirror as a unity and as a self. Such identification is fundamental, as it provides the individual with a perception of himself as a unity, and allows for the establishment of the correspondent equivalencies between the self and the image of the body that contains it:

---

1 Translated by Gyna Freire.

2 There are allusions to the necessity of using condoms, mentions of the risk of contracting HIV and the resulting fear of death. Ultimately, towards the end of the play, one of the protagonists is informed that one of their sporadic lovers has become infected, reactivating the specter of death.

> For the total form of his body, by which the subject anticipates the maturation of
> his power in a mirage, is given to him only as *Gestalt*, that is, in an exteriority in
> which, to be sure, this form is more constitutive than constituted, but in which,
> above all it appears to him as the contour of his statures that freezes it and in
> symmetry reserves it, in oppositions to the turbulent movements with which the
> subject feels he animates it. (Lacan, 2004: 4)

According to Lacan, the specular image plays a fundamental role in the formation
of the abstract self, which constitutes an ideal state; a "mold of all future
identifications" (Blasco, 1992: 7). Governed by this perception, the human body is
generally represented as a unity, constituting an image that suggests an equivalency
and reciprocity with a determined identity. This relationship is precisely what is
fractured in the analogy of love and human remains that Fraser posits, insinuating a
fragmented image of the corporeal in which the unity of the body and its humanity
are, at most, relative.

Imagining the body as a 'remain' is also present in other artistic disciplines. In
reviewing the representations of HIV in the visual arts, Juan Vicente Aliaga notes:

> Fragmented visions abound, split from a body that is almost inhuman, what
> is meant to be conveyed is its very condition as a *remnant*. Divided from the
> visual privilege, which it possessed in previous artistic periods, the corporeal is a
> symptom of the decomposition of the gaze. The body and death, or its nearness,
> go hand in hand. (Aliaga, 1993: 186-187)

This innovation that Aliaga notes in the treatment of images emphasizes not only
the growing importance that the body, as such, gains in these images, but also
the dissolution of the limits of representation and the clear tendency towards the
separation of the body into parts or 'remains'. The emergence of HIV/AIDS leads
to a transformation in the perception of the body, which corresponds to a number
of variables that also participate in the symbolic construction of the syndrome. As
such, the history of AIDS, its sexual transmission and the relation of the disease
with bodily fluids, is added to the stalwart anatomopathogical model, all of which
gives rise to an imaginary sectioning of the body:

> The body had become transformed into sinful, abject, and ill matter; a source
> of miasmas and fluids, and anal practices which religion and homophones
> condemned. It wasn't easy to reactivate it and put it into action. The massive
> use of new technologies weakened physical presence. Other devices came to
> represent it: electric diodes, videos, photographs and, in the nineties, net-art. The
> body was becoming digitalized bit by bit. (Aliaga, 2007: 73)

According to Aliaga, the human *soma* goes from being thought of as a unity that
contains the individual, to being imagined (and represented) as an aggregation
of parts and fluids, which are potentially discrete parts separate from the subject.

That "abject matter, source of miasmas and fluids" appears as a remnant or waste resulting from a process of decomposition that affects human corporeality, even denying its subjective dimension. The AIDS crisis provides a perception of the body as matter without affiliation, not only in relation to the "higher" human faculties (thought and conscience), but also with respect to the somatic processes which become ever more alien to the will of the self. According to Aliaga "AIDS has made of the world a carnal reality" (1993: 188), suggesting that such carnality expounds the least agreeable aspects of a bodily nature presenting the abject as "the true nature of love".

Readdressing the Lacanian image, representations of the body in times of AIDS would indicate a 'rupture of the mirror'. Such a rupture returns a decomposed fragmented image with which the self cannot possibly become identified. In relation to the fracture of the corporeal unity and its implications on a symbolic level, we find a connection with the Freudian concept of "the sinister" (*Unheimlich*) as an instance that 'breaks' the familiar and, in turn, makes it threatening. According to Freud, "*Unheimlich* would be all that which should have remained hidden, secret, but which has manifested itself' (1979: 17), a definition compatible with the idea previously mentioned of AIDS as that which uncovers the abject in human corporeality. On the other hand, if "the 'uncanny' is that class of the terrifying which leads back to something long known to us, once very familiar" (Freud, 1979: 12), the body, represented as a carnality separated from the self, would have just this effect, insofar as the familiar image would become foreign and unrecognizable.

Amongst the visual arts mentioned by Aliaga, as examples of the mutation of the corporal representations, Cindy Sherman's *Disgust pictures* (1987) and *Sex pictures* (1992), and the work of Robert Gober (we are referring to his 1991 pieces, most of them untitled) are particularly note-worthy. Both artists substitute the conventional configuration of the body with an accumulation of waste and isolated limbs – legs, feet, torsos – of an incomplete structure. Emblematic of this same tendency is the work of Andrés Serrano, particularly his photographs of bodily fluids such as blood, semen, urine and excrement (*Blood and semen* 1990 – , *Piss Christ* 1987 –, among others). If we accept Aliaga's proposition and we consider that one of the central characteristics of representations of the body in times of AIDS is the tendency towards fragmentation, then the *soma* appears portrayed as a wounded body, split and in a process of decomposition that ranges from estrangement to putrefaction. Although these associations are related to the sensible (and visible) manifestations of the illness, it is possible to venture that many elements intervene in conjuring up the presence of the uncanny or the abject in the AIDS stricken body. The physical deterioration and the somatic transformations caused by the illness give rise to a fracturing in the identification of the self with the image of the body itself. Simultaneously, this breach summons the figures of the "double" (Freud, 1979: 15) as a signal of the division of the self, in addition to facilitating a fragmented perception of the body as a conjunction of symptoms and lesions. Conversely, the illness also lends added visibility to the body as pure matter, subject to the ostensible processes of degradation and decomposition, and accentuating the abject dimension of the somatic. For José Miguel Cortés "The abject is the triumph of the body over the mind, the delirium, the loss of control, the deteriorated flesh, the flushed wastes" (1996: 199). Furthermore, this is related to the sudden emergence of death in a time where it is consistently denied; the appearance of HIV/AIDS implies a reactivation of mortality, a factor that had a bearing on the mutation of the representations of the body (sick or healthy) that emerged at this time.[3]

On the other hand, the insistence with which the human body appears as a location and privileged reference of discourses also suggests the impossibility of representation of the sick body. José Miguel Cortés expresses the following in this respect: The body, as such, has become something impossible, its unity has cracked. The drives, desires and frustrations which inhabit its interior have given place to a schizophrenic and fragmented being to whom the recovery of lost unity becomes an impossible task (1996: 237). Following these premises, we will analyze how, in some Latin American plays, there is an attempt to recover the subject-*soma* unity of the affected body through the use of language while, at the same time, this becomes a failed undertaking as it exposes the instability of the imagined body in relation to the illness.

Fragmented bodies

The idea of the sectioned body is exceptionally illustrated in the work of American artist Robert Gober, where the fragment is depicted as a fundamental element in the representation of the body that abandons the unity of the human to become a remnant of an unrecoverable presence. In 1990, Gober begins to work on sculptures based on fragments of masculine bodies emerging from walls. In these, humanity is presented as an absurd section, illustrating "the human being transformed, product of illness or warfare, into an invalid body, in an inert yet still alive being" (Cortés, 1996: 213). A certain agitation and concern is generated by those mutilated limbs that still seem to be alive; a contradiction that incites the viewer to wonder about the missing parts of that body, hidden, perhaps, on the other side of the wall. Gober chiefly focuses on legs and torsos, fractions of bodies not conventionally associated to markers of identity, which suggests that the violent event which fractured those bodies has made them indistinguishable in their damage and fragility. Cortés comments that these pieces are:

> Eulogies to a weak, sick, humiliated and mutilated body. The world has fallen
> (we do know not how) cutting the body and leaving its pieces at different sides

---

3   This is exemplarily evident in the importance that symptoms and physical sensations acquire in the texts which address HIV, especially in some autobiographical narrations like Sarduy's *Beach birds* or Hervé Guibert's *To the friend who did not save my life.*

of a wall. There are multiple influences and references: personal (childhood memories), social and affective (friends passed away because of AIDS), artistic and cultural (works of other artists, the wax museum, the morgues). (1996: 209)

HIV does not function as the sole discourse. Nevertheless, it becomes clear that the AIDS crisis in the U.S. is a landmark which conditions the gaze of the artists with respect to the body and its representations; "if they are not sick, they know someone who is or they are coping with the loss of someone who was sick. For me, death has temporarily relocated to New York. And many artists whom I know are finding ways in which to express that" (Gober cited by Cortés, 1996: 213). The specificities of the corporeal representations in the works of Gober serve us as a point of departure for the analysis of the Cuban plays *Pájaros de la playa (Beachbirds)* by Nelda Castillo and *Sangre (Blood)* by Yunior García.

Pájaros de la playa by Nelda Castillo

The play is a theatrical adaptation of the homonymous novel written by Severo Sarduy. It premiered in 2004 by the *El ciervo encantado* in Havana, directed by Nelda Castillo; the publication of the text takes place that same year in the periodical *Tablas*, vol. LXXVI pp. VI-VIII. Constructed over sequences portrayed in the original text, the play almost eliminates the narrative component of the novel. The playwright does away with the fable and articulates the dramatic text privileging concepts and sensations in a fragmentary way. As so often happens in some autobiographical novels about the illness, there is an insistence on the description of the bodies as conjunctions of painful symptoms that, in their turn, can be read as fragments of a subject in the process of deterioration.

The text elaborated by Castillo proposes a constant present in which declarations and descriptions of a "being in one's body" seem to extend beyond the limits of fiction. The director eliminates the anecdotes of *Siempreviva* (Always alive), *Caballo* (Horse) and *Caimán* (Alligator), and retains as central characters three indistinguishable patients who complain about their symptoms without actually naming their malady – exactly as it occurs in Sarduy's novel. Castillo engages in a dilution of subjectivities, leaving merely the voices and bodies in a state of deterioration that continuously enumerate their suffering and useless medications:

Patient 1: Painkillers, antihistamines, antiemetics.
[...]
Patient 1: My gums are bleeding.
Patient 2: Here I spy.
Patient 1: Scabies.
Patient 2: Apathy.
Patient 1: Sarcoma.
Patient 2: Frustration.

Patient 1: Boils.
Patient 2: Fear.
Patient 1: Spots.
Patient 2: Fear of hurting oneself, fear of cutting your nails (VI).

Symptoms, lesions, medications and states of mind appear as part of the same; fragments of the body and life hunted by disease. This enumeration tends to undo the organized hierarchy of the above-mentioned elements, giving pain, organs and cures equal importance and suggesting the disintegration of the individual in a cluster of chemicals and flesh. The vestiges of identity that peer out from the text appear as conditioned by the somatic, exerting it over moods and emotions. "Apathy", "frustration", and "fear" appear linked to the manifestations of the infirm body confirming that, in the universe presented, all is governed by the stimuli of the body in pain:

Patient 1: I surprise myself evoking a body, a lithe body that swims in a blue-tiledpool, black bathing suit, firm buttocks, he dives in and ends in a cannon ball, the fresh water splashes me.

Patient 3: This jumble of defeated tendons, flaccid and weary (VII).

Above, we see one of the few references to a healthy body, projected imaginarily, as both an object of desire and as a physical state that is desired. The "firm buttocks" and the "fresh water" offer a sharp contrast to the "jumble of defeated tendons" described by the speaker.

The concept of "other in me" (200: 90) coined by Eugenia Vilela to describe the presence of disease in the work of Hervé Guibert manifests itself in Sarduy's novel and in Castillo's adaptation, where illness is perceived as an invasion, origin of foreignness and otherness, "Patient 1: I am God, I am a hero, I am demon and I am the world. Which is a lovely way of saying what I am not, that I am not" (VIII). The 'not being' signals the consciousness of the transition to death, a process which has made the subject leave behind who he was in order to become a non-human; disintegrating into illness. Vilela characterizes this phenomenon as a conversion of the somatic into the subjective, which suggests that the discourse – in these types of texts – would be enunciated by the body and no longer by subjectivity anchored in reason:

Faced with the reality of the pain of the body, of illness in so far as *other in me*, the works of *self-fiction* – for example the literature about AIDS, in which we find the work of Hervé Guibert – come about as modes of resistance through which the body ceases being an object and becomes and constitutes itself into a subject. (2000: 90)

Insofar as the staging is concerned, a photographic register permits us to see a stage inhabited by three semi-naked actors that manipulate large plastic sheets. Given that the language refers obsessively to the physical, the production installs the corporality of the actors as the real stage of the plot. Bodies rid of individualizing elements pronounce the words that remit to that exhibited flesh as the core of all subsequent events. While the discourse refers to the symptoms, the materiality of the actors provides a stage appropriated by the illness that invades everything; "Patient 2: You sink into fevers, shivers and fainting spells and you keep on living" (VIII).

It would seem that illness has transformed these characters into a sequence of declarations that forge the past life and the present agony with the experience of pain. Oddly enough, it is only the anguish produced by an imminent death that seems to escape the enunciation of the pained corporeality, point from which a hint of resistance and attachment to the irrecoverable past is expressed, "Wait. Don't go. Let's end this night with grandeur. So many books that no one has ever read, so much passion that has never been assuaged by anybody. Wait, don't go" (VIII).

Sangre, by Yunior García[4]

This play is organized into eleven episodes structured around "*sangre*" (blood) in all its possibilities: filiation, transfusions, HIV transmission, sexual relations and family bonds. The idea of the fragmented body manifests itself in the structure of the play, sequenced in scenes titled with the names of the characters. Each segment presents a conflict related to blood or another bodily fluid, organized in an episodic manner in which each episode is linked to the totality, but also functions autonomously. Blood and semen operate as the nucleus of the plot in such a manner that the anecdote depends on the movement of these substances that, travelling from one body to another, activate the conflict in each scene. This is already announced in the first scene where a chorus reveals that, as an evil omen, great quantities of blood have occupied the Almendares River:

> The Almendares River awakened full of blood
> The press hasn't said a word
> They say that the blood belongs to those who still have hope
> And to those that have lost it forever
> They say that it is a plague/a curse
> An omen/A settling of scores
> Since it awakened full of blood
> The Almendares does not stink
> No one has dared stain it

---

4   *Sangre* premiered in 2007 and was published in 2008 within a collective volume entitled *Teatro cubano actual: Novísimos dramaturgos cubanos* in Havana.

> The river has become a place of worship
> Consecrated ground
> A place of penitence (369)

This image begins a series of scenes that problematize the relationship between desire, will and body – concepts that appear linked to the flow of bodily fluids. These scenes discuss, among other things, the advisability of a blood transfusion in a family of Jehovah's Witnesses, the possibility of HIV transmission in a sexual relation and the implications of maternity/paternity in instances of rape. In each case, an analogy is established between interpersonal relationships and the movement of fluids. These elements acquire meaning and moral significance while simultaneously operating as metaphors for desire, aggressiveness and love.

The separation between body and subject in this play works as a central element given that the author develops conflicts around the tensions between corporality and subjectivity. Such is the case in scene three in which Sara, pregnant as a product of rape, must confront her desire for maternity with the resentment against her aggressor and the sterility of her husband. Semen acquires autonomy with respect to the circumstances of the rape while working to project the uneasiness of Sara's husband:

> David: I only thought of one thing. That man's fertile semen in your womb. You
> think I don't want a son, Sara? I'm dying to have one. But I can't. The child that
> you're expecting isn't mine. And I won't be its father. (377)

David states that he does not feel affected by his wife's rape, but the presence of the 'fertile semen' of another man in her body posits the movement of bodily liquids as a destabilizing agent that contradicts the will of the subjects. In this and other scenes, semen is invested with symbolic connotations and with some reproductive power that exceeds the will of the characters. This can also be seen in scene seven:

> Isaac: I killed my mother. *(Silence.)* They wanted to give her blood. I demanded
> that they look for other alternatives, that our values didn't allow us to accept a
> blood transfusion; but they didn't listen. I got her out of the hospital and I hid
> her in a small workshop near the Almendares River. By midday she was already
> dead. I left her there, lying on top of a broken armchair, with her eyes half-open
> and her mouth dry. (393)

The possibility of the displacement of blood gains such an importance that it incites a man to let his own mother die, and although religious beliefs justify his actions, it is blood – and not faith – which lies at the root of the conflict.

Both blood and semen acquire a metaphoric significance in a double direction: they presuppose sexual desire and vital impulse – forces that appear to be conflictive and unmanageable. The mother who dies because of blood loss; Sara that aborts by hitting her womb and bleeding; Debora who dies of leukemia leaving behind her son in the care of Raquel, all of these situations demonstrate how blood ultimately occupies an uncontrollable space[5] in corporeality that appears as fearsome and disquieting. Similarly, semen is presented as linked to risky or violent sexual behavior, as is the case of Sara's rape, or in the scene between Judit and Pablo, which presupposes a risk of HIV infection:

> Judit removes her blouse. Pablo observes her for a few seconds and then begins to caress her. He kisses her. At first, slowly, and then with more ardor. Finally he sets her away from him.
> Pablo: I can't.
> Judit: Kiss me.
> Pablo: I'm ill.
> Judit: I know.
> Pablo: You don't know what it is. What it means. Of course I like you, I want you. But I won't put you at risk. Leave me alone.
> Judit: You won't be able to convince me.
> Pablo: Please, leave me alone.
> Pause.
> Judit: Alright, Pablo. But I'll be back. Hopefully you'll realize that this way, maybe, you're hurting me more. Bye.
> Judit puts her blouse on. Exits the tub. Tries to leave (386-387).

This scene illustrates a coincidence between fluids and desires, both associated with the danger of propagating illness. Later, this parallel reappears in a framework that combines desire, the possibility of infection and the ability to manage the risks inherent to the uninhibited circulation of affections:

> David: Does she know you're sick?
> Pablo: She knows and she doesn't care.

---

   5   In previous periods we find texts in which blood becomes a quasi-protagonist, Bram Stoker's *Dracula*, for example. In this narration love, death and eternity are combined in a subversive act. In spite of this, in vampire literature blood does not exist separated from the monster and it does not presuppose a sense of risk in itself. It is interesting to note the resurgence of the vampire narrative and film after the appearance of HIV/AIDS. Elements like blood, eroticism, transgression and the bite (as a metaphor for penetration) are reorganized in the 80s to produce a new generation of vampires whose relationship with blood and desire is different from that of their predecessors. Vampirism, at the turn of the century, is a group activity which is transmitted to others through the bite, alluding to HIV transmission through sexual activity. The new vampires form communities that exist in an intermediate state between life and death as they search for victims to 'convert'. This relationship has been investigated by Aurea Ortiz Villeta in *El arte latex: reflexiones, imagenes y sida*. [Exhibited from April 4 - June 4, 2006. Sala Thesaurus. La Nau, Carrer Universitat]. Valencia: Universitat de València La Nau, 2006.

David: You're crazy.

Pablo: Maybe

David: End it. You could go to jail. Or worse, if that girl's parents find out they're going to kill you.

Pablo: Don't tell me what I have to do!

David: What if you give it to her?

Pablo: Did I give it to you? I know how to take care of another person. I won't let anything happen to her.

David: What right do you think you have...?

Pablo: I have the right. I'm not dead. I'm not a decrepit invalid. I'm not vegetating in a bed. I have the right to fall in love with whomever. Whomever I want! I'm not misleading anybody (405).

This scene is the only one proposing the possibility of controlling the destabilizing power of the bodily fluids, given that in other instances they seem to move in direct opposition to the will of the characters.

It is possible to establish a link between the protagonism of bodily fluids and the appearance of HIV/AIDS, an event that contributes to the association between blood, contamination and danger. This infectious and conflictive potential has precedents in real life (cases of infection by transfusions) which confer upon blood an autonomous value from the bodies in which it dwells and the subjects through which it circulates.

Decomposing bodies

In 1987, Cindy Sherman presents the series *Disgust Pictures*,[6] in which she utilizes inanimate objects to compose, 'portraits', as in her previous works, In them, there is hardly anything that we would recognize as human; the references to identity are lost in the useless remains of objects or food which suggest, if anything at all, a decomposing matter. According to Cortés, in these works:

> Identity is completely perturbed, neither limits nor spaces are respected; the borders between the interior and the exterior have disappeared, the body has exploded and its pieces become confused, in a viscous and putrid totality with food and objects [...] Filthiness, violence, sex and death converge in photographs (*Untitled* 179, 1987) marked by the terrible AIDS pandemic, used condoms, bananas, carrots and other phallic instruments share the stage with a being that is only partially visible, whose gender is not apparent. (1996: 187)

---

6 The series *Sex Pictures*, from 1992, portrays human bodies with fragments of dolls, plastic objects, and so on. Cortés refers to this series and *Disgust Pictures* when he comments upon the disintegration of the body in this phase of Sherman's work.

If we consider that Sherman always photographs human bodies, we see that in *Disgust Pictures* these appear reduced to the materials that (de)compose them, and we are able to discern the undoing of a pre-established hierarchy of the parts (which are now unrecognizable), which is derived into an absolute dehumanization of the somatic. Here we are dealing with bodies that once existed as such but they are now captured by the camera as dissolved presences, barely evoked by the waste that they have generated. Commenting on *Sex Pictures* in 1992, Sherman states:

> I didn't want to make a discrete gay image or a heterosexual couple. I wanted to make it ambiguous so you wouldn't know whether it was a woman's nose or a man's nose that's right under the genitals of that man. AIDS was also an issue I wanted to address. There are no actual condoms – but allusions to condoms. Part of the terror I wanted to imply in the sexuality of the images is very much from the fear of AIDS and the terror that it engenders in the sexuality of our culture. (Lichtenstein, 1992: 88)

It is possible to establish a correspondence between the images present in Sherman's work and the descriptions of the physical present in some plays. The bodies tend to be represented as material remnants of a fateful process of degradation that, in some cases, corresponds univocally to AIDS and, on other occasions, is related to processes of moral deprivation or the tragic becoming of a sequence of events. Blood and semen reappear, now as stains, remains or simple filth that signals a state of decomposition, emerging as the spoils of an organism previously alive and functional.

Sudario, by Roberto Yeras

Sudario (Shroud) premiered on 5 July 2008 in the "Argos Teatro" by the *Versus Teatro* company in Havana, Cuba. The play (which remains unpublished) presents an unnamed female character, leaving as an HIV-treatment inpatient from a hospital; she walks about the city hoping to meet somebody that would keep her company. The portrait of HIV positive subjects appears here burdened with moral discourses imposed over a character that contains many of the stigmas imaginarily associated with HIV. Often, the protagonist is named as "foul", "vermin", "unwasted carrion" – terms which allude to her body and character, her faults as a mother and her addiction to drugs.

The idea of decomposition appears repeatedly:

> Tomorrow I'll be rotting. Slowly. The worms. My useless skin. One farewell. (2)

The motif is repeated consistently throughout the text:

I'll decompose slowly (there), with all these chemicals I have inside me. Which,
right now, fight for my life, I don't know why. (4)

The scene portrayed in Yeras's play, as Sherman's images, is populated by
decomposing bodies:

He was thin, the poor guy. He almost couldn't move, or talk. They didn't have
a wake for him. It was all rot. Like me. Only that I'm still alive. I don't know
why, if it is true. (6)

The abundance of references to bodily fluids acquires a striking quality
and, contrary to what occurs in García's work, they do not function as conflict
mobilizers but as remnants and trash. If in *Sangre*, fluids can be seen as 'living
liquids' (given that they generate action and appear to have autonomy), in this text
the exact opposite occurs: fluids are left as testimonies to a human past; they are
as 'dead liquids' whose presence is no more than a trail of destructive actions and
processes:

I'm sincere, the only thing I want to see is the milk run over this glob of flesh. I
want it on my tits, on my back, on my legs, on my arms, in my womb. I want it
to be drowned in it and after, I want to be left alone to sleep hours and hours. (5)

Besides naming her body a "glob of flesh", the character refers to semen ("milk")
as a fluid that is shed over non-fertile surfaces; additionally expressing a desire for
annihilation and abandon, in which the body is imagined as a tomb of liquids that
kill and suffocate. The protagonist describes herself as being stained by the wastes
of foreign bodies and her own, suggesting a devaluation of her human condition:

I'm a time bomb, dynamite without a sound. Fouled by sex, shat on. My legs
hurt, they hurt a lot. Maybe the best thing would be to throw myself in front of
a car. (1)

You stopped being you. To become the filth that I am. You picked me up from
the park, vomited and full of the milk of others, all over my body. (2)

The woman says she has been 'vomited on', condition that underlines the
idea of the dissolution of the body into excremental matter. The same concept
simultaneously makes reference to being stained by the wastes of others, which
in turn is complemented by the being "fouled by sex, shat on" or "full of the
milk of others", conferring upon her the quality of receptacle of the detritus of
unknown men.

The persistent relationship between sex and the process of disintegration is
striking. The descriptions of sexual conduct reiterate equally, disease, excess and
sin, suggesting the possibility of interpreting AIDS as a punishment, therefore

generating a negative myth of the erotic and its consequences. The character constructed by Yeras presents sexual desire exacerbated to the extreme, exemplarily expressed in the necessity to be splattered with semen "on my tits, on my back, on my legs". This extrapolation of desire remits to the concept of the 'hypertelic', according to Sarduy's proposition;[7] a desire that extends itself beyond its own finality towards paroxysm, or until the configuration of a monstrous construction by fault of excess that manifests itself in the transformation of eroticism into a death drive.

The exacerbation of the sexual impulse presents itself as inexplicable, fundamentally because the expression of such a desire is not accompanied by any reference to pleasure – a concept completely absent in the play. In that sense, we can consider this character as hypertelic, in that it moves beyond any end to suggest the fantasy of an almost literal dissolution into the fluids and wastes of an anonymous 'other'. The reduction of the human into pure materiality that, in its degradation, comes to represent itself as excrement, configures, in this case, an abject space, following Kristeva (1989), in which the absence of limits is extended to all of the spheres of the self, announcing an irrevocable process of disintegration.

Anatomía de un viaje (Anatomy of a Journey), by Marcos Purroy[8]

The play, of a realist tone with poetic elements, is organized into three scenes denominated "Stations", in a game in which each action is linked to the parts of a trip. The central characters are three young adults facing conflictive situations (divorce, HIV-positivity and the upbringing of a child), a portrait of a generation confronting its failures and frustrations. This text establishes certain analogous relationships between distinct physical conditions such as an unwanted pregnancy, an abortion or eroticism confronted with HIV-positivity. Such equivalencies suggest, once again, the tendency to represent corporality within instable spheres in process of disintegration. In this sense, one of the most significant fragments is the following:

---

7   Sarduy develops this concept in chapter two of *La Simulación* (The simulation). Here he characterizes the hipertelic as an aesthetic quality linked to an impulse of excess which verges on the sublime, whilst also implying the dissolution of the limits of the subject: "They are Hipertelic: They have gone further than their ends, as if a lethal impulse of supplement, simulation and gusto had, from an origin, marked beforehand by a lack of moderation, inscribed itself upon their nature" (1999: 1293).

8   This play premiered on November 16, 1990 in the "Rajatabla" venue in Caracas, Venezuela. Marcos Purroy, along with Johnny Gavlosky and Elio Palencia, will be, in time, considered the first Venezuelan playwrights to tackle the matter of AIDS in a rigorous manner, motivating with their productions other dramatists to write plays on this subject.

Alejandra: I learned that they didn't teach me death and detachment, the rails of
the metro, the smell of an antiseptic room next to the shine of sharpened knives
to remove a son, anal penetration, Kaposi Sarcoma, slit wrists, a putrid stomach
and flesh hanging off a bone... And that is happiness! Believe me! It's the only
fucking thing there is! (11)

Suggesting a certain equivalency between abortion (associated with "sharpened
knives"), anal penetration and Kaposi Sarcoma, the parallelism endows all of
these elements with negative connotations: anal penetration is associated with
aggression; abortion is forced upon the mother (rip a child from its mother by
merit of knives) and AIDS symptoms are depicted as homologous to suicide (cut
veins). Here, contrary to that observed in Yeras's text, the author uses diverse
imagery in relation to somatic harm, without insisting specifically on only one
symptom or process. The physical appears affected equally by the idea of the
illness, decomposition, infection or aggression; all of these concepts appear as
forces that attack bodies and push them towards their disintegration.

Purroy reunites multiple evocative images of somatic harm to compose a
representation of the contemporary body as a damaged organism. In the following
quote, one of the characters exposes the distinct components of this damaged
corporality, and again, diverse descriptive elements belonging to diverse orders
are put forth:

Alejandra: Look, Carlota... flesh is... skin that disintegrates... it is
immunodeficiency... Flesh is a one-month old fetus... destroyed, removed by a
teaspoon... It is a skin that is decomposing... Flesh is not having the defenses
for a cold... it is a hide clinging to a bone. (31)

The symptoms of immune-deficiency are associated to an abortion ('a fetus of one
month, destroyed'), appealing to the idea of a life interrupted. The body is named
as a flesh that wastes away, defining flesh and skin as the limits of the subject.
Purroy proposes that the illness (and the abortion as its specular image) generates a
process of de-subjectivation activated by the end of the flesh. Alejandra, meanwhile,
describes her circumstances as an end of herself and of her environment; defenses
are down, the skin wastes and becomes "hide clinging to a bone", the flesh ends
and, with it, the possibility of the future (the fetus); subjectivity is then confronted
with the fragility that threatens to disintegrate everything. The destabilization of
the subject at the root of the disintegration of the body occupies an important space
in this play, corroborated by the following:

Gabriel: Do you know what it would be like to have Kaposi Sarcoma? A type
of gorgeous blue cancer on your skin?... And the inflamed glands?... And a
mycosis, I mean, fungus in your throat?... *(He grabs his throat)* The anguish, the
despair, death over life, resignation. Having to beat off everyday because you're
afraid of screwing and feeling the pained moans of a passionate night; running

out the door when someone says I love you and you want to make love to him; thinking that I won't age and that I need to love and be loved. (26)

The body is then thought of and reduced to the manifestations of immunodeficiency. The character sees himself as the sum of the symptoms caused by opportunistic infections, along with his awareness of another effect of HIV: the impossibility of love. Sex seems impossible and Gabriel anticipates the despair that frustrated desire will bring. The fears associated with the transmission of the virus acquire increasing relevance; Alejandra expresses the horror that her brother's infected body causes her:

> Alejandra: [...] It's hiding my razor, buying two soap dishes, thinking about the need to write my initials on the silverware, plates, glasses, it's being afraid of kissing your own brother and greeting him, instead, with a pat on the back... Disinfecting the bathroom... finding money God knows where for treatments... boiling his sheets and wanting to hang a little bell around his neck so that I can take off when he gets near me...(31)

In this play, the idea of decomposition does not reunite all of the representations of the body; on the contrary, fragility confronted with illness is expressed through various images that occupy several intermediate spaces between the categories that we have established. The concept of wound, for example, takes on a certain prominence; descriptions of bodily deterioration point to the presence of sores which manifest themselves as points of contact between the damaged interior and an exterior that might very well contaminate or be contaminated. In the previous excerpt, Gabriel imagines his future symptoms, where repeated references are made to lesions that affect the skin. Here the skin is understood as the space that separates the inside and the outside of the subject. In this sense, the "fungus in my throat", the glands and Karposi Sarcoma are presented as abnormal openings that have the ability to connect the exterior world with the disintegrating body.

Los caminos que conducen a los ataúdes (The paths leading to coffins), by Alejandro Urdapilleta

The association between the 'wound' and the lesions caused by Karposi Sarcoma also appear in *Los caminos que conducen a los ataúdes*, by Alejandro Urdapilleta, included in his anthology *Vagones transportan humo.*[9] The text does not contain

---

9   First published in 2000, the book is a compilation of theatrical works produced by the author from 1985 to 1999, most of which were staged during the same period. The texts do not incorporate stage directions nor do they indicate actors or voices; they are, for the most part, fragments and poems that function as materials for the staging, leaving space for the director's input.

HIV in World Cultures

direct references to HIV, although there are veiled hints related to the subject. In the following fragment we shall see how allusions to the malady are, in good part, produced in relation to the presence of a wound:

> Do you see this wound?
> here
> in the middle
> it's an old wound
> a red mark
> a bite
> a stab, a nip
> like a red wine stain
> nothing gets it out
> it is the secret spoken in glances between brothers
> in the darkness of the bushes
> should I show it to you?
> See?
> I cover it quickly for fear of contagion
> my body will be blue before time
> would raise me two or three meters above ground
> and I would begin vanishing, twirling
> like the smoke of a boat out to sea (205).

The distinct modes of this wound encapsulate multiple significations; it is a mark, a scar of "a stab, a nip", it is permanent and "nothing gets it out", but it is also the sign through which the "brothers" recognize each other in an understanding look. The wound is also 'ancient', 'contagious', or rather, susceptible to contagion, a sign of future fragility or a premature death, implicit in the possibility of a body "blue before its time".

This brief text explores the possible meanings of the wound as an indicator of HIV. Its visibility operates as a sign of belonging to a group and remits, as is to be expected, to Karposi Sarcoma, in so far as it is accompanied by the reference to secret spaces for homosexual sex ("in the darkness of the bushes") and the complicity inherent to such spaces. On the other hand, the relationship between that old wound and a vulnerable body is made present by the mentioning of a possible fading away ('floating above ground'), which evokes an approaching death. The text continues:

> The paths that take you to the coffins
> have been blocked by sea urchins
> Where have they gone, the men
> that went to war?
> On holiday through the battlefield?
> to swing from the bones?

between shrieks and bombs?
Where did they go
with all that iron
and knives?
and why did they make that face?
why were they offended? (206-207)

The absence of the fable points towards meanings and implications devoid of moral condemnation. Through a fractured language, the author composes a text rich in sensorial and visual references. A possibly painful event crosses this layout; a route, whose endpoint is death, becomes littered with thorny obstacles and a certain awe created by offenses and absences. Urdampilleta wonders as to the whereabouts of those who are gone: the sick are named as those who "went to war"; the landscape is populated by unequivocal signs of painful deaths; the explosion of bombs, the shrieks, bones and the field of the dead, are equated to the experience of the illness that has twisted the route marked by the "paths leading to coffins".

Poisonous bodies: demonization of the transmission of the virus

In 2005, the AIDS Agency of France launched a campaign for HIV prevention in which a man is portrayed having sex with a human-sized scorpion. A second photo, aimed at a feminine audience, depicts a giant tarantula practicing oral sex on a woman. Undoubtedly the images are effective; they communicate to the audience that it is possible to have sexual relations with a dangerous creature that can, during coitus, inoculate its sexual partner with a fatal poison. Nevertheless, it becomes increasingly worrying that, in order to recommend 'safe sex', it becomes necessary to personify that risk in the form of a giant arachnid, considering in the image, that the monstrous creature stands as a substitute for the HIV-positive person. The appeal is accomplished, in this case, at the expense of the demonization of the carrier of HIV, where s/he comes to personify the virus.

The same operation appears at work in some of the plays we have analyzed, where the infection takes on a protagonic role. In the following texts the representation of the moment of sexual transmission is reiteratively portrayed as an aggressive and purposeful action, and if not directly criminal, it is mediated by the bad faith actions of someone who knows himself to be infected. All of which implies, as it is clear in the image we have discussed, a conceptualization of the body of an HIV-positive person as a lethal weapon.

Unicornios (Unicorns), by Aldo Miyashiro[10]

The story develops the complex relationship between Raúl and his adoptive son, Darío, who simultaneously develops a friendship with Raquel and Francis, two transsexual women. Raquel and Raúl are HIV-positive, both suffering from AIDS, who have resigned themselves to the idea of a premature death. A complex plot brings the characters to establish destructive and perverse relationships. Of all the plays studied, this text is the one that most clearly demonstrates the HIV-positive body as a weapon and, simultaneously, as a poisonous organism:

> FRANCIS: Is there someone who doesn't deserve to live?
> RAQUEL: There are many. Take Calo, for instance...I slept with him last night. Didn't he tell you?
> FRANCIS: No.
> RAQUEL: The idiot hollered, you would say (LAUGHS) he thought he was the world's greatest lover.
> FRANCIS: I don't think it's funny. Are you going to keep on sleeping with him?
> RAQUEL: Yes,... I'm dying Francis, but I'm not dying alone, I'll take down everyone who was a son of a bitch with me. Don't you remember everything that Calo did to me? How he used to get off on humiliating me? It's as if they'd given me a weapon, girl... screw me, I'll kill you. You're going to insult me Calo? Do you want to fuck sweetheart?... die you piece of shit.
> FRANCIS: It's not fair. Calo isn't infected.
> RAQUEL: And neither are you.
> FRANCIS: What does that mean?
> RAQUEL: If I've slept with a hundred men, you've slept with a thousand. And I was so careful with those hundred... I don't even know who gave it to me, or how or when it was... Is that fair? What the fuck is fair?... I hope that Calo is infected, that he suffers... he destroyed my self-esteem... I hope he breaks into itty bitty pieces... we were at it for a long time and the whole time I was praying to all of the saints that he would get it, I enjoyed it so much, I felt as if I would faint from so much pleasure and love that I felt for that man who once was mine... when...he finished he looked at me, self-satisfied, as always, and smiled... and he left. I laughed and I thought: "Smile, today you start dying"... I did everything I could, he won't be saved. I even bled. I don't want to die, but I will die... and I'm not going alone, it wouldn't be fair. (7)

The certainty with which Raquel affirms that she has "killed" her lover underlines the absolute confidence that she has in her body's infectious capacity. In spite of the fact that, ultimately, the audience is not made aware of the outcome, the playwright would seem to indicate that transmission has been successful. The play contains another scene, similar in theme; Raúl voluntarily infects Francis in a dark

---

10   Written and staged in Lima in 2003, the text remains unpublished.

theater hall where he convinces her to not use condoms exposing her to the virus. The consequences of this invitation are known later in the play:

> FRANCIS: I'm a carrier and I know when it was... the night that Miguel broke up with me... I never saw that man again, either... while I... Raquel was dying. I have hope, that the virus won't develop. (37)

As has been noted, transmission is depicted as a function of the body of the HIV-positive body used as a weapon, given that the character undertakes the task of infecting his/her sexual partner. Through the demonization of the infected person, Miyashiro presents two carriers with a potential for destruction and a complete indolence in relation to their actions. Additionally, Raquel takes pleasure in the possibility of burdening someone else with the illness. *Unicornios* presents various strategies which tend to demonize the HIV carrier as well as to promote the identification between illness and the sick. The HIV-positive person then becomes a predator and his behavior would seem to be that of a virus, whilst the receiver seems exempt of responsibility.

To these constructions of the body as weapon one should add the ambiguous characterization of the transgender characters that modify their gender identities in incoherent manners: Francis appears during the first half as a transsexual woman, and yet towards the end of the play we see her as a man, without any explanation. Raúl's case is no less strange: he is presented as a heterosexual, where later we come to find out that he maintains sadomasochistic relations with his adopted son, and later, as a corollary, he manifests a desire to become a woman. This conjunction of traits and 'inconsistent' behaviors would seem to equate dissidence against heteronormativity with a chaotic and perverse characteristic mostly associated to a tendency towards Thanatos and monstrosity. This relation is not a new one and it can be observed in previous literature that deals with homosexuality as a subject. Some relevant examples could be Thomas Mann's *Death in Venice*, Manuel Puig's *Kiss of the spider woman* and many of Tennessee Williams' plays. In them, homosexual characters appear hunted by a sort of fatal drive that derives from homosexual desire. Gay characters exhibit an evident predisposition to tragedy and death, which seems to evolve from symbolic associations between homosexuality and 'inversion'[11] (of heterosexuality). In this play, HIV seems to be connected with sexualities that are incomprehensible and doomed for failure, represented as erratic and self-destructive. The body of AIDS (the HIV positive individual) appears as a guilty body where the illness itself could also be read as the manifestation of an interior evil that tends to reproduce itself in the form of a lethal affection.

---

11   Judith Buttler elaborates on this subject in "Sexual inversions". In Stanton, Donna. *Discourses of Sexuality. From Aristotle to AIDS.* Ann Arbor (Michigan), The University of Michigan Press, 1992.

Curvas peligrosas y fuertes vientos (Dangerous curves and strong winds), by Marco Antonio Espinoza[12]

Curvas peligrosas focuses specially on the topic of the transmission of the virus, characterizing it as the result of asymmetrical power relations. The play is divided into two scenes, each one presenting Roland (a 50-year-old American male) in a hotel room with a different young Mexican man. On both occasions, it is strongly hinted that the young men engage in sexual relations with Roland because of money, and that the encounters are reiteratively becoming abusive. The man recounts his obsession with finding a former lover named Juan whom he refers to as "my jungle boy" or "my little Indian from the south". Through these monologues we come to discover that Roland acquired HIV through Juan, but he has not informed his new lovers of his condition. In the first scene, Alberto attempts to communicate to Roland that he is also HIV positive, information which Roland refuses to hear. In both scenes, the sexual relationship appears defined by the commercial transaction. In the first one, Alberto declares: "what I need are 20 pesos so that I can buy my school books" (129) and, in the second scene, Mauricio's financial need contrasts sharply with Roland's delusions:

> Mauricio: I already told you, my name's not Juan.
> Roland: It doesn't matter, the name doesn't matter.
> Mauricio: Just pay me now; I have to go back to the bar!
> Roland: I want you to come with me to Argentina, to "Tierra del Fuego". We can make love together, and then, when we're satisfied, I'll take a gun and shoot myself in the head. To the end of the world! Let's drink for that!
> Mauricio: I don't think so, you're nuts... I need my money! (134)

Transmission of the virus is linked to the abuse of power, evidenced by the complete disregard of the pain that one can inflict upon the other. Roland is uninterested in the identity of his partners, insisting on calling them by the name of his lost lover, which concurrently refers to the Mexican stereotype.

The author establishes a metaphoric connection to the North-South relationship on the American continent; the reference to sexual tourism contains a criticism of the domination that the most powerful zone in the area exerts over the poorest region, which is continuously reduced to images of the exotic and stereotypes about poverty ("you won't be hungry anymore... I'll feed you" (136)). The text charges the frequent simplifications of Latin America to pre-conceived standardized notions: the South, imagined as the end of the world (Tierra del Fuego) seems to be Roland's final destination:

---

12   Included in the second volume of the compilation *Teatro Gay* edited by Tomás Urtusástegui in 2002 in Mexico City.

Roland: (Perched over Mauricio as a father. He takes him by the shoulder. He hugs him. Sexuality is lost. Now nothing is the same.)

"Tierra del fuego" my dear Juan, my little Indian from the south... the name doesn't matter, it doesn't matter... Now you're safe... You won't ever feel hunger, I'll take care of you... I'll feed you... you'll live with me forever... hug me tight, we're going to be together, always together... my "jungle boy"... my little John. (136)

AIDS appears as complementary to this idea of the end of the world and announces that at the end of this voyage of no return Roland will drag down with him some "jungle boy":

Come with me, we'll be so happy, I'll take you on a trip, bigger than life. Look at my body (*he shows him an enormous discoloration (mark/spot) on his armpit*) It's the staining of the body, the shadow of the light. The marks of HIV/AIDS... don't be afraid. (135)

Although this text does not exhibit the aggressiveness present in Miyashiro's play, the dynamic in which the transmission is produced corresponds to similar precepts. Both plays present a character that voluntarily embarks upon the task of infecting his/her lovers, although in Espinoza's text what is sought is not so much punishment, as it is the fantasy of having company on one's deathbed. In that sense, we also see an identification between HIV and the carrier; Roland, whose conduct favors the propagation of the illness, seems to emulate the behavior of the virus, similarly to what occurs in Miyashiro's play.

We have recounted, panoramically, the representations of AIDS in relation to the bodily effects, which lead us to think about the forms of representing such bodies and the mechanisms through which they come into contact, (including the scene – veiled or not – of virus transmission). We believe that the emergence of this illness modifies not only a representational paradigm in literature, theatre and the visual arts; not only its symbolic mediation, but also the manner in which the somatic is understood in general terms, as well as the ways of experiencing corporeal realities, be they infected or uninfected.

The "being in the body" – and thereby, the "being in the world" – changes as a result of the epidemic. The very consciousness of flesh becomes threatening as well as it does the proximity with the body of an 'other'. This can be explained as a result of various elements surrounding the HIV/AIDS epidemic: in the early 80s, sex was finally relieved from some of its moral baggage; the birth control pill had freed people (especially women) from the fear of unwanted pregnancy, and medicine had conquered the cures for almost every venereal disease. On another front, wars had been physically relegated to distant locations, therefore in everyday life (in 'western' cultures, of course) the perception of one's bodily nature was a stable one. It is in this context that the emergence of AIDS takes place, subverting that previous feeling of stability in regards to corporeal experience.

The insistence with which the press presented the disease as one linked to minorities (immigrants, drug users, homosexuals and hemophiliacs) was effective in preserving the illusion that AIDS chooses alterity as its victim, but it also made alterity visible, presenting it as a menace and making its presence evident and fearsome. The 'tainted' and dangerous body of the 'other', adorned by preconceptions of hyperactive sexuality (gay men), contamination (drug users) and savage behavior (immigrants), became evermore present as the epidemic spread, reaching the 'general population'. At least until 1996 AIDS tended to be equated with premature and painful death, causing a sense of fear and discomfort related to the possibility of coming into contact with the illness. But ultimately, being in contact with AIDS is a fact of contemporary life. We can assert that it is not AIDS itself that transforms corporeal experiences, it is the awareness of carnality and instability that is triggered by the epidemic and by the way the governments and the media treated the subject. In any case, as we have tried to expose in the previous pages, the bodily experience changes considerably when confronted with the fear of extreme bodily changes and illness. These changes are made visible in a number of ways, dramatic literature being one of the many formats that allows us to observe the specificities of a constructed body image.

The representations of the body observed in these texts suggest a re-elaboration of bodily consciousness in at least two modalities: on the one hand, we see a tendency to represent the somatic as a fragmented matter which separates body from subjectivity (*Sangre, Pájaros de la playa*), leading to a representation of the body as flesh in a process of decomposition (*Sudario, Anatomía de un viaje, Los caminos que conducen a los ataúdes*) and a perception of the soma as an abject reality whilst maintaining fragility against the ravages of the illness. On the other hand, we can find that in the characterization of HIV transmission, the approach to this matter in the selected plays problematizes transmission exclusively through sex, ignoring all others forms. The insistence on representing HIV/AIDS as linked only to sex suggests that the epidemic unleashes a crisis – and even a sense of panic – about one's own carnality and intimate relations between bodies that go much beyond the constraints of the illness.

In the plays we have examined here, we see a body (the character's own and the body of others) that ceases to be a safe space, either because of a perception of its fragility and tendency towards disintegration or because of the infectious potential which is attributed to it. Possibly, it is this phenomenon that brings about the fixation with the sexual transmission of the virus, given that such a route implies a greater intimacy with the 'other' (intimacy that could be interpreted as being betrayed by the infection).

As we have demonstrated, these two tendencies, imbricated in the representations of the body, are part of the same phenomenon: the re-articulation of bodily experiences as dangerous and threatening. In this light we can propose that these forms of representation of the body that seem to recur in the plays analyzed are also a symptom of new subjectivity. In this way, the representations of a body separated from the self, the depiction of the somatic in a state of decomposition, and the scenes emphasizing its infectious potential, are part of the very same constitution of the subject necessarily emerging from a feeling of vulnerability, where *"living in the body"* is a condition of the possibility to *live in the world.*

References

Aliaga, J.V. 1993. El lenguaje es un virus, in *De amor y de rabia: Acerca del arte y el sida*, edited by J.V. Aliaga and J.M. Cortés. Valencia: Universidad Politécnica, 13-29.

—— 2006. La elocuencia política del cuerpo. *Exitbook: revista de libros de arte y cultura visual*, Nº. 5: 60-75.

Blasco, J.M. 1993. El estadio del espejo: Introducción a la teoría de Lacan, in *7 conferencias del ciclo psicoanálisis a la vista previo a la clase inaugural del seminario Sigmund Freud: Clínica psicoanalítica*, edited by E. Gonzalez Martínez, M.A. Garrido, J. Luzón Cordero, M. Rovira Pascual, J.M. Blasco Comellas. Eivissa: June, 1-9.

Butler, J. 1992. Sexual Inversions, in *Discourses of Sexuality. From Aristotle to AIDS*, edited by D. Stanton. Ann Arbor (Michigan): The University of Michigan Press, 344-361.

Castillo, N. and Sarduy, S. 2004. Pájaros de la playa. *Tablas.* Vol. LXXVI: VI-VIII.

Cortés, J.M. 1996. *El cuerpo mutilado (La Angustia de Muerte en el Arte).* Valencia: Generalitat Valenciana. Conselleria de Cultura, Educació i Ciència. Direcció General de Museus i Belles Arts.

Direcció General de Museus i Belles Arts, Conselleria de Cultura , Educació i Ciencia.

Espinoza, M.A. Curvas peligrosas y fuertes vientos, in *Teatro Gay*, edited by A. Algarra, M.A. Espinoza, J. González Dávila, T. Urtusástegui and G. Yuclán. México DF: Editorial Pax México, 127-136.

Fraser, B. 1996. *Love and human remains.* London: Omnibus Press.

Freud, S. 1979. *Lo siniestro / Sigmund Freud. El hombre de la arena / E.T.A. Hoffmann*, translated by. L. López Ballesteros y de Torres and C. Bravo-Villasante. Barcelona: José J. de Olañeta.

García, Y. 2008. *Teatro cubano actual: Novísimos dramaturgos cubanos.* Havana: Ediciones Alarcos.

Kristeva, J. 1989. *Los poderes de la perversión.* Mexico DF: Siglo XXI Editores.

Lacan, J. 2004. *Ecrits.* New York: Norton and Company.

Lichtenstein, T. 1992. Interview with Cindy Sherman. *Journal of Contemporary Art.* Nº 5, Vol. 2 Fall: 84-88.

Miyashiro, A. *Unicornios.* Unedited. Play provided by the author.

Ortiz, Á. 2006. El sida en el cine. Lágrimas, lucha y melancolía, in *El arte látex: reflexión. imágenes y sida.* Valencia: Universidad de Valencia, 74-83.

Purroy, M. 1997. *Anatomía de un viaje.* Caracas: Fundarte.

Sarduy, S. 1999. La simulación, in *Sarduy, Severo. Obra Completa,* coordinated by G. Guerrero and F. Whal. Madrid, Barcelona, Lisbon, Paris, Mexico, Buenos Aires, Sao Paulo, Lima, Guatemala, San José: ALLCA XX.

Urdapilleta, A. 2008. *Vagones transportan humo.* Buenos Aires: Adriana Hidalgo Editora.

Vilela, E. 2000. Cuerpos escritos de dolor. *Revista Complutense de Educación.* Vol. 11, N° 2: 83-104.

Yeras, R. [unpublished] *Sudario.* Unedited. Play provided by author.

Chapter 5

Listening to Myself: Politics of AIDS Representation – a Personal Perspective

Richard Sawdon Smith

Representing Myself

Simon Watney starts the introduction of his book *Imagine Hope: AIDS and Gay Identity* (2000) with a disclaimer, "This book consists of a sequence of essays written about many different aspects of HIV/AIDS in the 1990s. It thus reflects something of my own involvement with the course of the epidemic, and makes no claims to represent anyone else's view or experience" (2000: 1). On one hand it may seem odd that someone who is seen by many as an authority and a voice of the AIDS epidemic should want to qualify his writing as that of a singular voice, but not so strange when we consider, as Marita Struken has pointed out in her book *Tangled Memories: The Vietnam war, the AIDS Epidemic, and the Politics of Remembering* that, "the politics of AIDS representation has centered on the issue of who speaks for people with AIDS and activists have consistently wrestled for control of the debate" (1997: 159).

Although one may read Struken's statement explicitly as a conflict between certain groups and particular institutions – be they medical, scientific, drug companies, the government, cultural institutions (such as museums and galleries), as well as more generally the media – the statement also implies that, within what we might loosely call an AIDS community, there is sensitivity to the rights, feelings and representations of others. The AIDS movement, a community of those affected by AIDS (although this should imply all of us, not just those living with HIV/AIDS), is made up of a myriad of different groups. Affiliation may well be based on sexuality, gender or ethnicity as well whether the virus was contracted through sex, intravenous drug use or blood transfusion, or those supporting and caring for people with HIV/AIDS, all of whom may have a different perspective on the epidemic. Although Struken and Watney were writing in the 1990s, these issues are still alive and sensitive today, with an added dimension of not just who is speaking for whom but also about the history of responses by these communities to the AIDS epidemic, in terms of who said and did what, or rather who spoke for whom. This was apparent in a response by Nelson Santos, the Executive Director of Visual AIDS, to a recent article, 'Toxic Beauty: The Art of Frank Moore' by Roberta Smith published in the 6 September 2012 edition of the *New York Times*. Santos writes that although it was a poignant review, there were some inaccuracies;

"Smith incorrectly states 'One of the first members of Visual Aids [sic], the artistic arm of Act Up [sic], he [Frank Moore] was instrumental in designing the looped red ribbon that became a symbol of the fight against AIDS" (www.visualaids. blogsot.co.uk).

Outlining what these two misconceptions are, primarily that "Visual AIDS was not the 'artistic arm of ACT UP'" (Santos 2012) and perhaps more significantly, it was the Visual AIDS Artists' Caucus that created the red ribbon (originally known as "The Ribbon Project") in 1991. The red ribbons should always be credited to the Visual AIDS Artists Caucus as a whole and not list any individual as the "creator" of the red ribbon. All of the members of the Visual AIDS Artist Caucus were instrumental in the design (Santos 2012).

Santos is quite particular about why he believes there is a need to correct these inaccuracies and highlight the work done by communities, because, as he says, "it is important to not conflate histories, or credit individuals over communities. Actions should not be re-written, ideas should not be lost and histories should not be silenced" (Santos 2012). These comments underline a fear that, for all the work done by people in the past for an appropriate representation of their communities, a fight to be listened to (highlighted by arguably one of the most memorable graphics of the last 30 years, *Silence = Death*), through time their voice would be lost, wrongly attributed or misrepresented.

So in the same way as Watney, I feel I should start with a disclaimer that in this chapter I represent no one but me – quite literally in the case of my photographic self-portraiture work, images that I have been making since the 1980s in response to the HIV epidemic and the loss of friends. As Watney (2012) confirms, "it's of the greatest importance that we speak on our own behalf, as best we can, not least because we are all surrounded by institutions which claim to represent us, but which are often merely recruiting the fictive idea of a constituency behind them to their own self-interest (including academic 'theory')".[1] My work became more personal/self-centred and reflective when I was diagnosed HIV positive in 1994 and turned the camera on myself (even more than usual) to explore the complex and varied thoughts that were going through my head. Thoughts that included the overwhelming negativity of society towards people who were HIV positive; the fear of the unknown; the emotions of facing potential death; foolishly looking for explanations and seeking some sort of truth, but ultimately trying to establish some sort of control over my own body and the invisible (to the naked eye) virus inside. Later many of those fears subsided, although not vanquished for good, replaced by trying to find balance and cohabitation with the virus, a form of reconciliation and an understanding and negotiation of the conflict of a newfound self. My work very much focusing on 'power/knowledge' relationships that deal with a conflict between individual and institution in terms of establishing one's personal identity and subjectivity. Even though I have been HIV positive for some 19 years now, the issues of disclosure – to whom and when – never goes away,

---

1   Email communication between the author and Simon Watney 15 November 2012.

but there, I've said it, I've come out in print, again. This might seem strange to treat this as an issue, considering my work, but it is never that simple. I don't know who might be reading this; how this information could be used or spread. Each time I talk about my work I have to consider the audience; how much I want to reveal to them, although on experience, the direct response is always positive. This immediately gets us into the area of identity politics and politics of (self) naming. There has always been a certain amount of risk associated with naming in the context of AIDS as Sturken writes, "issues of anonymity and stigma were particularly pronounced in the first years of the epidemic [...] naming oneself as a person with AIDS [...] constituted both a stand against discriminatory policies and an assertion of one's identity." (1997: 159). Again, the relevance of these words, written in the 1990s, is today still incredibly pertinent.

Over the summer of 2012 a number of articles appeared about 'coming out' as HIV positive. Shane Valentine, a young gay man in a self-penned article, which appeared in QX magazine entitled 'HIV + one year in!' wrote, "I also feel very strongly that until us positive guys stand up and speak out, HIV will remain in the closet! If we stop being afraid to speak out about it, then maybe it will begin to enter into the mainstream and start making people think twice before taking risks!" (Valentine 2012: 11). Valentine continued with what can only be called a rallying call to other HIV positive people, "be brave and believe that we can all make a difference be it small or large; collectively it can only make a positive impact!" (11). Around the same time as the Valentine article, the Australian 2000 Olympic silver medallist Ji Wallace decided to send a letter to the Star Observer to announce his HIV status, after another Olympian, Greg Louganis, spoke on air in an 'interview with Piers Morgan about his own HIV positive status. Wallace said he was 'inspired' to write because:

> I too am an Olympic medal winner living with HIV. I have never publicly disclosed this before but felt inspired by [the] interview [...] and by Anderson Cooper's 'coming out' letter last month describing 'value in being seen and heard' in the face of disturbing violence, bullying, persecution and condemnation by peers, colleagues, government officials and worst of all family and friends (www.starobserver.com.au: 2012).

He believed that he too had been a 'victim' of such atrocious behaviour but had been lucky enough to come through, continuing he thought, much in the same way as Valentine that "being seen does have value" and that "a voice does have value" (Idem). These are just a couple of many stories about coming out that can be found in print or online, with people also uploading videos on YouTube and other social media platforms. Alex Garner has even created a website, outaboutHIV.org, for uploading your own coming out videos, although by November 2012 his were still the only videos on the site. While great respect goes out to those who are able to speak up – and these passionate calls for coming out appear to offer very convincing arguments to create a more visible and audible acknowledgement of people living with HIV – it does not mean that it is appropriate action for everyone, not least if people find they do not have a safe and supportive environment around them, as Wallace admits he had. The struggle to find a sense of control with a diagnosis such as HIV permeates into all aspects of one's life, including the decision about who, when and how to tell others, as Watney writes: "the sense of control individuals can still exercise over their lives, without having to be *publicly* defined primarily in relation to only one aspect of them, however important that aspect may be to them *in private*"[2] (2000: 270). Sturken claims that this battle, the politics of AIDS representation on the issue of who speaks for people with AIDS, has "intersected with identity politics, the central tenets of which are proclaiming one's identity and declaring that identity as crucial to one's ability to speak" (1997: 159).

Garner (2012) during his video upload to outaboutHIV announces in a declaration of pride (but perhaps also to give his comments some authority) that "I am a gay man, I'm a Chicano and I'm HIV positive". Garner defining himself in terms of his sexuality, gender, ethnicity and HIV status as a position from which to speak and be listened to, and as such acquiring a political voice. He acknowledges that not everyone will feel comfortable in doing the same and so hopes that his self-naming will provide a source of inspiration and comfort to those that cannot. Sturken outlines debates in the 80s and 90s about self-naming that were crucial elements in discussions about the culture of "victimology" (2000: 160). The argument being that people living with HIV/AIDS should not be represented as victims, as this could be seen as derogatory, associated in people's minds with the inevitability of death rather than living, with pity and in some sense making the 'victim' complicit in their own fate. At the same time, identity politics also prompted accusations of marginalisation that embraced victimhood for political gain (Sturken 2000: 160-161). Garner (2012) does not use the word victim himself but right at the start of the video states, "I'm not ashamed and I'm not embarrassed", as a way to cut off thoughts of victimhood and pity. These debates about how language is used in a negative or positive manner are very familiar but worth mentioning in the context of Wallace's statement. Even though he mentions being a victim, he believes coming out is not about embracing any notion of being an AIDS victim, but as a position of strength that will make him and others less of a victim to the attitude and actions of society.

It appears then that the politics of representation of people with AIDS, issues around identity politics, (self) naming, victimology, are still alive today as much as they ever were. It is perhaps woeful that these debates still exist in the second decade of the 21st Century, 30 years into the epidemic, but they provide a background context to, rather than an explanation of, my own artistic practice. Importantly though, when Wallace comes out and mentions the "violence, bullying, persecution and condemnation" he and others experienced, he is challenging, in a Foucauldian sense, the power relations between the individual and the wider

---

2   Italics in the original.

society. It is this power/knowledge discourse, in Foucaultian terms, that becomes central to my own practice. As Sara Mills explains:

> by analysing the way that power is dispersed throughout society, Foucault enables one to see power as enacted in every interaction and hence as subject to resistance in each of those interactions. This makes power a much less stable element, since it can be challenged at any moment. (2003: 53)

When Valentine says "speak out about it, then maybe it will begin to enter into the mainstream", he too is recognising that there is resistance in everyday actions. The response to AIDS appears to me to play out Foucault's notion of power/knowledge relations as a site of resistance, if we understand Foucault's intent as Mills suggests "where there are imbalances of power relations between groups of people or between institutions/states, there will be a production of knowledge" (2003: 69). Those with power create all sorts of studies and investigations into those who do not have such a privileged position. Because of these institutional imbalances in power relations between, for example, heterosexuality and homosexuality, there are many books about the 'problems' of gay people but not about straights, just as there are many more studies of women than there are of men; of Black people than White, and so on. The same would be true when applied to issues of health and ill health, and in general, as Mills writes, "one could argue that anthropological study has been largely based on a study of those who are politically and economically marginal in relation to a Western metropolis" (2003: 69).

So while the imbalances of power relations between marginalised groups and institutions and the state were and are still being played out in response to the AIDS epidemic, it is clear that there was a difference as the force of the resistance also came from those with more political understanding and economic viability. People who might be considered as 'marginalised' groups made themselves as or even more knowledgeable about the virus, its effects and treatment, as any institution or their representative. It is these power/knowledge relations and responses that have influenced my own photographic practice. As an artist I work with what is around me, a very experiential and empirical approach to research. If we divide photographers into those who work from the personal and project out into the world, and those who go out into the world and bring it back to us, then I'm the former. While my work explores issues to do with living with AIDS, it was not the intention to make a political point about (self) naming or to comment on victimology, I am not putting myself forward as a role model. Although I understand that it may appear that outing myself, as with Valentine, Wallace and Garner, that I am using my status as a way of validating a position from which to speak about AIDS. I am also aware that this is a privileged position, from a safe and supportive environment, whether that is because of living in the UK with access to the National Health Service and free medication, in a secure academic job or surrounded by understanding friends and family. As Sturken points out, it is possible to speak without sentimentality from this position of a deeper engagement with philosophical questions of life's purpose and finitude, to even articulate it as a transformative experience (1997: 163). This experience is not the same for everyone; without access to proper health care it can just be another form of hardship and despair, as can the loss of so many friends or complications from medication (164). As Watney says, there are those who do not wish to be reduced to a diagnostic history, as there are those who live publicly with it (2000: 270). People will engage at different levels and this engagement will change over time. Watney sums this up neatly for me, and an approach that applies to issues in my own practice as an artist when he writes, "as with most things in life, for many the middle way is best, acknowledging HIV enough to take it seriously, and to be able to put up and sustain a fight, but not to the extent of letting it take over one's entire remaining life. This is not necessarily as easy as it may sound" (2000: 270).

But my work does not allow me to deny my HIV status. Even though I often talk about it in the third person, this figure in the images is a representation, a representation of ideas and thoughts I wish to explore, a character created to act out these expressions. I am and I am not the person in the photographs. Yes that is me, but I have created different personas that I inhabit as the subject of the photographs. Like many other HIV-positive people, life can often be divided in to pre and post-diagnosis, so fundamental is the shift in perception of ourselves. This is not a negative but a new perspective on our identity and to a certain extent our subjectivity – how we know, see, feel our body. This is when I developed the idea of *The Damaged Narcissist*, a series of self-portraits that explore this reforming and emerging new identity. I make no apology either, for identifying with the narcissist, even if the narcissist has had a rough time of it; often seen as a negative, the vain individual or the crude analysis of the 'homosexual' in love with his/her self-image, the same sex. If narcissism is taken as a negative, then a damaged narcissist is a double negative. Does this mean they cancel each other out and make a positive? Narcissism is, however, sometimes looked upon as a positive force; after all, we have to love ourselves before we can love others. If narcissism is about vanity, then why would I and other artists who are defined as ill want to turn the camera lens on ourselves? *The Damaged Narcissist* is a corruption of this vanity, a desire to express, but also control, one's concerns about an illness, to decipher this diseased and once potentially damaged body and make sense of a virus invisible to the naked eye. In this chapter I will explore these issues in more detail.

For now though, it is worth mentioning that I have created a new persona, *The Anatomical Man*, which required the tattooing of my body and has resulted in me looking at my life as pre and post-tattoo, as it has created a fundamental shift not only in my perception of self – almost as much as the HIV diagnosis – but how others perceive me as well. Another fundamental change that informs the work of *The Anatomical Man* is the introduction of highly active antiretroviral therapy (HAART) that has seen HIV redefined in medical circles – for those who have access to the medication – as a chronic rather than acute manageable disease. This creates another duality pre and post-drug treatment, where those on medication can expect a normal life expectancy, and with an undetectable viral load find it almost impossible to pass on the virus. *The Anatomical Man* sits quite firmly post-drugs, however, the persona is born out of a long-standing project called *Observe* in which I have documented photographically and through film the consistent, regular and repetitive trips to the clinic to have blood tests to screen for levels of ill health. This invasive but necessary procedure induces a small amount of pain, but through my work and perhaps fetishisation of the process, I have turned it into a ritual that my work now demands so that I can continue the project. In some ways, creating the work makes the nurse (their hands visible in the pictures) carrying out the blood test complicit not only in my own artistic practice but in possible masochism of subjection to the needle. This observation of health, looking for internal signs of the effect of the virus living in the body, as a barometer of perceived medical truth and evidence by the prick of a needle and the drawing of blood, led to another painful procedure: the tattooing (a process that also draws blood with the use of a needle) of medical illustrations depicting veins and arteries onto my body. I have therefore simultaneously collapsed the internal and external together on the surface of the skin. Where I had once made the nurse complicit in my practice I now confuse them. This is not a mapping of my own veins and arteries but representations, anatomical drawings from the 1850s. I am playing with layers of the real and the imagined; I am no closer to knowing myself but have presented an alternative, another me.

One may question why would someone identify his self so publicly with HIV and so permanently as with the tattoos, and that would be hard to answer beyond the old adage of 'the personal is political'. HIV is still with us; there is no cure and so it is still permanent like tattoos. There are people who have used tattoos to identify their HIV status to warn or attract potential partners, such as the bio-hazard sign. However, my work explores a certain reality of living with HIV; a personal perspective, it is not a sign for others. Indeed, the images are all deliberately ambiguous in their potential meaning to the casual observer, to the extent that one may have had to read this chapter to fully know what my work represents.

Listening to Myself

Listening to Myself, the title of this chapter, refers to an image of mine from 2002, part of the *Damaged Narcissist* series, pre-tattoos. In fact it refers to a couple of images *Listening to Myself: Closed* and *Listening to Myself: Open*. They are photographic self-portraits, a naked torso set in a room that is fairly non-descript; the metallic Venetian blind behind the figure and white walls could be a bedroom as much as a hospital room. The figure, me, is listening to his own heartbeat through a stethoscope. Medical paraphernalia usually used by the doctor now promotes questions of appropriation, authority and ambiguity in my own hands. In one photograph the eyes are closed, in the other staring back at the viewer. It might also be worth noting that they form part of a triptych that includes *Looking at*

Myself: X-ray, in the same location but this time the figure is holding and looking at an x-ray of a skull up towards the ceiling, an x-ray of my own head. I do not look ill, in fact quite healthy. However, the image of a person who is ill is never neutral, or simply of a moment in time. Such images suggest a history before illness of how one came to be ill, a life pre-illness signalling there must have been a different body than the one shown to us at this moment. As well as making us reflect on a history prior to the photograph being taken it can also suggest a future, depending on the illness depicted, but all too often in the history of AIDS representation it is of a future that is assumed to indicate an early death. Obviously not all images of ill-health signal death, but they are seen as an 'other', not the normal way of being in the world. The assumption is that the person will get well and the body will change back to something to be considered as normal, healthy and good. It is often hard for us to reconcile the fact that our body has changed through illness and that with an incurable illness it is never going to return to the ideal or fantasy of the normal healthy body. The image of illness then, is always one in a state of flux, reflecting the continuous changes in our body. Although such a reading of an image can be a reflection of the subject's turmoil, it can potentially deny the subject of their identity because it's only recognised as transitory rather than real or actual body. Maybe this can be applied to the reading of any photograph if we believe they are a moment in time, but this is pronounced with images of the ill-body when constructed as other, different to the healthy norm.

In this chapter I wish to expand on the rationale for creating and naming the images *Listening to Myself* as a way of articulating issues of looking, as well as to consider why listening, especially when dealing with representations of AIDS that address concerns of meaning and trying to make sense of experiences of health, illness and disease, has been an important issue for many. A tension exists between the act of looking and the act of listening, as the former tends to suggest being active while the latter a passive position, even though it could be more productive. In our society, illness can come tainted with the notion of wrongdoing, a perception that the person who is ill has brought this upon his or herself; that illness is something bad and potentially we read this as the person being pathologically bad as well. The negative impact of such thoughts, so prevalent with AIDS, can be more crippling than the illness itself. Therefore the narrative of a picture can also include these negative assumptions, whether the author of the work intended them or not, and we have to be careful that we are not interpreting with predetermined assumptions. What I have tried to investigate through my own photographic practice, and articulate here, is this position of flux or ambiguity between the past and the future to create a present, to create a presence in the present that acknowledges the past and future but that also recognises this current body as mine and not as an abnormality to myself. Illness, I suggest, can help us to experience the world in a different way, and phenomenologically speaking, perceive the world in a different way through our new body. Rather than illness being totally detrimental, it can help us to gain greater knowledge and produce new insights into the world around us, helping us to understand and experience our own bodies better. A great source of inspiration in helping me to try to understand my relationship with illness was the work of British photographer, or cultural sniper as she liked to call herself, Jo Spence. 'Listening to myself' was a throw away comment made in passing by Spence when writing about her response to being hospitalised with breast cancer. Although I claim this was a throw away comment, as it was just a phrase in a sentence, it marked a significant turning point in her attitude to both her illness and her body. For me, her work highlights issues of control, and the power/knowledge relations at play in medical, scientific and state institutions.

The issues of control of one's own body is magnified with the diagnosis of ill health, a time when the physicality of the body forces itself into a subject's consciousness as never before, perhaps for the first time in such an intense way, creating a recognition of the body but almost immediately a misrecognition, not wishing to accept this ill-body as the self. Jacque Lacan suggests in his psychoanalytical proposal of the mirror stage[3] that the infant first sees and mis-recognises the reflection of a fragmented lived experience as a whole body in the mirror. However, I would suggest that the person with ill-health looks upon a diseased and damaged body as if the mirror is cracked, and does not recognise the body reflected as whole, as the self, but as fragmented or something alien. An alien body that if healed would return to the whole, healthy body of the previous self. Though if we believe this previous healthy self to be only a fantasy, or as Lacan says a 'specular image' of a wholeness – a wholeness that was mis-recognised – it is the ill body that reflects reality not experienced when healthy. I will return to these thoughts of the alien body later in relation to Drew Leder's phenomenological account of the absent body. Spence identified and incorporated this alien body into her own subjectivity by listening to herself, a way of coming to terms with her body not as self and other, that is, the dichotomies of healthy and unhealthy, good and bad, beautiful and ugly,[4] but as her body, wrestling control away from the medical profession in how she defined herself as a person. It is these elements that I have tried to incorporate into my own work. Spence chose to take a holistic view of her body, which is what she meant by listening to herself. But even she admitted this was never easy, as she writes in the *The Walking Wounded*, "it is sad that even though I had made a study of semiology, when my body 'spoke' to me

---

3   What I'm suggesting here is an interpretation of Jacque Lacan's mirror stage, as it represents a fundamental aspect of the structure of subjectivity. Lacan claims there is a tension between the young baby seeing a whole image in the mirror compared with its uncoordinated body, which is experienced as a fragmented body. An imaginary sense of mastery is created when the child identifies with the image as its own to resolve this tension. Lacan calls this the 'specular image' – the image of oneself that is simultaneously oneself and 'other'. For Lacan this is the basic reason for the power of the imaginary in the subject. See Lacan, Jacques (1994) *The Four Fundamental Concepts of Psycho-Analysis* London: Penguin.

4   For further detailed analysis of these dichotomies see, Gilman, Sander (1995) *Health and Illness*. London: Reaktion.

with her various 'signs and symptoms' I could not understand what was being 'said'" (Spence 1986: 215). Watney (2012) believes this is still very important "since the unconscious often has no other way of reaching us except by such forms of acting out, the full significance of which may take years and decades (if ever?) to become apparent."[5]

Spence was clear that her work was a way of trying to take control of the situation, in this case breast cancer, and that her photography work was about being able to have more control over her body and that this was part of a wider struggle for women to generally have more control. She was fully aware that she and other women should not be seen as victims: "the work is about the process of struggle when ill and acts as a metaphor for all struggle. I think we should represent the struggle for *becoming* well and not just throw up a new breed of victims and heroines" (Spence 1986: 209).[6] Spence's diagnosis of cancer runs parallel with the naming of AIDS and a new political movement of patient power coming out of the US, such as ACT UP, promoting a questioning of authority, the government, the church, the pharmaceutical industry and even the medical profession. Spence was fully aware of these debates and in fact was a close friend of Watney, attending many of the initial meetings of the AIDS & Photography group he set up, which led in time, amongst other things, to the Ecstatic Antibodies project. Watney, arguably one of Britain's most articulate and well know commentators on the AIDS crisis, was himself fully versed with the debates happening in the States at the time. Activists in New York City were themselves talking about listening, but their response was more plural than self-reflective. They were clear that if they wanted people to listen to them that they needed to make a noise, and what they feared was the opposite: not being listened to, or worse, to be silenced, to have their voice taken away, to be voiceless and therefore unrepresented. The most visible sign of the time was ACT UP's graphic text based symbol of 'Silence = Death' on top of a pink triangle, making obvious reference to the pink triangle that homosexuals were made to wear in Nazi concentration camps. But again it was not just about being listened to that ACT UP were concerned with, but also how PWA were being portrayed, how photographic representations could stereotype and stigmatise those with AIDS.

"STOP LOOKING AT US; START LISTENING TO US", was the chant from the streets of New York outside the Museum of Modern Art (MOMA) when it exhibited the work of Nicholas Nixon, a story that appears to have found its way into AIDS folklore. Perhaps so many of us are familiar with this story because evidence of the flyers people handed out at the time still exist, which had printed in capital letters at the top (the literary way of shouting) "NO MORE PICTURES WITHOUT CONTEXT". The stereotype that was made visible in Nixon's photographs that activists were afraid of, persisted for years and perhaps still does today: very stark, striking images in black and white of individuals

---

5   Email conversation between the author and Simon Watney 15 November 2012.
6   Italics in original.

– men – looking incredibly ill and thin, with gaunt eyes, on their death bed, alone. The demand printed in the flyer was for more positive images of PWAs and although, in all fairness, the request was for a greater range of images that better reflected people's life experiences of ill-health than the singular story that made newspaper headlines or got exhibited in major galleries, trying to replace one stereotype with another does not necessarily help increase understanding of the issues. The danger is that it also expects photography to be at the heart of being able to reveal some hidden truth about AIDS and perhaps create meaning out of illness through visual representation. The suggestion in the text of STOP LOOKING AT US; START LISTENING TO US is that photography has in some way silenced the subject rather than giving voice to them. This idea is a recurring theme throughout my chapter but there was a different thought by some early photographic pioneers who believed that they just had to listen to the photograph to hear some truth not evident to the naked eye. One such practitioner was Dr Hugh Diamond who not only documented the insane at the Surrey Asylum in the 1850s but also believed that it had the power to heal certain cases of mental ill health. To improve the patients' condition they were posed and dressed to appear 'normal'. In his paper delivered to the Royal Society in 1856, Diamond claim that, "the photographer [...] needs in many cases no aid from any language of his own, but prefers rather to listen, with the picture before him, to the silent but telling language of nature (1976: 19).

Diamond was just one of many early pioneers such as another Englishman Sir Francis Galton and the Frenchman, Alphonse Bertillon. They had the same purpose at the end of the 1800s/ beginning of the 1900s of detecting within European society patterns of bodily evidence of deviation from 'normality', particularly the 'criminal', although they took two very different approaches. Galton invented a system of composite portraits that used various multiple layers of photographic negatives detailing facial characteristics to determine a biological 'type'. Bertillon constructed a more elaborate and detailed filing system. Records were kept of individuals within a 'macroscopic aggregate' that eventually led to conformation of the criminal by a photographic representation. This system built up an enormous archive of statistics and photographs that were aimed at identifying repeat offenders, as opposed to Galton's biological type, predisposed to crime by 'nature'. Galton has been credited as the founder of eugenics and, as such, his use of photography to seek 'betterment' in the heredity development of race cannot be underestimated. The pseudo sciences of physiognomy, the judgement of character from facial features, and phrenology, the judgement of mental functions from the shape and size of the skull (a crude early attempt at neurology), are closely linked in their reliance on visual features of the head as a guide to categorising types of people. Photographers armed with social statistics, and aided by an almost universal belief in society that photography revealed an undeniable truth, sought to provide a visual record that described the deviant and in turn the normal, in this case the normal being the law-abiding body, but the same can be applied to an idea of the healthy body. Stuart Marshall has pointed out that this idea of the norm, "particularly when coupled with the concept of the 'natural', was to become one of the most important reference points for describing the relationship between the individual and society from the mid-nineteenth century up to the present day" (1990: 25). Roberta McGrath has also forcefully indicated, when writing about issues of health and photography, that we must beware of confusing the natural with that which is cultural and ideas that place "nature above history" (1990: 142).

The prime example is Henry Fox Talbot's description of photography in 1844, as the 'pencil of nature'; the effect of light on specially coated paper to produce images without the aid of the artist's pencil. The photograph is not described as replicating nature but replicating the hand of the artists, a point that seems to have been missed by so many during the development of photography. It is important to recognise that it is the hand that takes the photograph and the set of beliefs and prejudices, or simple ignorance, attached to the hand that indicates how the image should be read. It is work by people such as Spence that has tried to find alternatives to these well-established views on how the ill should be photographed. At play here is the power/knowledge discourse as discussed in the introduction. Writing in *Ecstatic Antibodies: Resisting the AIDS mythology*, Marshall marks out quite clearly that it was through these early medical photographic studies following in the traditions of Galton, that male homosexuals first became visible, although the medical project was designed to try and record the notion of sexual deviancy, and as Marshal continues, "thus the male homosexual, defined only and utterly by his sexuality which saturates his very being, was delivered to the camera, for the medical profession and for society itself. The regulation of homosexuality and disease were irretrievably woven together in the domain of the photographic image" (1990, P28). It is here that Marshall also claims some of the first homosexual politics were first mapped out, and such politics became even more relevant when AIDS was seen as a gay disease, as the calls to stop being looked at and start being listened to testify.

The Absent Alien-body

It is through this medical discourse that a definition of the 'Other' has been formed, primarily around what the healthy are not; illness as the antithesis or absence of health. The healthy body is the 'norm', and 'abnormal' bodies, the 'sexual deviant' included, are generally not considered the subject for photography unless for medical and scientific reasons, as mentioned in the previous section. But as Marshal says "the sexual and social identities 'discovered' in this process were in fact constructed by it" (1990: 26), resulting in the construction of an institutional gaze deciding what the problem is and how to deal with it. The process of classifying and categorizing types through photography actually silencing the subject; subjects are made visible but they have no voice. A definition of 'normal' is always considered by what it is perceived not to be: the 'abnormal'. As with power/knowledge relations, the body that is absent to us, that is never under investigation, is the healthy body. Drew Leder has argued, in his book *The Absent Body*, that absence is necessary for functioning in the world. It would be impossible to live while considering every movement and positioning of our body especially if we were to try and comprehend the internal at the same time. Generally it could be argued that awareness of our bodies appears to be, at the very best, temporal; we function in society by being unaware of our own body, at least for certain sections of society considered to be normal and healthy. Leder sums up the body's tendency to disappear from awareness and action with the terms "ecstatic" whereby the body projects outside of itself into the world, and "recessive", when the body falls back from its own conscious perception and control. In addition he also points out that the body simply "moves off to the side" (1990: 69) when surface parts of it are not in action.

In response to these ideas I created a body of work called *Absent Body: The Photographic Stain*, where a naked male figure is covered in white body paint from head to toe so that the identity of the individual is not so apparent. He is shot against the corner of a white brick studio, a generic representation of the/ an institution; white on white, the figure and his identity disappearing into the institutional surroundings. But as the series goes on the figure draws at first the outline of their body in blood red on the wall and fills it in to create a silhouette (Figure 5.1). At the feet of the silhouette the cable release is visible to indicate this is a self-portrait. Simply, the figure is trying to carve out their sense of self on the institutional walls and, in terms of illness, assimilating the other – the alien body of ill health – into their own identity by clearly recognizing and representing it. The most interesting analysis by Leder in relation to this work is when he considers what he calls the 'dysappearing body'. The conspiracy of silence we adopt about our own body is broken when it becomes diseased or damaged, but even then we may not relate to this broken body as ours. He writes, "insofar as the body seizes our awareness particularly at times of disturbance, it can come to appear 'Other' and opposed to the self" (1990: 70). This aspect has been crucial for many people confronted with their own illness. If we understand the body to be absent while healthy, forced into consciousness, the effects can be traumatic beyond the conditions of ill health. Not only would this have to take into account notions of the repressed, but also the effects of social and cultural histories on the body, such as the stigma associated with AIDS.

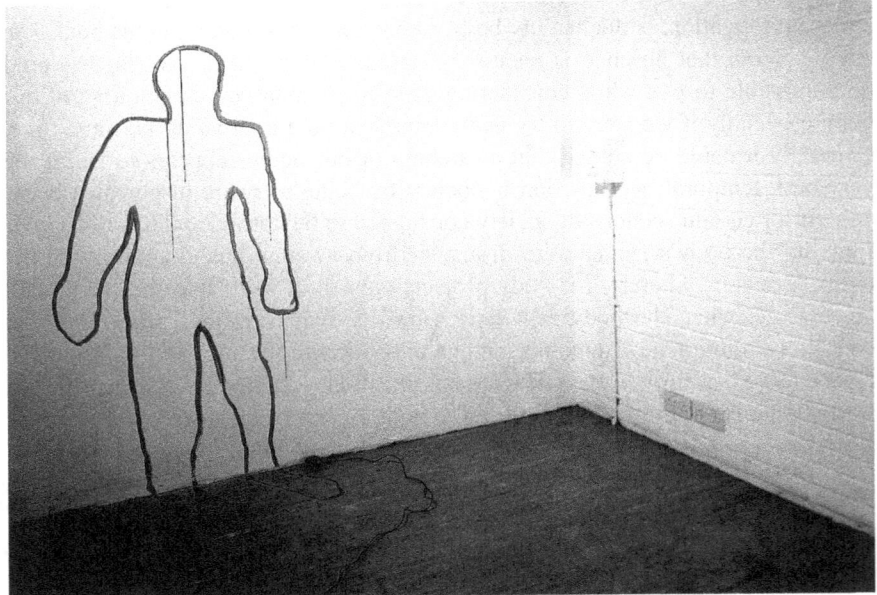

Figure 5.1 Absent Body: The Photographic Stain

Watney (2012) believes that 'body image' still "remains such a fertile area of exploration, based on the often hidden psychic reality of the body, a reality created from memories which are often for good reason repressed." Watney continues that "for many of us HIV re-enacts all sorts of dark things about our relationships to our bodies and desires."[7] For Leder it is when the body becomes diseased or damaged that it seizes our attention, and the attention of others, most strongly. The body forces itself into our consciousness at times of dysfunction and that comfortable absence is lost. It dys-appears; that is, appears in a dysfunctional state. The body is now perceived but experienced as other, creating a dys-juncture with 'normal' bodily state of dys-appearance (Leder 1990). Although this goes some way to understanding the shock of confrontation with the body when diseased or damaged, Leder's is a regional ontology of the body – how alienation of the body from the self occurs. As Leder puts it, "the body is no longer alien-as-forgotten, but precisely as re-membered, a sharp searing presence threatening the self" (Leder 1990: 91). It is possible to draw a parallel here between this 're-membered' body, as the fractured one that breaks the Lacanian mirror stage, and the fantasy of the whole or healthy body. But Spence believes that her experience of ill-health, or more precisely her treatment in hospital, highlighted the fact that the female body is always objectified and fractured, "just as the female body is fragmented and colonized by advertisers [...] so it is similarly fought over by competitors

---

7   Email conversation between author and Simon Watney 15 November 2012.

for its medical 'cure'. There are no departments of 'whole body' medicine in any hospitals I have ever attended. The concept is quite alien at any institutional level" (1986: 155).

Leder's phenomenological account of the body has drawn a response from a number of sociologists (Schildrick 1996: 3, Williams 1998: 77, Corker 1999: 77, Overboe 1999: 27) who have questioned the extent to which his theories can be implemented. They argue that, although all bodies have the potential of corporeal irruption into consciousness, the being of any body that is 'Other' heightens the threat and therefore it is not simply the possibility of the broken body that disrupts the boundaries of the transcendent subject. While Leder's analysis describes a certain universal structuring of bodily experience, it does not recognise that apprehension of the body, or lack thereof, is shaped in a thousand ways by one's material, social and cultural environment, as well as by the body's capacity for pleasure. To suggest that our body is absent from daily consciousness does not fully recognise what it is to be a woman, or black, or old, or disabled, or gay, in the society we live in. However, it is precisely these groups that feel they are invisible in a heterosexual, white, male, middle class society. That they have a lack of representation and when they are represented visually it is only to be subjugated, to be classified and categorized, stereotyped by certain images and not listened to.

In the Archive

At the height of paranoia about the potential of an AIDS epidemic there were calls for not just people with AIDS but all gay men to be quarantined, put away to protect the rest of society. This language replicates the very same actions of the late 1800s discussed before, and would need to involve a system of identifying, of making visible those people it then intended to vanish and silence. The same process can be seen as one way in which the medical image of the 'abnormal' body is quarantined to the safety of the archive in an act of what McGrath has called "representational liquidation" (1995: 99). As in the previous example, those who are underrepresented are made visible but only so that they can be classified and categorized, whether that is the criminal or the person with AIDS or the gay man. As an artist I have tried to describe and document my personal response to living with AIDS through photographing myself, so that I am able to make visible my experiences. As part of this process and looking for similar work – a desire not to be so isolated – I undertook research in the Visual AIDS Frank Moore Archive Project in New York City, where a whole host of artists and photographers have slides of their work, many creating self-portraits as narratives that provide moving personal histories in the face of illness that are an inspiration to many around the world. Making public these personal histories means that the artists are in fact outing themselves as HIV positive, and, even in a more supposedly 'tolerant' society, this outing could be read as a political act in its own right. Yet, I cannot help but try and articulate some concerns, my ambivalence or perhaps ambiguity about the notion of an archive for living artists. To some extent my issues are not necessarily with this particular archive but with the function of archives, which, by their very nature, categorise and classify images, and in turn people, by predefined concepts of identity, often articulated as 'other'. To have my work accepted, I had to go through the process (at least in my mind) of identifying myself as a HIV positive artist. This in fact is the only criteria for acceptance into the archive; there are no qualitative decisions made about the art. There are of course other archives around the world that have defined categories, for example, Black Artists, or Women Artists.

Obviously one does not preclude the other, and there may already exist an archive for HIV positive, Black Women Artists. The flip side is the archive for healthy white male artists. There are of course hundreds of these, only they are not described in these terms and they do not come under the same sort of scrutiny. The creation of specific archives is born from some form of political decision, an identified need for a particular archive, which in turn can politicise the work by association and to a predetermined agenda that had not been intended by the artist. The work in the archive might be by a HIV positive person but it does not follow that the work is about HIV. We can understand that, as many artists were dying as a result of AIDS, the Visual AIDS Frank Moore Archive Project was established to try and find somewhere where the work could be preserved, so as not lost to the world. As the life expectancy of people living with HIV/AIDS has increased, so has remit of the archive. Evolving from this precept, the Visual AIDS Organisation, with the archive being just one part of it, has taken on many other functions. It moves from a passive archiving role to an active role, the role of activist in terms of its advocacy work for HIV awareness. Rather than the art work itself, the work of the archive is the predominant political act here. Invited guest curators who select work, who normally reflect their individual agendas, and their own readings and interpretations of the work, extend this act. The choice of work may be included in a show whose themes the artist had never considered before. While the archive is open for everyone to visit and look at the work, the public/ visible face of the archive is the monthly-curated virtual exhibitions. I am not criticising nor suggesting this is a negative, but highlighting that the artist often has the least influence in the process of how their work is read.

It is at this point that I decided to create a site-specific work of art that could be called an interruption into the archive, both physically and psychologically. The series *In the Archive* is a series of photographs of me, naked, simulating the act of viewing the archive as if I might be a researcher or curator – which I am and have been – but on this occasion, act out the role I perform. I already exist in the archive – my images are located there – and through the act of photographing myself, I am physically in the archive again and at the same time reproducing myself as these images are reproduced to be placed back in the archive for the next researcher or curator to view (Figure 5.2). I believe this repetition starts to illuminate something of the uncanny inherent in photographs of the HIV/AIDS body, the body photographed as other, as an alien diseased body and yet the self. My desire

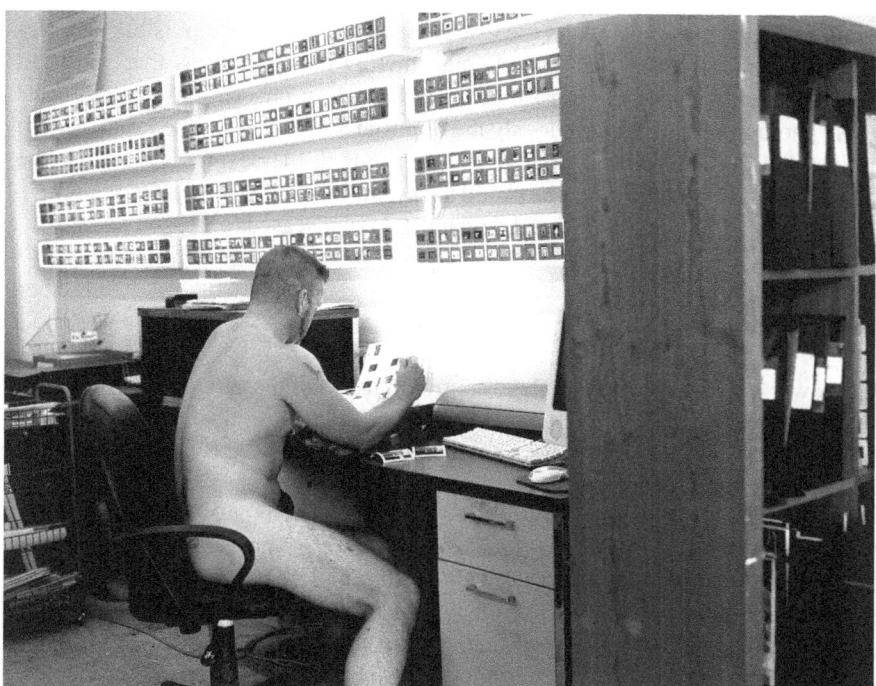

Figure 5.2 In the Archive

is that when the next person to come along views this project in situ, that a form of recognition happens in terms of their own body and my body, the AIDS body, being witnessed as they sit or stand contemplating the theme of their research, looking at the slides of work on display which now contain these very images. My level of ambiguity with the notion of an archive is perhaps predicated by the concerns mentioned earlier about the use of photography in medical institutions to classify the homosexual as a sexual deviant. The politicisation of the photographic portrait has been dominant in certain academic writing dealing with issues of control over the production and dissemination of images, and has been at the heart of debates for many artists and writers since the late 1960s. In particular, much has been done to question the validity of uses of photography in nineteenth century institutions as the social and cultural history of photography has been continuously rewritten. Many writers[8] have explored the relationship between photography and power, concerned with representation as a fundamental tool in control of the

---

8 See, Tagg, J. (1984) *The Burden of Representation*, London and Basingstoke: Macmillan, Green, D. (1985) 'On Foucault: Disciplinary Power and Photography', *Camerawork*, no. 32, Sekula, A. (1986) 'The Body and the Archive', October, Vol. 39, Evans, J. (1988) 'The Iron Cage of Visibility', Ten 8, no. 29.

criminal, the sexual deviant and the diseased body. These often invisible histories have been exiled to the archive and controlled by the institutions that produced them, with limited access to those outside of the institution, especially the subjects of the photographs. This is obviously the opposite to the work of the Frank Moore Project Archive; it is not an archive of the criminal, the sexual deviant and the diseased, although some might be proud to say, in an ironic fashion, it is an archive of work by the criminal, the sexual deviant and the diseased.

Recover/Discover

The power of representations and the control of usage of those representations was recognised very early on in AIDS activist work in line with this thinking coming out of the academy, especially how photographic portraits had come to symbolise, that is, stereotype, in the press and media, the AIDS body as singular, dying and looking incredibly thin and ill, as was objected to in the Nixon MOMA exhibition. As I have mentioned earlier, the replacing of negative images with positive ones potentially replaces one stereotype with another and does not speak of the true experience of people who have been diagnosed with a life threatening illness. My own work treads an in-between ground, resting somewhere between ambivalence and ambiguity rather than positive representations, as I have tried to articulate with work in the archive. I am ambiguous about my illness, not about the illness that has killed friends and lovers and many millions of others around the world, but the one I live with that has not killed me yet. My work is quite different from other earlier artists confronting living with AIDS that I deeply admire, such as David Wojnarowicz, who wrote with such passion and anger about his experiences of being gay and HIV positive in America, in that it is very introspective. In part, this ambivalence I mention is articulated in my photography by creating different personas so that I can distance myself from the image and at the same time feel that I'm controlling living with AIDS. In an interview with photographer Jason Evans published in 'They Shoot Homos Don't They?' magazine, I explained that HIV brought my emotions closer to the surface, and at the same time it gave me even more of a sense of distance. In challenging me on 'A Distance From What?' I simply explained a distance from the world and expanded further by saying "it's critical, it's mental, and it's physical. It's a distance from lovers, it's a distance from getting too involved" (2008). Although this has led to a sense of not being-in-the-world, my ambivalence extends to the fact that a potentially life threating virus has given focus to my art and in turn my life, to the point that it is hard to imagine life without being HIV positive. The virus has made me consider myself anew but at the same time made me question, through my photography, a perceived threat of a loss of identity, a struggle to describe an identity and subjectivity that is not solely defined by AIDS, but where I know that the medication I take is what has allowed me to live a full and productive life.

In 2008 I created a body of work that appears to politicise its message simply by the mode of production as fly posters, free of slogans apart from the title of 'Art Pos(*t*)er / Aids Pos(*t*)er. The project is a hybrid work, editing together work from different series of photographs produced over a six-year period from 2002-2008 that were originally intended for the gallery but now produced in a format that potentially suggests some form of subversion beyond the gallery wall onto the street. Yet again there is an ambiguity, as the work suggests no particular political message on first reading, unlike the earlier work of ACT UP. Sitting my fly posters on the street amongst advertising for all sorts of events and commodities could be read as some sort of posturing. While direct comparisons are, maybe, not useful, particularly as the Art Pos(t)ers / Aids Pos(t)er series was produced in a time that effective medication had become readily available to those who could afford it and so there is not the same sense of urgency, the series differs from the early activists work in that it highlights the plight or concerns of an individual rather than speaking for a community, and it celebrates the portrait rather than relying on text-based graphics. It differs from the work of Nixon, not because it does not show an emancipated figure but because it is self-portraiture, the patient controlling the image, creating more complex narratives. But of course, when Nixon's work was shown at MOMA there was not the range of such effective drugs so readily available as there are now. The series of posters as with the *In the Archive* series also includes images that are questioning and reflective on my own position in the AIDS community, as in the image *Red Ribbon*, where a large ribbon is wrapped around the torso and the eyes (Figure 5.3). As mentioned at the start of this chapter, the Visual AIDS Artists' Caucus created the red ribbon as a symbol of remembrance for those who have died of AIDS related illnesses, visualising that loss, and also as a tool to highlight the need for further action. In the photograph the symbolism is clear: a large, red ribbon blinding the self, but its interpretation is open. Is the figured burdened by the memory of so many loved ones lost, or does it represent a personal memorial? Has the person become defined by their illness? Does it highlight the fact that stigma around AIDS still exists? Has the ribbon become such a powerful symbol that the people it was intended to represent are not recognised? Has it become sign rather than substance? Is it just another logo that drug companies can stick on their advertising to suggest that they care? It could be all of these things. As with submitting work to the Visual AIDS Archive, creating a series of self-portraits that can be posted around town has created a situation of outing myself as a HIV positive in a very public way, beyond the gallery wall or academia. Individually the works are ambiguous enough for people to question the intention but together create a clearer narrative of exploring different aspects of living with AIDS. The majority do make explicit reference to the medical, and suggest a vulnerability of the doctor's authority in the power/ knowledge relationship between doctor and patient, institution and individual. They do appear to propose the idea of taking control and responsibility for one's own health; listening to myself. Yet they still offer no solution, no ultimate truth. The image *Recover / Discover: Red* – where the unwrapping of the bandages

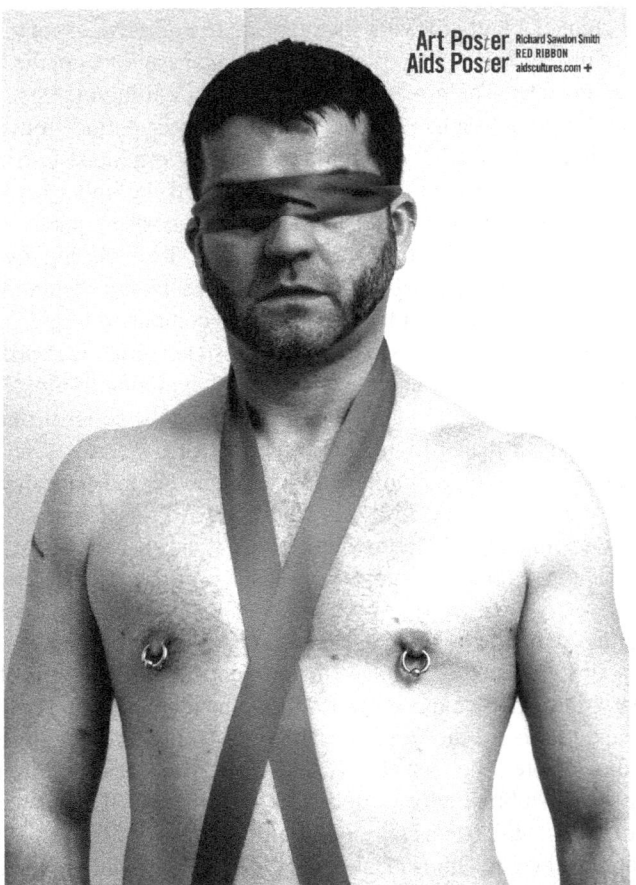

Figure 5.3 The Red Ribbon

reveal yet another layer of bandages – was produced in response to the writing of Akira Mizuta Lippit, which helped summarise my concerns of trying to make sense of AIDS, of trying to find meaning in it:

> In the register of health, recovery refers to the process of healing, of restoring the body to a phantasmatic condition of wholeness. Recovery, the act of recovering, however, also initiates a semiotic chain that includes covering, that is concealing, as well as discovering. In fact, the tension between recovery and discovery informs the scientific drive. For scientific practice praxis is always torn between the desire to recover the totality of natural phenomena and to disrupt that closure with new discoveries, new ruptures. (1994: 6)

The 'phantasmatic condition of wholeness' appeals to me in the same way that we can talk about the Lacanian mirror stage or the 're-membered' body of Leder. Illness underlines the fact that we live a fractured life and the idea of wholeness is the fantasy. Lippit explains this further when he asserts:

> Every surface can be torn to reveal another surface, another plane of intensity. The result of such manic layering [...] leaves the viewer searching for a non-existent essence, constantly suspicious of the infinite surface. With each layer that is peeled away there appears to be another to take its place, rather than revealing an essence of the body we merely add to it another layer or fragment. (1994: 7)

Conclusion

In the case of an incurable disease there will never be a return to a previous whole. Maybe recognition of a new wholeness, one where the multiplicity of the fractured body or that the 'dysappearing' body is recognised; a new body created by listening to oneself for greater understanding. However, what Lippit's article helps us to realise is that there is no truth to be found, only the desire to keep on looking for one. Within the search for new discoveries there is always the potential for error as Foucault writes in the introduction to George Canguilhem's (1998) *The Normal and the Pathological*, "for at life's most basic level, the play of code and decoding leaves room for chance, which, before being disease, deficit or monstrosity, is something like perturbation in the information system, something like a "mistake [...] In the extreme, life is what is capable of error" (1998: 21/22). Put another way, life gives way to chance, and Foucault reads this as "error is at the root of what makes human thought and history" (1998: 22). This is not intended in any way to diminish the loss and hardship people have suffered and still suffer due to AIDS or to justify its existence. As a long-term survivor, perhaps my work is still caught in a cycle of trying to make sense of life, continuously looking for this 'non-existent essence', believing that if illness is articulated as natural (if not more so than being healthy), it can help us learn about life. When the red ribbon was first created it encapsulated a time identified by Douglas Crimp as Mourning and Militancy. Now we are in a time that is less definable, Sturken calling it a "second wave" claiming, "in its omnipresence and in the relentlessness of its cultural analysis, AIDS has in some sense been normalized, by which I mean that it no longer is a crisis or emergency situation but rather is part of the everyday" (1997: 164).

Although thinking about this second wave in terms of an era of 'post-suffragist', as proposed by my colleague Alan Beck,[9] does help to try and articulate the sort of ambiguity present in my work. Suffrage, to mean the right to vote, has obvious

---

9 Alan Beck author of *The Unspeakable act: 'performing' AIDS Deaths* in email conversation May 2007.

parallels with the Women's Rights movement and with women being given the right to vote in the 1920s in America and the UK. I am sure many women would say today that they are still not treated equally, but while some might still keep on the good fight, the majority of people assume things are okay. The same could be said with AIDS; there is medication but it is not a cure. My most recent work, *The Anatomical Man* (Figure 5.4), the tattooing of veins and arteries on to my arms, was as a direct result of having to continuously go for blood tests, as mentioned previously. The tattoos are not a trace of my own veins but medical anatomical drawings from the 1800s. Representations that might have been used in medical diagnosis and as such open to interpretation and error. The work is very much about living with the virus, making visible not just the workings of the internal body but the routines of medical observation that check that the medication is working, as well as looking for signs of potential side effects. The daily meds. The three monthly intrusive needles. All a reminder that life is reliant on these interventions. The message of urgency so vibrantly articulate in the militant work of earlier activists may not be needed now and battles seem to have been won, but inequality still exists. The case studies of people outing themselves as HIV positive and the issues surrounding this action highlighted at the start of this chapter demonstrates that there is still incredible stigma associated with AIDS. This does appear to be a very sad state of affairs and one wonders how far we have come in the last 30 years and why so many of the references here that refer back to writings from the 1980s and 90s still seem relevant today. Although I believe illness can help us to understand about being in the world, and if we listen to ourselves we can pass that information on and help others, it also seems fitting to finish with a quote from Marshall written as long ago as 1990:

> Only through these media [performance, visual arts, video, films, printed media] is there a possibility of [...] producing radically different conceptualisations of the body, disease and health. In this way it is possible to produce new representations that offer new possibilities for identification, which speak complex, difficult and contradictory experiences of AIDS. (1990: 36)

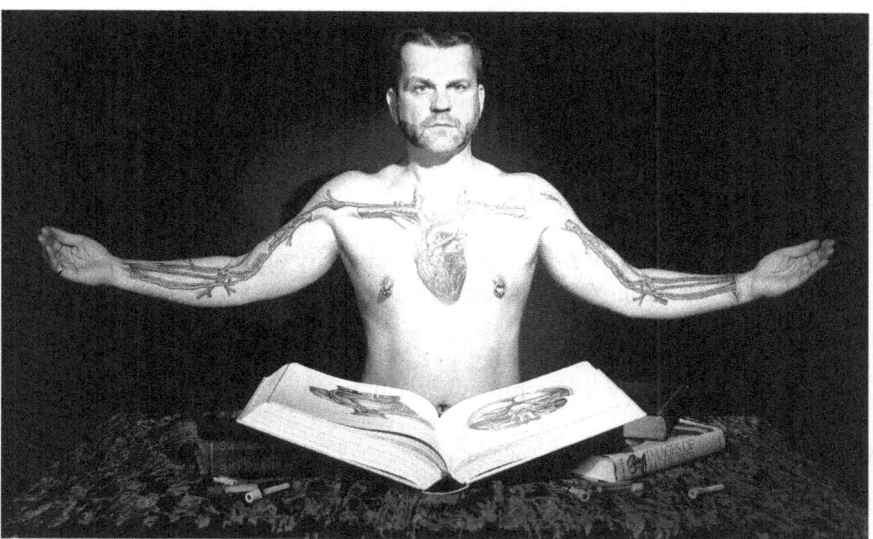

Figure 5.4 The Anatomical Man

References

Burton-Bradley, R. 2012. *Aussie Olympian reveals HIV status*. The Star Observer [online, 8 August]. Available at http://www.starobserver.com.au/news/australia-news/new-south-wales-news/2012/08/08/aussie-olympian-reveals-hiv-status/82378 [accessed: 9 May 2012].

Canguilhem, G. 1998. *The Normal and the Pathological*. New York: Zone Books (Translated by Carolyn R. Fawcett in collaboration with Robert S. Cohen).

Corker, M. 1999. 'Disability' – The Unwelcome Ghost at the Banquet... and the Conspiracy of Normality. *Body and Society*, Vol. 5 (4): 75-83.

Crimp, D. 1989. Mourning and Militancy. *October*, Vol. 53: 3-18.

Crimp, D. and Rolston, A. 1990. *AIDSDemoGraphics*. Seattle: Bay Press.

Diamond, H. 1976. On the application of Photography to the Physiognomic and Mental phenomena of Insanity, in *The Face of Madness*, edited by G. Sander. New York: Brunner/Mazel, 17-34.

Evans, Jason. 2008. So Who is that Guy? *They Shoot Homos Don't They!*, No. 5, August, 14-21.

Evans, Jessica. 1988. The Iron Cage of Visibility. *Ten 8*, no. 29: 38-51.

Foster, H. 1996. Obscene, Abject, Trauma. *October*. Vol. 78: 106-124.

Foucault, M. 1973. *Birth of the Clinic*. New York: Pantheon.

Foucault, M. 1991. *Discipline and Punish: The Birth of the Prison*. London: Penguin.

Frith, W. 1994. Jo Spence: Narratives of Dis-Ease. *Versus*, January/April.

Garner, A. 2012. *Alex Garner*. outaboutHIV.org [Online, 28 June]. Available at http://www.outabouthiv.org/2012/06/28/alex/ [accessed: 30 November 2012].

Gilman, S. 1995. *Health and Illness*. London: Reaktion.

Green, D. 1985. On Foucault: Disciplinary Power and Photography. *Camerawork*, no. 32: 6-9.

Lacan, J. 1994. *The Four Fundamental Concepts of Psycho-Analysis*. London: Penguin.

Leder, D. 1990. *The Absent Body*. Chicago: University of Chicago Press.

Lippit, A.M. 1994. The X-Ray Files: Alien-ated Bodies in Contemporary Art. *Afterimage*, December, 6-7.

Marshall, S. 1990. Picturing Deviancy, in *Ecstatic Antibodies: Resisting the AIDS Mythology*, edited by T. Boffin and S. Gupta. London: Rivers Oram Press, 19-36.

McGrath, R. 1990. Dangerous Liaisons: Health, Disease and Representation, in *Ecstatic Antibodies: Resisting the AIDS Mythology*, edited by T. Boffin and S. Gupta. London: Rivers Oram Press, 142-155.

McGrath, R. 1995. Geographies of the Body and the Histories of Photography. *Camera Austria International*, 51-52.

Mills, S. 2003. *Michel Foucault*. London and New York: Routledge.

Overboe, J. 1999. Difference in Itself: Validating Disabled People's Lived Experience. *Body and Society*, Vol. 5 (4): 17-29.

Santos, N. 2012. *Where Anxieties (and Misconceptions) Roam*. [Online: Visual AIDS, 7 September]. Available at http://visualaids.blogspot.co.uk/2012/09/where-anxieties-and-misconceptions-roam.html [accessed: 10 September 2012].

Sawdon Smith, R. 2004. Exiles of Normality: Photography and the Representations of Diseased Bodies, in *Cultures of Exile: Images of Displacement*, edited by W. Everett and P. Wagstaff. New York and Oxford: Berghahn: 153-174.

Sekula, A. 1986. The Body and the Archive. *October*, Vol. 39: 3-64.

Shildrick, M. 1996. Posthumanism and the Monstrous Body. *Body and Society*. Vol. 2 (1): 1-15.

Smith, R. 2012. Where Anxieties Roam 'Toxic Beauty: The Art of Frank Moore' at N.Y.U. *The New York Times*. [Online, 6 September]. Available at http://www.nytimes.com/2012/09/07/arts/design/toxic-beauty-the-art-of-frank-moore-at-nyu.html?_r=2&adxnnl=1&adxnnlx=1353351683-hjsUwsiBuGUvNihCYYwHRQ [accessed: 10 September 2012].

Spence, J. 1986. *Putting Myself in the Picture: a Political, Personal and Photographic Autobiography*. London: Camden Press.

Spence, J. 1990. No I can't do that, my Consultant wouldn't like it. *Silent Health: Women, Health and Representation*. London: Camerawork.

Struken, M. 1997. *Tangled Memories: The Vietnam War, the AIDS Epidemic, and the Politics of Remembering*. London and Los Angeles: University of California Press.

Tagg, J. 1984. *The Burden of Representation*. London and Basingstoke: Macmillan.

Valentine, S. 2012. HIV + One Year in!. *QX magazine*, no. 911, 23 August, 10-11.

Watney, S. 2000. *Imaging Hope: AIDS and Gay Identity*. London: Routledge.
Williams, S. 1998. Bodily Dys-Order: Desire, Excess and the Transgression of Corporeal Boundaries. *Body and Society.* Vol. 4 (2): 59-82.
Wojnarowicz, D. 1992. *Close to the Knives: A Memoir of Disintegration*. London: Serpent's Tail.

Chapter 6
Who Dies? Transformations in Derek Jarman's Last Films

Paul Attinello

It may be idiosyncratic that certain topics in my research on the artistic culture that grew up around AIDS in the 1980s and 1990s involve responses to questions or problems that confused or exasperated my younger self. Thus, my research on rage and paranoia in music about AIDS reflects an ongoing argument over appropriate emotional reactions in a Los Angeles HIV-positive writers' workshop during the late 1980s; my general decision to research a wide range of artistic responses (rather than only the politically assertive ones) reflects my disappointment with ACT-UP's ideological limitations in the early 1990s. Looking at Derek Jarman's last films brings back a memory of standing in a San Francisco bookstore in 1992, looking at stacks of his then new manifesto *At Your Own Risk: A Saint's Testament* (Jarman 1992); I remember being furious at the vanity, the sheer hubris, that I read into this title. As though there were not masses of people less famous, less creatively successful, even poorer than Jarman, who were also sick, in pain, dying... but of course I can now easily understand such resentment, and how it was fueled by my own vanity, fear and despair.

But dealing with Jarman's films and writings is, in any case, not always easy. Often seemingly headstrong and quarrelsome, his diaries and personal writings reflect an admirable empathy as much as they do egotism and an anger generated out of what sometimes seem deliberate misreadings of the intentions of others (especially other artists, and especially those who might be seen as his competitors). Over time, as I have watched his films and read books by and about him, I have started to see a Jarman I might not have been able to understand back in 1992: one who was certainly furious about his own illness and treatment, yet one whose empathy – for the suffering not only of a large circle of friends and acquaintances, but also of a much wider world of people who were dying – could be, in its own way, immense.

***

Jarman's last films – *The Garden* in 1990, *Edward II* in 1991 and *Blue* in 1993 – combine musical and narrative gestures to negotiate a complex and varied territory full of history, memory, fantasy and insight. Their maps outline personal and artistic constructions of empathy, as opposed to more direct identification; violence and death, as opposed to love and rescue; and a politicized resistance fueled by rage, as opposed to a larger acceptance of the existential inevitabilities of death. This territory is not, however, as open-ended as it may seem – although the various stories and scenes appear to be scattered across a broad range of cultural references, they ultimately focus on Jarman's increasingly intense experience of the AIDS crisis and its concomitant grief, illness and confrontation with death. If *The Garden* foreshadows death and *Blue* accepts it, the crucial exposure of an intricate knot of fantasy and reality happens in *Edward II* when, at the end of that film, musical and rhetorical sleight of hand transforms the king and his murderer[1] into Jarman and his lover/rescuer. This transformation, which was altered in mid-shoot from the original script, appears to be a response to Jarman's increasingly severe health crises and his unwillingness – with that of his friends and collaborators – to give up hope.

The then young Simon Fisher Turner's musical scores for these films – collages created with the director's encouragement – emphasize a wide range of experimental styles and ideas, all related to various trends of the 1980s; these experiments parallel Jarman's approach, as he uses quasi-musical processes to construct his avant-garde narratives. Aural elements also help to construct Jarman's insistent fusion of social and physical violence with AIDS, and ultimately, after the climactic turn of *Edward II*, everything is transformed into a purified sound world of meditative gongs for the image-less, death-driven *Blue*.

***

It is worth briefly articulating the timeline of Jarman's life and work as it connects with the history of AIDS, as they are increasingly entwined toward the end of his life. Jarman was born in 1942 and started studies at the prestigious Slade art school in 1963; in the 1970s he began to make short films while working in other media, as well as designing sets for such films as Ken Russell's The Devils (1971). His first feature film was Sebastiane (1976), with its entangled nexus of naked beauty, gay eroticism, violence and death, followed by Jubilee (1978) and The Tempest (1979). At this point his techniques and artistic intentions were rapidly changing, and he would constantly cross-connect various aesthetic and political ideals with sharp attacks on homophobia and oppression. In 1981, references to the conditions that would be identified as AIDS first appeared in the gay press. Art works in various genres started focusing on AIDS in late 1982 and 1983; in 1985, Jarman's film The Angelic Conversation included his first public reference to AIDS. The expanding AIDS crisis created an increasingly vast artistic response between 1984 and 1989, and Jarman was increasingly involved in a great deal of political activism during this time. In 1986, he acquired what was to become Prospect Cottage in Dungeness, and began to plant its famous garden – a garden which appeared in several of the last films, and which represented another means

---

1   Jarman derives his characters from the play by Christopher Marlowe, as well as from history and legend.

of being creative, as well as a quiet retreat from the frustrations of film funding and collaboration.

Jarman himself was diagnosed with AIDS in 1988, during the filming of *The Last of England* (also released in 1988); from this point until his death, most of his work referred to AIDS in some way. *War Requiem* (1989), a commission to film Benjamin Britten's famous cantata, suggested connections between soldiers and gay men, as well as between the deaths caused by two world wars and those caused by AIDS. *The Garden* (1990) referred more specifically to AIDS as one of its central subjects; its dreamlike nature emphasizes symbolic and the emotional arenas, where AIDS has so much more impact than the merely medical or political. In 1991, as Jarman became increasingly ill and began to have problems with his eyesight, he created the performance piece *Symphonie Monotone*, a source of the material that eventually became *Blue* and *Chroma*; he completed his most famous and approachable film, *Edward II*, in the same year. The abovementioned polemic *At Your Own Risk: A Saint's Testament* appeared in 1992; in 1993 he created *Wittgenstein*, the most important of his late films that does not refer to AIDS. Later that year, he released his final film, *Blue*, and in June he wrote the related book *Chroma*; these were his last completed major works, and he died in February of 1994.

***

Jarman is, of course, as crucial to avant-garde film about AIDS as Diamanda Galás is to avant-garde music on the same theme. His work is, however, a complex matter, if for no other reason than because Jarman often treated AIDS as merely one (admittedly central) pillar of an extended structure of homophobia, violence, oppression and Thatcherite conservatism – not necessarily because all of these things are logically or historically linked, but because he saw them as elements in a network of emotional and experiential connections. *Sebastiane* (1976) – his first film – already positions the gay man as a tragically abused martyr, and the fluid, even chaotic, complex of topics and referents in films, starting with *The Angelic Conversation* (1985), suggests a world struck by AIDS (among other things). But it is more sensible to discuss AIDS as a significant background, and occasionally foregrounded, aspect of *The Garden* (1990) and *Edward II* (1991). More directly and importantly, AIDS is certainly at the center of his final film *Blue* (1993). These films are also notable for their many significant musical scenes and gestures, not to mention the nearly musical pacing and continuity of all the later films.

Before he made these final three films, a transitional commission suggested later developments. *War Requiem* (1989), a filmed meditation on Benjamin Britten's cantata of the same name, was made soon after Jarman first learned that he was HIV-positive. It seems evident that it is emotionally linked to his feelings about AIDS – through images of dying and intimately affectionate men, of grief and of mourning, and of politicized brutality – although the published shooting script/diary (Jarman 1989) never mentions the word. The final words of the epilogue Jarman appended to the script do, however, suggest its impending resonance:

the *War Requiem* I heard in 1963 seemed shockingly arbitrary. I hope that my film has a similar feeling of discomfort. Perfectly crafted films exclude the chance encounter that stops you in your tracks. I like rough edges…. Like a stone cast in a silent pond. This mirrors the thrill I experienced as a child casting a stone into still water […] I throw this film into the water, lest we forget. (1989, 47)

The Garden (1990) was undoubtedly a relief for Jarman; in some ways a revisioning of the Passion in terms of gay love, violence and AIDS, it was free of the strictures of an existing artistic work, or of anxious and opinionated backers. As Michael O'Pray (1996) points out, it is a psychodrama, a personal journey through the unconscious that uses a variety of found and invented materials as elements in a narrative collage. The brilliant score by Turner is similarly a collage; its directed changes in mood help to keep the otherwise nonlinear material in line. Turner, who has maintained a notable career as a genre-crossing composer and recording artist under several names (including SFT and The King of Luxembourg), was evidently given significant encouragement and room to experiment in all of his work with Jarman; his investment in contemporary styles such as minimalism, punk and electronica is manifested throughout.

Most of *The Garden* is wordless, although a few notable voice-overs foreshadow the poetic meditations on death that make up much of *Blue*. As a result, music is often emphatically central; in fact, one experiences much of the film as driven, paced and organized by a fluid dreamscape of music. Just as the musical styles sometimes suggest the minimalistic melanges of Michael Nyman or Mike Oldfield, so the film technique at times resembles *Koyaanisqatsi* (1982) and the other Reggio films created with Philip Glass. There is also a wide range of musical pastiche and quotations, from melancholy neo-Baroque suspension-filled strings to a lip-sync satire of Audrey Hepburn's *Think Pink*. Most of the instrumental music, performed by the innovative Balanescu Quartet, is mixed with (or imitates) electronics; in fact, the many intrusions of mechanical noises, slow glissandi and gradually changing textures suggest influences from a wide range of electronic processes.

From the beginning, *The Garden* seems to be Jarman's dream in his cottage, looking at a cross as well as out through the window at his Dungeness garden (Jarman 1995). The title refers both to Eden and to that famous garden, which he constructed in the last years of his life. A strange combination of plants and objects, art and nature in a peculiar synthesis, it is also featured in the *War Requiem*. During the time he was creating *The Garden*, Jarman was influenced by James Hillman, the Jungian analyst who created a transcendentally intense 'archetypal' psychology. Jarman states, "I can sit for half an hour with a book – novels die in my hands. I'm left with poetry. History, biography, or a new James Hillman will keep me concentrating" (1991, 78).[2] This journal entry from May 14 1989 may refer to Hillman's *A Blue Fire* (1989), published that same year (though

---

2   Despite its subtitle, this book includes journals only for 1989 and part of 1990.

it is not clear whether Jarman means "new" as in newly published, or as in newly acquired by him). If he does mean *A Blue Fire*, connections to the film are easy to see – chapter headings include 'Many Gods, Many Persons', 'Imaginal Practice: Greeting the Angel', 'Mythology as Family', and 'The Divine Face of Things'. An entry a month later indicates that he is treating the psychological importance of these images with equal seriousness when he states, "I only go the cinema now out of friendship or nostalgia. I cannot watch anything that is not based on its author's life. Acting, camerawork, all the paraphernalia, bring me little pleasure without the element of autobiography" (1991a, 102-3).

Very much a nocturne, *The Garden* is dreamlike, poetic, reflective and beautifully filmed; episodes such as the musical glasses played by a row of elderly women emphasize the formal, ritualistic nature of the whole. At the same time, there are abrupt cuts and violent scenes – this is also a movie about homophobia, madness and violence. For Jarman, however, AIDS is really an instance of violent homophobia. He saw it chiefly as an attack on him and on all gay men, focusing more on the surrounding social and political responses than on the disease and its processes, as did many others at the time.

It would be improbably complicated to describe the scenes of the film, and many of its musical turns are more focused on underlining the drama of the Passion or emphasizing gay or homophobic cultural/political positions than they are on anything related to AIDS. However, several musical references are worth mentioning. The most violent scene – set in an Italian police canteen, where the insults of the Passion are recreated through an ugly realism without music – decamps into a complex, schizoid solo for electric guitar, alternatively enraged and meditative. A borrowed recording of Russian choral music appears behind the apocalyptic climax, reconnecting it to the film's religious archetypes and their black-and-white resonances. The gentle final elegy, after the speech beginning "I walk in this garden, holding the hands of dead friends / Old age came quickly for my frosted generation / Cold, cold, cold, they died so silently", evolves into a music/film relationship similar to that of the Glass/Reggio trilogy that began with *Koyaanisqatsi*. This 1980s abstract musical style mourns and comforts after the tragedies of homophobia and violence, and prefigures the emotional structures and gestures of Jarman's last films. In an interview Jarman associated it with his own preparations for death – "I felt elegiac making it, I built the garden and then sat there wondering whether I would be there next year to enjoy it" (1992, 107) – and O'Pray believes that Jarman identifies himself as Christ (O'Pray 1996, 102-3).

All of the drama of this film is connected to gay men as tragic dying 'Christ' figures, as in *Sebastiane*. However, because Jarman was thinking specifically about AIDS while making *The Garden*, the tortured and dying men are implicitly dying not only of violence, but also of the virus. Because Jarman, in common with many activists in the 1980s and early 1990s, regarded deaths by AIDS as products of the implicit violence of government inaction, and also because the figure of Christ is more of a tragic symbol than a reality, we are expected to reflect on both of these ways that gay men can be killed. The Passion-oriented death scenes, grouped on the commercial DVD under the subtitle 'Tears for the Dead', are therefore generalized by the final spoken elegy to apply to all gay men.

***

Although *Edward II* (1991) also contains sequences of surreal transformations, it is altogether sharper-edged than *The Garden*. Nearly every scene involves concrete references to the modern world outside the film as well as to Marlowe's play, and to a kaleidoscope of attendant historical events and legends. Turner's score is similarly more focused and restrained; although there is a range of Medieval and Renaissance pastiches, plus patches of orchestral baroque and even cheesy jazz organ, most of the score is constructed in 'set pieces' built on traditional musical forms that have clear beginnings and endings. The early scenes emphasize the darkly energetic physical eroticism of Edward and Gaveston: at the beginning of the film, two young men fuck on a bed in the background as Gaveston drinks coffee and speculates about returning to court. Later, as Edward and Gaveston kiss and play with each other on the throne, two intense male dancers from the radical London troupe DV8 enter and perform an athletically aggressive *pas de deux* that suggests fighting as much as passion, finally kissing one another in an echo of the principals.

The published screenplay includes notes and reflections by Jarman, Tilda Swinton and Associate Director Ken Butler that frequently mention the Director's increasing fragility and debilitating illnesses during filming, however the film itself includes no direct references to AIDS. Nevertheless, there are a number of oblique references, especially Annie Lennox's cover of 'Every Time We Say Good-Bye', the same Cole Porter song she performed for the AIDS benefit CD and video collection *Red Hot + Blue* (1990). Jarman had already directed that first video (Jarman 1991a, 62); the use of his own home movies from childhood, though in line with retrospective techniques in many of his films, seems to have a particular meaning in that music video, as it suggests that Lennox is mourning an already dead or dying Jarman. Of course, when the cover reappears in the film, it is only 'about' Edward's painful obligation yet again to exile his beloved Gaveston. The accompaniment swells from a piano to add an accordion, becomes romantically passionate, and they dance and kiss. However, the musical connection implies the underlying identity of king and director, which will be borne out in the film's final scenes. Even more significant are dramatic encounters with members of OutRage, a London-based gay activist organization, who, with a few of the Sisters of Perpetual Indulgence, represent Edward's supporters in a climactic riot. The passionate rage of the demonstrators is counterpointed by the brutal anonymity of the helmeted police, who pound nightsticks on their shields in an intimidating display of fascist violence; both are counterpointed with a speech by a malevolently smarmy Queen Isabella (Tilda Swinton), wherein she dismisses the protesters using the measured and disdainful intonations of Margaret Thatcher. OutRage returns at the end of the film for a scene that recreates the mourning tableau typical at the end of an

Elizabethan tragedy, when minor characters universalize the audience's responses to the deaths of major ones. These scenes are among the most emotionally intense in the film – though they are played by non-speaking extras – partly because of the noise, the silence and the music, and also because of the real and personal commitment embodied by these demonstrators who represent, and also actually are, beings immersed in a political war over both expressive freedom and personal survival.

The film's ending brings up a great deal of powerful resonance that is focused in several directions. A happy ending, based on the legend that Edward escaped to become a hermit in Europe, is contrary to Marlowe's original play (and to Bertolt Brecht's rewritten version (1994)) as well as to the screenplay, as it existed before the final scenes were filmed. Jarman and his collaborators agreed, during the last days of filming, that having the prince mourn his father and imprison the traitors did not work for them anymore. Thus, the legendary violent death by poker – probably the most horrific such scene to appear on stage before the Jacobeans – is mitigated to become merely Edward's nightmare (or perhaps a vision?); in any case, something imagined that does not 'really' happen in the context of the story. And Lightborn, the famous jailer and murderer of the originals, becomes a secret agent of freedom, too deeply in love with his king to kill him. Played by Kevin Collins, Jarman's partner from 1987 until his death, the film's Lightborn is transmuted from a malign killer into a warmly masculine, working-class lover – one who not only refuses to murder the king, but who flings the horrific and symbolic poker into a pool of water, extinguishing its threat. The Freudian poker vanishes and love conquers – a love that may involve real sexual organs, but not red-hot evisceration. Some of these final scenes were reconceived and directed at a time when Jarman was especially ill; he did not even come to the studio on the day the poker scene was shot. Is it necessary to point out that the original dramatic death may have seemed less and less attractive to an increasingly sick man, as well as to his many friends on the set (which perhaps explains this happy ending, if it needs explaining).

The brief but intense epilogue, which moves the film solidly into a contemporary reality as well as establishing a firm emotional connection between everyone involved (including the film's spectators), was thus vastly changed from the original script, which simply focused on the prince as the new king.[3] Edward's final speech is drawn from three separate couplets out of Marlowe's Act V, Scene 1; such a blenderized Marlowe results in a meaning remarkably different from that of the original play. Marlowe is, of course, always thornier and angrier, more

---

3   The published script (Jarman 1991b) explains all these changes, but shows somewhat more confusion; although the alterations are noted and explained, there are several versions of the ending (but all with the same 'blenderized' lines from Marlowe). The scenes marked Sequence 73 and 75 are not in their filmed order, and the final Sequence 82 was staged differently, as noticed in pages 150, 154, 168; only the completed film seems to be entirely clear in its intentions.

nearly-Jacobean in some ways than the more familiar Shakespearean model. The original sources are all from Marlowe's Act V, Scene I (this first passage consists of lines 23–31). The entire scene is emotionally chaotic: Edward, having lost Gaveston, faces losing the war, his crown and his life, and he rants and rages in lines that are petty, accusing and increasingly incoherent:

> *Edward:* …But when I call to mind I am a king,
> Methinks I should revenge me of the wrongs
> That Mortimer and Isabel have done.
> **But what are kings, when regiment is gone,**
> **But perfect shadows in a sunshine day?**[4]
> My nobles rule; I bear the name of king;
> I wear the crown; but am controll'd by them,
> By Mortimer, and my unconstant queen,
> Who spots my nuptial bed with infamy…

A vindictive and chaotic tantrum, where the boldface lines convey a poisonous despair. But Jarman will reuse them in an unexpected way. The next excerpt, lines 106-113, progresses further into the king's disintegration:

> *Edward:* …Yet stay, for rather than I'll look on them,
> Hear, hear! *[gives crown to the Bishop]* Now, sweet God of heaven,
> Make me despise this transitory pomp,
> And sit for aye enthronised in heaven!
> **Come, death, & with thy fingers close my eyes,**
> **Or, if I live, let me forget myself!**
> *Bishop:* My lord –
> *Edward:* Call me not lord. Away, out of my sight!
> Ah, pardon me. Grief makes me lunatic…

Even the furiously sarcastic Edward recognizes that raw terror is causing him to lose his balance. At the end of the scene, in lines 149-54, despair wins out:

> *Edward:* Mine enemies hath pitied my estate,
> And that's the cause that I am now remov'd.
> *Berkeley:* And thinks your Grace that Berkeley will be cruel?
> *Edward:* **I know not; but of this I am assur'd,**
> **That death ends all, and I can die but once.**
> Leicester, farewell.
> *Leicester:* Not yet, my lord; I'll bear you on your way.
> *[Exeunt; change scene]*

---

4   Emphasis added.

Jarman's reconstruction uses the three original (boldface) couplets exactly as written, but removing their original contexts completely changes the meaning. They join to form, in rapid, passionate sequence, a vision of evanescence; a dismissal of death and an invitation to it, all in the context of a virtually Buddhist transcendence of life and emotion (Marlowe 1969, 508-12). The final words, spoken by Edward over gently shimmering electronics and boys' voices, are thus reconnected and transformed into a statement by Jarman himself, in his persona as a dying man:

	Line no.
"But what are Kings, when regiment is gone,	28
But perfect shadows in a sunshine day?	29
I know not, but of this I am assured,	152
That death ends all, and I can die but once.	153
Come Death, and with thy fingers close my eyes.	110
Or, if I live, let me forget myself."	111

During these words, instead of Marlowe's final scene (where Edward's son establishes his authority after his father's death), we see a group of activists, quiet and stationary; white t-shirts made to glow with reflected light, accompanied by a shimmering memorial music. This music remakes them into angels of mourning: mourning their fallen activist comrades; mourning their friends lost to AIDS; mourning Edward; even mourning – in anticipation – Jarman himself. The placement of a harp glissando and swelling boys' voices in the middle of the next-to-last line emphasizes the invocational "Come Death", ultimately allowing it to represent Jarman's own passionate move from fear to acceptance.

***

There could hardly be a more sound-oriented film than *Blue*; it is, in fact, made almost entirely of sound, the visual element reduced to a blue screen, one not even intended to reflect the material reality of film (as are some abstract films). When, after several showings, the original blue film loop started to show scratches (contrast, for instance, the materially filmic quality of the famous opening sequence of Ingmar Bergman's *Persona*), Jarman had it replaced with a blue gel that would show no marks. As Jarman's last major film, it is imbued with the problems of his final illness, and this blue blankness is an obvious reference to Jarman's cytomegalovirus-based blindness, as well as to his metaphorical expectations of death. But it also fuses these with his increased fascination with simple colors, as in *Wittgenstein* (the commissioned film from 1993, just before this one) and *Chroma* (a published journal (1994)), as well as his response to a documentary about Yves Klein. *Blue* is based on *Symphonie Monotone*, a performance work created and performed by Jarman and Tilda Swinton for an AIDS benefit screening of *The Garden* in January 1991.[5] The film is seventy-five minutes long and although it can be purchased on video media, for obvious reasons there has been much wider distribution of the audio CD, which is slightly shorter.

Blue is a fascinating work, though it is less a film than a piece of autobiographical performance art – perhaps more like the monologues of Karen Finley, Tim Miller and other 1980s performance artists than anything else.[6] Ranging over the war in Bosnia; medical clinics in London; sexuality and remembered bedrooms; coffee houses; funerals of friends; intense or parodic political manifestoes establishing political and existential stances, and personal meditations on daily life and impending death, the general tone is introverted, closer to that of Jarman's journals than his other films. There are moments when the music and monologue become more spectacular or more symbolic, but they are for the most part fleeting, transitory, hallucinatory. The opening gongs, for instance, refer to Jarman's increased interest in Buddhism in his last years, and thus suggest his sharpened awareness of problems of existence and eternity. Although Jarman's voice represents a central identity throughout the film, Tilda Swinton's voice appears as an alter ego (as it may have been in the original performance work). Other voices are generally only briefly heard, and they come from 'outside', representing (as

---

5   I am dubious about O'Pray's (1996, 201) identification of the text as mostly made of quotations; there are even fewer quotations in the later version. Perhaps O'Pray is thinking of the many 'conventional' phrases that are used as a sort of takeoff ramp to start the piece, as they are in most of the sections of *Chroma*.

6   Because *Blue* is more sound art than film, it is useful to consider Richard Foreman's surreal polemic *Film is Evil, Radio is Good* (Foreman 1987), wherein a chorus of young radio station employees (led by a protagonist who is disconcertingly named Paul Antonelli) announces: "When something goes through the ear, it goes straight to the heart. But when it goes through the eye, it's the brain that gets it, and that's the bad news [...] [W]hat you see, i.e. film, you tend to believe. Bad, bad, bad. But what goes in through the ear, you supplement with your own creative imagining [...] [W]hat hypnotizes the eye and so blinds you to possibilities of self-recognition is what we self-confidently proclaim as evil. Film is, therefore, essentially evil [...] [F]ilmmakers often go out into the world pretending to themselves that the world they are capturing on film becomes, thereby, their own personal property. Certainly not true [...] We might point out [...] that what [a listener] refers to could be thought of as an almost sexual exploitation of the material world by the invariably ego-obsessed maker[s] of practically all contemporary films." Although Foreman's arguments are overstated, partly for comic and partly for analytical purposes, Foreman admits in the play's introduction (Foreman 1987, 147-54) that he does think film can be a dangerous medium. Given Jarman's career-long focus on existential deconstructions of the more problematic aspects of film, it is perhaps not overreaching to suggest that this, his final major work, is yet another attempt to break away from the false consciousness usually represented by film.

do several sections of the musical score) an external, largely invisible world to which Jarman reacts. 'Blue' is also a character, a boy. He becomes an erotic lover, an idealized memory or vision, and also a figure who can represent Jarman to himself, but he inevitably dies at the end, with Jarman himself saying, "I place a delphinium, Blue, upon your grave."

There are beautifully calm or sad passages, angry passages, and several unexpectedly and violently funny outbursts:

> I am a mannish
> Muff diving
> Size queen
> With bad attitude
> An arse licking
> Psychofag
> Molesting the flies of privacy
> Balling lesbian boys
> A perverted heterodemon
> Crossing purpose with death. (Jarman 1994, 118-19)

For the film, the first three lines of the poem are barked in the butchest of masculine voices, but then three women's voices take over in Andrews Sisters chords to complete the stanza, falling in pitch and energy until its last fatal word. Throughout the film, the continuity of both text and soundscape is more emotional than it is narrative or logical, but the whole hangs together through its dreamlike quality, gelling with a sense that the newly blinded Jarman is exploring his inner world, with only occasional references to outside stimuli. In fact, the focus is ultimately on blindness. There is a sense that this blindness is equivalent to the death for which it is forewarning; that, for Jarman, the loss of sight is his first experience of the end, an entrance into a limbo where he starts to accept a death that seems to have already occurred.

The text is actually all from a single chapter of the book *Chroma* – admittedly one of the longer chapters, there titled 'Into the Blue' – but the drifting stream-of-consciousness of thoughts, experiences, memories, quotes and styles is similar to that explored in other chapters, which also speak, as do most writings on AIDS, of death (for instance in 'White Lies', the first chapter) and its link to sex. A journal entry explains the Cagean origins of this structure and gives earlier titles for the project: "*Blueprint* becomes *Bliss* – dedicated to St. Rita of Cascia, patron of lost causes. Into the blue. Wandered through the bookshops and bought *The Book of Changes* to construct the script" (Jarman 1991a, 87). One can imagine that there might have been a series of color films by Jarman if he had had more time. In the published book, the copyright page says that the chapter 'Into the Blue' is "taken from" the film. This suggests that the performance piece came first; the film was then based on that, and finally, the book used 'Into the Blue' as the nucleus for an expansion of the ideas of the film, combined with material derived from Jarman's long-term habit of journal writing. The dating explains this: the performance piece took place in January 1991; the film was completed and premiered in March 1993 (Jarman 2000, 320, 322); the book's subtitle states that it was written in June 1993; Jarman died in February 1994, and the book's publication date is 1994. The published text has many sections that are not in the film and follows more coherent lines of development and associations of ideas, words, experiences. But however one compares sources, the order of this collage of texts was rearranged fairly freely for each version.

In the book, the end of the final chapter 'Translucence' is a poem that says farewell to a ghost named Mr Seethrough, who has changed his sex and become a woman; the lapidary diction of farewell and the suggestive Buddhism of the last line recalls the Japanese tradition of writing death poems as suggested by Hoffman (1986):

> As she disappears
> I toast my ghost
> In acqua vitae
> Luminous presence
> Here and gone. (Jarman 1994, 151).

That is the final farewell of the book, though it joins a series of farewell deaths that go back – perhaps to *Sebastiane* in 1976 – as well as forward to the farewell gongs of *Blue*:

> I fill this room with the echo of many voices
> Who passed time here
> Voices unlocked from the blue of the long dried paint
> The sun comes and floods this empty room
> I call it my room
> My room has welcomed many summers
> Embraced laughter and tears
> Can it fill itself with your laughter
> Each word a sunbeam
> Glancing in the light
> This is the song of My Room.
>
> [David
> Howard
> Graham
> David
> Paul
> Derek
> Graham
> Howard
> David]

Blue stretches, yawns and is awake.[7]

Perhaps my old irritation at Jarman for what I read as egotism was merely another example of me missing the point, of making incorrect assumptions. Throughout Jarman's work, relationships, journals, it seems clear that he did not make much of a distinction between himself and the many with whom he identified: gay men and lesbians, ancient Buddhists, Roman martyrs, saints, the young, the angry, the frustrated, and, of course, the dying. The rapid, complex shifts back and forth in points of view, identities, defenses and attacks suggest this, and perhaps I should have read what I once thought was vanity as a championing of others through himself, and of himself through others.

If the eye is a camera, perhaps a series of transformation shots could be filmed, following each other in a slow-motion series; a transformation of soldiers dying in World War I into gay men dying of AIDS; a transformation of Christ into a man attacked and humiliated by laughing policemen; transformations of Tilda into Mary, of Edward II into Jarman; of externalized rage about death, about blindness, about war, about violence, repression and inequality, into an internalized identification, even a kind of defiant acceptance. And finally, a transformation shot that turns Jarman, in his garden, into everyone who dies: into blue...

Filmography

The Angelic Conversation (dir. Derek Jarman, 1985).
Blue (dir. Derek Jarman, 1993).
The Devils (dir. Ken Russell, 1971).
Edward II (dir. Derek Jarman, 1991).
The Garden (dir. Derek Jarman, 1990).
Jubilee (dir. Derek Jarman, 1977).
The Last of England (dir. Derek Jarman, 1988).
Red Hot + Blue [video collection] (dir. Percy Adlon et al, 1990).
Sebastiane (dir. Derek Jarman, 1976).
The Tempest (dir. Derek Jarman, 1979).
War Requiem (dir. Derek Jarman, 1989).
Wittgenstein (dir. Derek Jarman, 1993).
'Qatsi Trilogy' (dir. Godfrey Reggio): *Koyaanisqatsi* (1982); *Powaqqatsi* (1988); *Naqoyqatsi* (2002).

---

7 Names in brackets are spoken on the soundtrack of *Blue*.

References

Brecht, B. 1994. *Edward II: A Chronicle Play*. New York: Grove Press.

Foreman, R. 1992. *Unbalancing Acts: Foundations for a Theater*. New York: Pantheon.

Hillman, J. 1989. *A Blue Fire: Selected Writings*. New York: Harper & Row.

Hoffman, Y., translator, 1986. *Japanese Death Poems written by Zen Monks and Haiku Poets on the Verge of Death*. Rutland, VTt: Tuttle.

Jarman, D. 1989. *War Requiem: The Film*. London: Faber & Faber.

Jarman, D. 1991a. *Modern Nature: The Journals of Derek Jarman*. London: Random House.

Jarman, D. 1991b. *Queer Edward II*. London: British Film Institute.

Jarman, D. 1992. *At Your Own Risk: A Saint's Testament*. London: Hutchinson.

Jarman, D. 1993. *Blue: A Film* [audio CD]. New York: Elektra.

Jarman, D. 1994. *Chroma: a Book of Colour – June '93*. London: Vintage.

Jarman, D. 1995. *Derek Jarman's Garden*. London: Thames & Hudson.

Jarman, D. 2000. *Smiling in Slow Motion*. London: Random House.

Marlowe, C. 1969. *The Complete Plays*. London: Penguin.

O'Pray, M. 1996. *Derek Jarman: Dreams of England*. London: British Film Institute.

Turner, S.F. 2013. *Simon Fisher Turner* [website]. http://www.simonfisherturner.com.

Chapter 7

Within the Limits of the Body: Artistic Images of HIV/AIDS in Spain and its Relation with the Cultural Industry

Rut Martín Hernández

The response by the world of art to the AIDS crisis in Spain is a clear reflection of a series of political, economic, social and cultural circumstances that define the country's context, which have markedly influenced the way in which artists, communities and groups have tackled this problem. Starting out with an analysis of the artistic images that have been generated in Spain, this chapter maps the issue through Spanish artists, works and exhibitions whose main topic is HIV/AIDS. From these it is possible to analyse the epidemic's complexity in the context of Spanish society; its mystifications; the sufferer's role, and the strategies and mechanisms needed to alleviate the negative effects of the disease, not only on the infected person's body but also on his/her social portrayal.

A study of visibility devices and the relationship between social manifestation and artistic manifestation reveals their scant impact on the cultural industry over a period of three decades during which HIV/AIDS art has not had an institutional impact consonant with the social impact of the epidemic. These works very seldom catch the eye of artistic institutions around the world – the ones that control their visibility – and therefore have lately become deeply engrossed in anything and everything to do with the changes that new technologies are incorporating into artistic languages. Works on HIV/AIDS, when they do not break away from the suitability criteria of museum collections and occupy public space, end up being reduced to peripheral exhibition circuits. On the clear occasions when they do make it directly onto the street, one can observe how media coverage of them is generally poor. It could be understood that artistic production about HIV/AIDS in Spain has been pretty poor, especially if one considers the influence it has had artistically in other countries such as the USA, UK and Canada, where the problems it has raised from a social, political and cultural point of view has had a clear impact on the contemporary art scene.

It was not until the number of sufferers had grown large enough that artists took to reflecting on the problem in their works. Writer Alberto Cardín was the first person on the Spanish cultural scene to acknowledge that he was HIV-positive in 1985, the same year that he wrote one of the landmark works on AIDS in Spain, entitled *AIDS: Biblical curse or deadly disease?* (1985), in which he tried to dismantle the symbolism associated with this disease. There followed other writings such as *AIDS: alternative approaches* (Cardín 1991), which analysed the patient's need to go from being a passive subject to being an active one, and a few more in which HIV/AIDS, although less explicitly, was always present. In *The close and the distant* (Cardín 1990) HIV/AIDS emerges as a fundamental factor in establishing new ways of relating to others.

The artistic images that broach this subject are metaphorical in origin, unlike in other countries where collective struggle and communicational strategies have dominated the portrayal of HIV/AIDS. Thus, individual experience is configured as a starting point for establishing a broader social context in which the echoes of intimate personal stories resonate, often told in the first person. Paul Julian Smith (1996) picks up on this trend that is trying to recreate itself in the physical marks of the disease, so as to incorporate acceptance of death, with the "fatal strategies" of Baudrillard (1983):

> while North Americans have responded to the epidemic above all with rage, the Spanish response has been one of love. I will suggest that this love is indeed compatible with the fatal strategy and manifests itself in the recurrent motifs of the remainder and the prosthesis: the former suggests a respect for the body and its products in their very abjection, even unto death; the latter suggests a supplement to the body, which permeates its once hermetic membranes, breaching the boundary between self and other. (1996: 104)

The exploration of the portrayal of the disease and the portrayal of the body in contemporary art are similarly configured as open lines by these types of image, closely connected with the subject.

One factor that has influenced how Spanish artists and authors have approached the HIV/AIDS crisis is the political situation that Spain found itself in at the outbreak of the epidemic. The recent transition to democracy fostered a climate of optimism centred on a positive attitude to the freedoms which had been won, one after another, and which represented a radical advance compared with past times. Society was not prepared for what HIV/AIDS would entail; a new conception of sexual practices and identitary issues that were seen as a step backwards, since they were reminiscent of the repressive discourses of earlier periods. The Spaniards' instinct was more to push the problem away and label it as someone else's than to question the moral stances of the discourses that relied upon these analogies. This caused considerable delay in 'owning' HIV/AIDS as a problem squarely within society, and therefore in taking effective measures. It is worth mentioning that, even today, Spanish society has still not begun to interiorise the HIV/AIDS crisis as its own problem.

Spain does not share the United States' tradition of grassroots social rights movements. Thus, Spanish artists have found it difficult to juggle aesthetics with the taking of a political stance, which is a specific feature of many U.S. creations and an issue that lends direct impact to works that set out to contradict the construction of the disease and to inform and educate people about preventing HIV. Alfonso Almagro explains that:

> although in our country artistic creation introduced a hitherto non-existent public debate and entailed a rethink of its own limits and ability to influence the social, we talked about life, love and death and in so doing we couldn't sacrifice the aesthetic, much less marry it up with the political, even knowing as we did that the aesthetic is also an ideological stance towards death; it's also a political stance. (2006: 70)

Conversely, most North American actions and undertakings were carried out by a strong homosexual community that united to form a platform from which to denounce the homophobia, sexism and racism that were behind the discourse on HIV/AIDS, and to demand political and healthcare measures that would serve to keep the epidemic in check and enhance sufferers' lives. The assertion of sexual identity has only happened in Spain since democracy, around the same time as the first AIDS cases. There had not been time to form strong action groups as they were still concentrating their efforts on ending sex discrimination, which had already been overcome in the United States at that time by those groups of homosexual activists who were grappling with the epidemic.

The lack of objective information about the virus and its association with particular social groups supported the firmly entrenched idea of 'high-risk groups', which still prevails in some societies and has entailed serious consequences. Until the number of sufferers had grown large enough, hardly any plastic works broached the problem directly. Much of the responsibility for this assumption – that the disease is something which only affects others – lies with the press and the media, which, from the time the epidemic broke out, focussed on particular matters that reinforced that assumption.

Key artistic images in the portrayal of HIV/AIDS in Spain

HIV/AIDS in Spain can be approached in diverse ways in relation to the arts. Pepe Espaliú heralded and set the scene for the other artists who later delved deeper into this problem using plastic language. Espaliú became the key figure in art about HIV/AIDS in Spain. He went public about being HIV-positive in 1992, at the same time as he presented *Carrying*, one of the first and most iconic Spanish artistic manifestations on the topic. His contributions to the HIV/AIDS discourse marked a before-and-after in the matter. His "*AIDS-created*" works, as he himself called them, were the turning point that helped configure the subsequent artistic treatment of the disease. The time that elapsed between his being diagnosed and dying was very short, but very fruitful in terms of manifestations and undertakings, and he used it to produce a legacy of high artistic and social value.[1] During that time, Espaliú became vocal about life through a sufferer's eyes, giving interviews, 'working' the media and publishing articles on the topic. Likewise, his works emphasised sufferers' isolation and the need for a change of attitude towards them, while also reflecting on the psychological, physical and social consequences of the disease through bare, metaphor-laden plastic language.

Other authors such as Pepe Miralles, Jesús Martínez Oliva and Javier Codesal have also constructed very personal discourses on the topic, which have run through all their works and offered people a highly committed view on the issue. Pepe Miralles may be regarded as the Spanish artist who has most consistently shared his thoughts on HIV/AIDS in his works, which are rounded off with a theoretical and curatorial labour on the subject. In a language very characteristic of an activist, he hits out directly and explicitly against imposed morality; questions the problems associated with HIV/AIDS and calls for carriers and sufferers to be more accepted, better informed and to have more opportunities to socialise. In Pepe Miralles' words, "thinking about the disease is a constant necessity, a job we cannot turn aside from. And one of the best ways to mitigate the other effects of the disease" (1996). For their part, Jesús Martínez Oliva and Javier Codesal handle the topic of HIV/AIDS as a consequence of the characteristics of their own productions, not as an end in itself, but they think actively about the construction of the visual language and how it is able to directly impact the social portrayal of the disease and the consequent inclusion of carriers and sufferers.

On the other hand, there are authors who have dealt with HIV in their works indirectly or just sporadically, approaching the topic from a perhaps more serene, more metaphorical viewpoint, personalising the feelings of loss, of not being understood, of fragility and social exclusion, and at variance with the aberrant images used by the media. These artists' relationships with the virus are linked to other considerations such as the body; identity; the gender struggle; sexuality; visibility and otherness. Although on these occasions HIV/AIDS is present in various ways, but not as a single traceable theme, these creations enable the complexity of HIV/AIDS to be seen from different viewpoints and they open up new ways of thinking, which, despite being only on the fringe of that complexity, help one understand the nuances associated with it. This is true of the work of Águeda Bañón, Alberto García-Alix, Alejandra Orejas, Alex Francés, Alicia Lamarca, Ana Navarrete, Ex – Cupidas Group, Eduardo Nave, Eduardo Sepúlveda Guillén, Enrique Lista, Evarit Navarro and Bia Santos, Fernando Bellver, Frederic Amat, Genín Andrada, Girlswholikeporno, Guillermo Paneque, Guillermo Valverde, Jana Jaleo, Javier Flores, Javier Pérez, Josu Sarasua, Mercedes Carbonell, Mili Sánchez, José María Baez, María José Belbel, Mur - ur Vindel, Paco de la Torre,

---

1   It was when he was diagnosed that Pepe Espaliú began to tackle the subject of HIV/ AIDS in his works.

Patricia Gómez, Pedro G. Romero, Pilar Albarracín, Rosalía Banet, Sonia Guisado and Zush, along with many other artists who have approached this topic with the clear intention of counteracting the images that have made AIDS into, as Susan Sontag (1988) pointed out, a metaphor-laden disease.

On the other hand, there are those groups which stand out, through collective authorship, that have used artistic-activist strategies in their struggle against AIDS. We must realise from the outset that these artists' works are not the standard works that have been done in general on the topic in Spain. Instead, they constitute an honourable exception that has made it possible to enjoy some effective and suggestive creations which express this problem's complexity. While activist art in Spain has not had the forcefulness and impact gained in the United States, it is nonetheless true that the nineties saw the emergence of a higher number of creations whose forcefulness was based on subversive strategies that focussed on gender issues.

It is within this context of demands that seek to do away with single, imposed identities that a good part of the struggle against Spanish HIV/AIDS takes place. Using strategies similar to those employed by identity-based activist movements, these groups likewise perform a job of an ideological character and have a marked political and social agenda that attempts to alleviate the marginalisation of carriers and sufferers, and to build interdisciplinary support networks. Strongly influenced by American activism, the space in which they carry out their actions is the public space, where they can interact more directly with society. Their language lends itself to a speedy, explicit reading, facilitating identification with the highest number of people possible, in contrast with the cryptic language characteristic of government institutions.

One of the main Spanish artistic/activist groups was *The Carrying Society*. It was strongly influenced by Pepe Espaliú, founder of the group, and was the outcome of a workshop he led at ArteLeku. Another influential figure in the various groups that he was a member of was Pepe Miralles. He was involved in specific projects such as the *1st December Project*, those carried out by the *Local Neutral* group, *Social AIDS Project/1* and *Social AIDS Project/2*. Similarly, campaigning by groups whose interests lay more broadly in the struggle for gender freedom should also be mentioned; in this case the groundwork done by *La Radical Gay* and *LSD,* which, in the struggle against HIV/AIDS, served as an engine for the Madrid activism of the nineties. Equally important was the work done for the struggle against HIV/AIDS by Spanish identity-based associations, groups and organisations, which, on many occasions, have incubated local-action anti-AIDS groups.

Points of cohesion. Specificities of HIV/AIDS art

In any case, and even though works about HIV/AIDS represent too low a percentage of the total number of national artistic manifestations, these artists try to make it clear that, as José Luís Brea clearly asserts:

> AIDS is none other than the terrible effect produced in citizens' lives by the
> inadequate defining of the culture of a time, of an age – our age. AIDS is
> actually the brutal damage that the out-and-out poverty of vision of the State-
> administered world does to us who inhabit it. It's "their" disease, as we, all of us,
> have to bear it. Yes, it's the disease of a social body that, now badly constituted,
> no longer serves us as a model for building our own, or even for keeping it in one
> piece, so as to be able to inhabit it – as organic. (www.accpar.org 1995)

Their conceptual ideas, on the majority of occasions, stem from an active social
commitment. Sometimes they are expressed in direct and explicit language and at
other times they take on an intimate appearance not without crudeness, making use
of the symbolic and the metaphorical, but always attempting to boost action and
persuade people that getting involved is the only way to truly portray the disease.
One of their common features is that they begin with questioning as an argument
of artistic creation and, from that point on, they explore new forms of portrayal:
can art enhance the ability to think? Would this ability to think change our modus
operandi in tackling AIDS? These are questions that Spanish artists seem to ask
themselves in their pieces. Juan de Nieves muses about these types of creations by
suggesting that:

> they begin with a private action and, through the artist's own decision, they
> are then transferred into the sphere of the public, since the categoricalness of
> what is happening (to us) pushes aside the barriers of delicacy. To speak words
> in response to facts is to do more than to say or state, since to the former –
> mechanical and verbal – has to be added the quality of being willing to get
> involved in what is said. [...] In general, the use of words as a denouncement,
> or as a wake-up call to stimulate thinking, is one of the ways that has least
> impregnated the Spanish art scene. Anyhow, whether through slothfulness or out
> of a lack of commitment, even fewer are the undertakings that use the word as a
> medium for questioning the social reality. (1994)

The interest that these works take in breaking the boundaries of the disease –
which hem in its sufferers – is one of the engines that questions the trend of the
inaptly named *welfare systems*. One which attempts to exclude any kind of anomaly
that detracts from the market laws which inundate all aspects of the public sphere.
Many of these artists work with the body as a reflection; the wounded, fragmented
body takes on all its symbolic overtones to become the icon par excellence from
which to structure the other elements; "every wounded identity needs a haven of
peace and light in which to see with its eyes closed, smell the acids of its galaxy
with its nose blocked and listen to its soft sounds even with its ears plugged"
(Buján 2001: 53).

Despite the conceptual and formal differences of the work produced in Spain
about HIV/AIDS there are a series of characteristics that have influenced its
evolution over these three decades. From the turn of the Twenty-first Century

onwards there no longer exists such a direct identification of AIDS with death; the urgency and subversion that prevailed in the nineties has given way to a discourse that once again connects the disease with the sphere of the private, moving it away from the public. In contrast with Alberto Mira's statement "pain is private, AIDS is a public problem; opinions of AIDS are generated in a public sphere, and it is here that they can be altered" (1993: 154); the urgency of Douglas Crimp's affirmation: "We don't need a cultural renaissance, we need cultural practices actively participating in the struggle against AIDS" (1987: 7), and Pepe Miralles' rhetorical question "are there artists who still think it's time to go to sleep?" (1994), it seems that Spanish artists have let themselves be dampened down by Spanish society's loss of interest, aided by and reflected in the fact that the media give the topic hardly any attention. It seems that talking about AIDS is not in vogue now. As Manuel Clot asserts

> The outbreak of the AIDS crisis was, for art, the militant reclaiming of the possibilities of the directly political in its practice and in its form, bridging the frontiers between artists, works and the public, causing overspill between the spheres of the social, the behavioural, the individual and the artistic, and filing down the thickly ridged joints between genders, styles and ways of being [...] In that context of upheaval and changes, the work of art begins to emerge as a powerful example of a discourse situated on the fringe of the hegemonic power domain. (1997: 78)

In the process of normalisation that the topic of AIDS is undergoing in developed countries in general and, by extension, in Spain, we come across a different discourse than the silence that prevailed in the first stage; the voices that are keeping up the struggle are not getting heard or given the social support they should be. The strategies for struggle used up to now, despite having a low impact on public opinion, go more unnoticed – if that were possible – and are not easily understood. It should not be forgotten that many of those people who were actively struggling against AIDS in Spain have died, and with them has disappeared a vital way of understanding art and the disease; an effective way of proposing vehicles of change that will give rise to different views, which will get people out of this 'lazy' way of understanding how existence operates in contemporary society.

Impact of artistic images about HIV/AIDS in the Spanish cultural industry: Dissemination and visibility devices

One thing worth noticing is that, for the most part, the number of artists who have dealt with the topic of HIV/AIDS have had to do it without the support of the artistic institutions. Critic David Pérez wonders "up to what point is it possible, from within the system itself, to create art that aims to place us *beyond* that very system?" (1997: 29). Museums and contemporary art centres have taken no interest in a topic that has significantly shaped contemporary artistic language by giving a new vision of the body and its fragility, and a revival of protest strategies and codes that impact the public, the political and the social. Espaliú put it this way:

> Even though AIDS is affecting world culture profoundly, there isn't a single cultural institution in this country that has done anything at all for it. How is it possible that these people who devote their energies and our money to mediocre exhibitions, to tacky productions, don't spend a single cent on anything to do with one of the most topical current themes in the art world? (1992: 56)

Along the same lines, it is odd that the more one tries to impact the social, the less institutional recognition one gets.

The functionality of the museum space had already been called into question in the seventies when economic pressures, along with a failure to tackle social problems and the emergence of artistic manifestations that took place beyond the museum (performances, happenings, actions, public undertakings and so on) set the scene for an unprecedented crisis in the international museum sphere. With the advent of AIDS, this crisis came to the forefront once again, since art institutions were unable to create representational policies suited to society's needs and, paraphrasing Theodor Adorno, they turned these centres into mausoleums in which the institutionalisation of the art experience entailed its separation from its context and from life.

There is a stark contrast between the proliferation of contemporary art centres that are seen throughout Spain, posing as venues for a new, more accessible vision of the artistic event, and their lack of interest in topics that are outside 'the currently recognised' and 'the normative'. All these infrastructures could allow themselves to have an impact on specific local problems or on questions that are not broached by the 'big temples' of art, and which would vest them with their own personality. However, these behaviours are mostly conspicuous by their absence. In the words of Crimp:

> what museums set out to do in the late sixties, to be important in the social sphere, was not carried out well, since the museum's purpose had been to offer itself as a venue for an art divorced from daily life. Now that there are cultural manifestations that are finally beginning to move away from the walls of the museum and to articulate a specific relationship between aesthetic production and social life, the museum will enter upon a new phase in its history. Its walls will be the symbol of the division between two kinds of contemporary art: one alive, and the other dead. (1989: 66)

While it is true that certain strategies would lose all their force and conviction by being confined within the walls of a museum, it is also true that works on HIV/AIDS do not all share the same features. Beyond the almost perennially present social aspect, they could be considered by the institution with a view to creating a discourse that would get them out of their marginal and peripheral position, and give them a voice and visibility by breaking the barriers of silence and concealment. Moreover, museums could encourage, promote and subsidise works carried out in the public space or other spaces that would make it possible to approach the art event from a less narrow perspective and thereby rise above mere contemplation as the spectator's only relationship with the work of art. Creations outside of the 'white cube' atmosphere favoured by museums of art would in turn become part of their programmes and would extend their reach. As such, they would be more in line with the post-modern condition that pays attention to the demands of involvement, expansion and context-dependence of current artistic manifestations, thereby favouring interdependence between the various fields of knowledge and the different artistic languages.

Trends in 'committed art' in Spain have not evolved in the same way as in other countries where, from the nineties onwards, they began to acquire something of a museum-suitable character. There, the interest of a certain sector of the art world in politico-social issues enabled the carrying out of a series of initiatives that made it possible to give a voice to those people who demanded the right to be different. Here, in reality, there are very few artists who have taken up the reins in this regard and boldly broken the parameters of institutional normativity to make politically different and committed pieces. Nonetheless, it must be emphasised that the few who have done so have made very valuable contributions. It should be borne in mind that "it is understood by now that all art is ideological and all art is used politically by the right or the left, with the conscious and unconscious assent of the artist" (Lippard, 2000: 479). The lack of commitment to, or interest in, the social reality of the time is also a political stance. The act of not including art about AIDS in cultural agendas is more than a deliberate oversight; it is a stance towards the world, towards artistic practices and the relationship between art and the spectator.

Among the exhibitions organised by institutions and art centres, various kinds of initiative can be discerned. The most common have been those that try to fundraise for AIDS research and sufferer support. These are normally exhibitions whose works do not focus directly on the HIV/AIDS problem, or provide explicit food for thought about the situation that the disease is bringing about; they tend to be more in the nature of donations by authors that help draw in the public (and their money), but do not engage them personally. They perform a useful function, but they also highlight what many artists and groups who are working on this topic are fighting against, that is, that the responsibility of fostering research and setting up support networks should be performed by public institutions and not by private initiatives. From the artistic point of view, they lack the intention to perform critical and iconographic analysis and are influenced by the lack of coherence that arises out of the fact that, conceptually, they are designed for a purpose that is not embodied in either the choice of a specific work or the specific topic for which they have been planned.

Meanwhile there are those initiatives that try to show the impact of AIDS; they concentrate on representational policies; they are designed to display a vision of works that arise out of the need to think about the more complex aspects of HIV, and they publicly raise questions that will encourage self-questioning by the spectator. These exhibitions – which are pretty scarce in Spain – try as a whole to create a discourse which, going beyond the artistic institution, conceptualising it and disseminating it amongst the public, serves as a starting point for making waves that will trigger an open debate about AIDS. As Alfonso Almagro rightly states:

> When a creation about the disease is being planned, it will never entail confronting the disease itself, but rather its muteness and invisibility at public and State level. The battle will be against the social construction that has been made out of the AIDS crisis and the way in which that crisis has been handled. Moreover, this will mean that art will not only take a stance on this problem, but will also aim to make an impact on the social (2006: 50).

It is these types of exhibition that are going to contribute somewhat to the discourse about HIV/AIDS, through works that handle the topic with the complexity it deserves and with a curatorial discourse that boosts this effect so as to succeed in bringing these fuller and more critical visions to Spanish society.

During the eighties there was no exhibition that, besides raising funds, deeply depicted what AIDS stood for in Spanish society and culture. This moment is characterised by the fact that media interest and social panic were at their peak. When international institutions were beginning to give it some of their attention with initiatives such as *Let the Record Show* in 1987 at the New Museum of Contemporary Art in New York, the *Art against AIDS* project in San Francisco in 1988, and Gran Fury's participation in the Venice Biennale in 1990, the Spanish art world stayed completely on the sidelines of this problem. The first initiatives to take the problem a bit more seriously did not emerge until the following decade, which also coincided with the period when the disease was having a greater impact; annual infection rates were still rising and a disconcerting situation of epidemic proportions was coming about.

High-profile exhibitions about HIV/AIDS in Spain

The first exhibitions held in Spain related to the issue of HIV/AIDS were *Members Only* in Barcelona in 1993, and the individual collection *AIDS Days* by Javier Codesal at Gallery XXI in Madrid in that same year. *Members Only* was conceived as a comment on contemporary sexuality, although some of the pieces exhibited dealt specifically with the topic of AIDS. Organised by Ruth Turner in collaboration with the Carles Poy Gallery, it included over 180 works by various artists. In parallel, they also produced a document to inform the public about HIV/

AIDS. The event was aimed at raising society's awareness on the topic of AIDS and also serving as a vehicle for information and prevention. That same year, the Trayecto Gallery in Vitoria hosted the *Virusemia* exhibition, which also intended to show the AIDS crisis from the viewpoint of artistic creation, and the collection *Sida: Entre l'art y la inforamció* (AIDS: Between art and information) that took place at the Sala Museu in Valencia.

Juan de Nieves' initiative for the University of Santiago the following year, 1994, was a serious and committed attempt to tackle the subject. Under the title *AIDS: decision and action*, which made its intention clear from the outset, this collection brought together works by Javier Codesal, The Carrying Society, Jesús Martínez Oliva, Pepe Espaliú and Alejandra Orejas. Organised by the Vice-Rectorate for Cultural Policy of the University of Santiago de Compostela and held in the University's Pazo de Fonseca (Fonseca Palace), four of the selected works were created especially for the event. In the words of Juan de Nieves:

> AIDS: a pandemic that is on everyone's lips. Liable to be judged and metaphorised. Stubbornly believing that "it couldn't happen to me", we refuse to investigate its complexities and we run away from the commitment that it calls for. To all questions of social disorder – AIDS creates a state of marked discrimination – we reply with pride through gestures of convenient solidarity, derived from a half-learned social behaviour (1994).

This exhibition was conceived from a viewpoint of social and active commitment which aimed to boost action and persuade people that getting involved is the only way to represent the disease accurately. All the works deployed a demanding and forceful tone in their messages which, explicit and critical of the official rhetoric, set out to transform apathy into taking an interest, and opinions into speaking out. In 1995, *50 artists against AIDS* was held in Seville, and *Art and AIDS* in the Esfera Azul Gallery in Valencia. The following year saw *Art against AIDS* at the Royal Exhibition Hall in Madrid. These exhibitions, despite setting out to create a specific vision, lacked the necessary force to be able to create a discourse of their own that would contribute something significant to the subject.

At around the same time, in 1996, another high-profile exhibition was inaugurated: *Thinking about AIDS*, curated by Pepe Miralles, considered by then as one of the most knowledgeable artists on the topic in Spain. This exhibition, held in A. Lambert's Art Space in Xàbia, involved artists such as Javier Codesal, Jesús Martinez Oliva and Visual Documentation Workshop, which had already dealt with this issue previously, along with another series of authors to whom it was suggested they explore the complexity of the disease from their position in the plastic arts territory. Neither Alex Francés, Helena Cabello, Ana Carceller nor Pilar Albarracín had dealt with this subject before, although their work is centred on issues such as gender identity, which are directly related to some of the overtones that the HIV problem brings out. As Isabel Tejada states, "the identification of the disease with certain biological differences or with certain sexual lifestyles means that these individuals are imagined to be the disease's hypothesis, its representation, the disease itself. While there is still one heterosexual person convinced that AIDS is not something he or she might get, this viral and social crisis will continue" (1996). Several notions such as getting a check-up; images for prevention; being committed; self-pleasuring, and vexations, crop up in works that investigate the complexity of being seropositive. From the body's viscera and fluids; showing the boundaries of the body; the inner workings, to making the spectator more aware of the many undercurrents running beneath the representation of the sufferer and the carrier; of the symbolic connotations that turn a physical disease into a social disease.

At the turn of the century there was a considerable fall in the number of such initiatives, largely because the media's interest had flagged by then. Even so, there were two exhibitions in particular that are of interest because they covered the changed mindset that led to the HAART therapies being included, and made it possible to observe those modifications in the thinking and behaviour of sufferers and society. Following its discovery, the disease evolved unevenly depending on the geographical, political and economic setting. There was a need to analyse that evolution too from the point of view of artistic manifestations. It made no sense to foster a discourse on AIDS in Spain that showed the lack of understanding of the eighties or the urgency of the nineties. At this new stage it became necessary to continue focussing on the symbolic representation of the disease, which unfortunately had changed very little, while dealing with it from another perspective. Since there was no such direct identification with death, the concepts of loss and grief were less present, and those concepts morphed into issues of the fragility of the body as it tried to cope with the side effects of the medications. The characteristics of the diseased body had changed; the lipodystrophy alluded to a different type of marked corporeality and this was reflected in the iconography associated with the disease.

In 2001, *Identidades feridas: da arte na doenza* (Wounded Identities: On Art in Infirmity) opened at the Laxeiro Foundation in Vigo. Curated by Xosé Manuel Buxán, it set out to comment on diseases in general and AIDS in particular. Organised to mark World AIDS Day (1st December) and with the collaboration of LEGAIS (Vigo Lesbian and Gay Group), this exhibition displayed the work of María Xosé Ares, María Jesús Fariña Busto, Dolores Gálvez, Lucía Gómez Fernández, Ernesto González Torterolo, Enrique Lista, Juan Carlos Meana Martínez, Alex Mene, Jorge Migota Dago, Mart Riv and Sara Sapetti. All of them young artists in training, who had not felt the urgency that the AIDS crisis aroused in the society of the eighties and nineties. As Javier Buján concedes, "most of the time, a disease is a closed world that doesn't exist outside the group of sufferers. [...] So disease is reduced to specialist circles" (2001: 48). What emerges is an attempt to offer a contemporary view of the topic and set down potential names of artists who are beginning to work on a crisis whose end is still not in sight. Curator Xosé M. Buxán was attempting what was done a decade earlier by Juan Vicente Aliaga and José Miguel García Cortés in their book *Of love and rage. About art and AIDS* (1993), and Juan de Nieves in *AIDS: decision and action* (1994), in which they advocated a series of artists whose works on the topic had already gone down in the plastic history of the virus in Spain.

The last of the high-profile exhibitions put on up to the present is *El arte láte(x) (Latex Art)*, curated by Judith Navarro García and Sofía Barrón Abad with with coordination by Norberto Piqueras[2] and organised by the University of Valencia's Vice-Rectorate of Culture in 2006. From April to June, the Thesaurus Hall in the La Nau building hosted one of the most important themed events held in Spain. Of particular interest was the curatorial discourse, in which pieces by Spanish and international artists were presented to create a global and multidisciplinary discourse on the HIV/AIDS problem. The selection of works was carefully chosen to include both pieces from earlier decades (Pepe Espaliú, Javier Codesal, Liliana Maresca and Alejandro Kuropatwa) and more current pieces (Antuan, Patricia Gómez, Fernando Bellver, Paco de la Torre, Alicia Lamarca, Eduardo Nave and Pepe Miralles) so as to give a vision of how the portrayal of HIV/AIDS, and the conceptual aims that have been at the forefront at each particular time, have evolved.

As part of this exhibition, two audio-visual pieces were presented; one in documentary format devoted to HIV/AIDS prevention, and the other a montage of scenes from motion pictures whose purpose was to introduce spectators to part of the most interesting North American, Latin American and European filmography produced on the topic of AIDS. The theme song of the montage was "She's called AIDS" by Spanish rapper Prodigal Son: "I've a disease that bleeds away my life; she was born, grows in me, breathes and feels alive, she's called AIDS, and doesn't act nice with anyone else 'cause she wants us to be together for the rest of our days". Without a doubt this was a key art exhibition on AIDS in Spain; fearless, committed and highly suggestive. With consummate skill it combined plastic creations with action, the deepest metaphorical thinking and the most direct and specific information. One of its most successful features was the global approach on which it was built and which offered the spectator a vision of the multiple facets and aspects associated with HIV/AIDS, handling its problem with all the complexity and importance that it definitely deserves.

Another high-profile initiative took place at the Faculty of Fine Arts in Valencia, under the title *SIDA ací i ara. No et Quedes als núvols* (AIDS here and now. Don't stay with your head in the clouds) in December 2006, curated by José Luis Cueto, Pepe Miralles and Ramón Espacio. Then in its third year, it was organised in collaboration with Calcsicova (the coordinating organization for associations engaged in the struggle against AIDS in the Valencian Community). Youthful creators and a lot of imagination helped ensure the success of its projects and works, which combined a ludic undertone with a commentary on the topic of HIV/AIDS. José Luis Cueto wrote, "with each year's call for submissions we offer the

---

2   The author thanks the coordinator and curators of the exhibition for making themselves available and helping her gather information and documents on the topic.

opportunity to make a commitment to aesthetics and ethics matters and to subject them to critical thinking about the world, about the meaning of our work as artistic producers. Responses have to include a real involvement with social relations and the responsibilities that these bring with them" (2006: 6). The exhibition's most remarkable feature is its ability to keep going year after year, which goes to show how involved the lecturers at the Faculty of Fine Arts of Valencia are with this problem. Bearing in mind that the best professionals who have tackled the subject, both from a theoretical point of view and through their works, come from this university, the writer must remark on how their sustained efforts are helping to keep the discourse on HIV in the public eye, and how important this fact is. In so far as this experience is laid on for the benefit of the new generations of creators who are tackling the subject, it is giving rise to a critical mass of artists who are the ones that will analyse the current position of the epidemic and the implications and changes that occur as time goes on.

Along the same lines comes the exhibition *Exprésate* (Express Yourself), recently opened at the Faculty of Fine Arts of Madrid under the curatorship of Aris Papagueorguiu, Manuel Barbero and Tomás Zarza, in cooperation with Apoyo Positivo (Positive Support) and CESIDA (the Spanish Coordinating Organization for HIV/AIDS). This exhibition presents the work of students from the Faculty of Fine Arts of the Complutense University of Madrid and of the Felipe II Centre for Higher Studies, whose approach to the problem focuses critically on the social portrayal of the disease and on the need to keep attention focussed on a problem that is still very much present.

AIDS and art have also been paired as an adjunct to other Spanish exhibitions that have dealt with broader subject matters. Generally, this subject has been handled by curators who are also deeply involved with issues of gender identity. Exhibitions such as *El rostro velado: travestismo e identidad en el arte* (The veiled face: transvestism and identity in art), *Micropolíticas. Arte y Cotidianidad* (Micropolitics. Art and Daily Life), *Transgenéricos* (Transgender People), *100%*, *Héroes Caídos* (Fallen Heroes), *Visibles* (Visible People), *Fugas subversivas: reflexiones híbridas sobre la(s) indentidad(es)* (Subversive flight: hybrid reflections on identity/ies) and *Radicales Libres* (Free Radicals) have included in their selections works that deal specifically with HIV/AIDS and that invite viewers to think about the identification of AIDS with homosexuality. The discourse that is constructed on this topic questions this identification – one that has steadily gained strength since the early stages of the epidemic – and the way in which it has influenced the homophobia that is still present in many social strata.

There have been few occasions when it has been possible in Spain to look deeply at the work of international artists and groups who have made a name for themselves in the struggle against HIV/AIDS. In the nineties, the Santa Mónica Art Centre in Barcelona held two exhibitions. The first one, in 1992, presented the work of the group General Idea, made up of A.A Bronson, Felix Partz and Jorge Zontal. The group was formed in 1967 and disbanded in 1994 when two of its members, Zontal and Partz, died from AIDS-related diseases. Inspired by feminist movements and gay liberation fronts, and by the writings of authors such as Lévi-Strauss, Roland Barthes and Marshall McLuhan, they forcefully attacked the capitalist market with their multiple collectively-authored pieces. Their interests ranged from topics such as alternative sexual identity; explicit criticism of the art business, to the role of the media and the AIDS crisis – always through creations that called for the spectator's participation. General Idea was one of the first to incorporate the HIV/AIDS topic into their work. In 1987 they appropriated Robert Indiana's painting "LOVE" to create the AIDS logo, which featured in many of their works. Fifteen years later, in 2007, the Andalusian Contemporary Art Centre presented their work again in a retrospective that included works dating from 1967 to 1995, and also featured the group's own magazine, *File*, with contributions from some of the most radical and heterodox figures on the international art scene in recent decades, including groups such as Art Language, writers such as William Burroughs, and bands such as Talking Heads and The Residents.

The second exhibition by the Santa Mónica Art Centre was *Domini Public* (Public Domain) in 1994. This exhibition brought together groups of artists connected with AIDS activism such as Gran Fury and Material Group, along with other groups such as the Guerrilla Girls, Peter Dunne and Loraine Leeson, Carole Condé and Karl Beveridge, Jo Spence, Dan Graham and Jeff Wall. Another interesting piece, also in Barcelona, was the mural painted by Keith Haring in the Raval neighbourhood in 1989. The artist left his mark in the syringes and condoms that he painted on a long wall in Salvador Seguí Square where, at the time, drugs used to be exchanged, traded and consumed. Before the wall was demolished the mural was copied onto another wall next to the Barcelona Museum of Contemporary Art in a move that largely deactivated the spirit of Haring's original work.

In 1992 the Queen Sofía Art Centre Museum in Madrid presented the work of Robert Gober; twenty-two pieces representing body parts, washstands, urinals and drains. In 2002 the Velázquez Palace in Madrid, during the PhotoEspaña festival, exhibited the first major retrospective of the work of the North American photographer Nan Goldin in Europe. The 350 works included her *Cookie Mueller portfolio*, in which she portrays her friend over a thirteen-year period, up to her death from AIDS in 1989. Félix González Torres' work was shown at the exhibition held in the Galician Contemporary Art Centre from 12 December 1995 to 9 March 1996. Another important exhibition was *Epílogo. Lugares de la memoria* (Epilogue. Places of memory). Organised by the Contemporary Art Space of Castellón in 2001, it included Félix González Torres' iconic work *Sin título* (Untitled) 1991, in which spectators could observe the enormous empty bed that was exhibited in New York in 1991.

It could be deduced from what is set out here that, in spite of the impact of the AIDS epidemic in Spain,[3] the response by the art world has been relatively patchy

---

3 According to the AIDS Epidemiological Surveillance Report for Spain by the National Epidemiology Centre (30 June 2011 Update) published in November 2011, "Since

and, apart from a few exceptions, the dissemination of pieces on the topic has been hampered by a lack of visibility and continuity in time. Using art-related languages, the artists and groups that have dealt with the problems that the epidemic has posed have emphasised the need to end the negative social portrayal of the disease. One that has led to discrimination against, and concealment of, carriers and sufferers, as well as the need to help with prevention and the dissemination of biomedical advances, and to give multidisciplinary support to sufferers. Their artistic strategies and mechanisms of action plainly show that they are right about the need to talk openly about the disease and what it entails, either via direct language inherited from North American activism or in a more poetical and introspective language.

A parallel can be drawn between the way Spanish society treats sufferers and carriers and the attention that Spanish artistic institutions pay to artistic manifestations addressing the topic. Pepe Miralles comments in this regard:

> the art system has undervalued its social impact, this being a non-grata topic for exhibition curators, gallery owners and art critics alike, who have never understood what the relationship is between art and AIDS – perhaps because they don't understand either what the connection is between AIDS and heterosexuality. The silence characteristic within Spanish art is an outcome of the effectiveness of the homophobic discourses that have been constructed out of the pandemic. (2001: 199)

One wonders whether the situation with the epidemic would have been different had artistic institutions given visibility to creations that called into question prejudices about HIV/AIDS, and informed people about how it is actually transmitted, so as to dispel the false myths that have markedly influenced the risk-taking actions by a sector of the population who thought they were out of reach of infection. These creations, alone and in isolation, cannot alleviate a problem whose solution depends on multidisciplinary intervention, but maybe they could have helped change risky behaviours. It was not until over a decade after AIDS emerged that the earliest reactions were discernible – more than enough time to have included the topic of HIV/AIDS in the cultural agendas of Spanish artistic bodies. This silence reveals a kind of undercover censorship which, although not explicit, does reduce and limit certain expressions that are then consigned to the periphery, to the fringes of a market that does not include them in its system of hierarchies.

Three decades on, the way of tackling AIDS has changed, and we have cause to be grateful for all the artistic initiatives that are still valiantly reminding society that the baggage of symbolism and stigma that surrounds HIV/AIDS is still very much present. A baggage which, unfortunately, has not kept pace with scientific advances, and HIV/AIDS – although not a death sentence in developed

---

the outbreak of the epidemic a total of 80,827 cases of AIDS have been notified. (…). The rate of new HIV diagnoses is similar to other Western European countries, but above the average for the European Union as a whole".

countries – is still a disease with deep and far-reaching physical effects. There are still unresolved questions. Artists, as a cog in the machine but nevertheless an important one, can, through their works, projects and actions, contribute to enhance the strategies that will make it possible to rise to the challenges that the evolution of AIDS brings with it.[4]

References

Brea, J.L. 1995. Sida: El cuerpo inorgánico. *Acción Paralela* (Online), n° 1. Available at: http://www.accpar.org/numero1/sida.htm (accessed: 16 June 2012).

Buxán Bran, X.M. 2001. *Identidades feridas: da arte na doenza* (Laxeiro Foundation: 21 December 2001 - 16 January 2002). Vigo: Laxeiro Foundation.

Cardín, A. 1985. *SIDA: ¿Maldición bíblica o enfermedad letal?* Barcelona: Laertes.

Cardín, A. 1990. *Lo próximo y lo ajeno*. Barcelona: Icaria.

Cardín, A. 1991. *SIDA: enfoques alternativos*. Barcelona: Laertes.

Clot, M. 1997. Los pronombres de Sodoma (Tradición de la ausencia como síntoma postmoderno), in *Del arte impuro. Entre lo público y lo privado*, edited by P. David. Valencia: Generalitat Valenciana, 57-68.

Crimp, D. 1987. Introduction to the Winter 1987 issue of the journal *October*, dedicated entirely to the AIDS crisis and entitled *AIDS: Cultural Analysis/ Cultural Activism*. The issue was reprinted in book form in 1988. MIT Press: Cambridge, 3-16 (1987 edition).

Crimp, D. 1989. *De vuelta al museo sin paredes. Arena Journal*. N° 1 (February), 61-66.

Cueto, J.L. 2006. Art, sida y visibilitat, in *Sida ací i ara. No et Quedes als núvols* (Joseph Renal Hall. Faculty of Fine Arts. December 2006), edited by Cueto, J.L., Miralles, P. and Espacio, R. Valencia: Universidad Politécnica de Valencia.

Espaliú, P, 1992. La Fuerza del SIDA. *El Europeo*. 43.

Lippard, L.R. cited by Guash, A.M. 2000. *El arte último del s.XX. Del posmodernismo a lo multicultural*. Madrid: Alianza.

Mira, A. 1993. Esta noche....SIDA, in *De amor y rabia: acerca del arte y el Sida*, edited by J.V. Aliaga and J.M.G. Corté. Valencia: Universidad Politécnica de Valencia, 145-166.

Miralles, P. 1994. Sobre arte, compromiso y sida. *Universitas* supplement. *Uno más uno* journal (Mexico City). N° 18 (16 May).

---

4 An early version of this chapter was published in *Revista de Artes Plásticas, Estética, Diseño e Imagen. Bellas Artes*. 2012. n°12. La Laguna: Servicio de Publicaciones de la Universidad de La Laguna: pp. 91-113 (*Plastic Arts, Aesthetics, Design and Image Journal*. Fine Arts. 2012. No. 12. La Laguna: Publications Section of the University of La Laguna.)

Miralles, P. 1996. *Pensar la sida* (Epai d'Art A. Lambert: 19 April – 11 May 1996). Xábia: Espai d'Art A. Lambert.

Miralles, P. 2001. Chico seropositivo busca.... Sobre sexualidad y el Sida, in *Miradas sobre la sexualidad en el arte y la literatura del siglo XX en Francia y España*, edited by J.V. Aliaga. Valencia: Universidad Politécnica de Valencia, 191-200.

Nieves, J. 1994. *SIDA: pronunciamento e acción* (Galician)/*Sida: pronunciamiento y acción* (Spanish) *(Pazo de Fonseca: from 8 to 28 July 1994*. Santiago de Compostela: Universidad. Vicerrectorado de Política Cultural.

Pérez, D. 1997. Del arte autorreflexivo al arte transitivo, del arte transitivo al arte recíproco, in *Del arte impuro. Entre lo público y lo privado*, edited by P. Davi., Valencia: Generalitat Valenciana, 19-38.

Río Almagro, A. 2006. Para que no me olvides...Cotidianeidad y reivindicación en los tiempos del sida en el Estado Español, in *El arte látex: reflexión, imagen y sida* (La Nau building, Thesaurus Hall: April-June 2006), edited by S. Barrón Abad and J. Navarro García. Valencia: Universidad de Valencia, 46-73.

Smith, P.J. 1996. *Vision Machines: Cinema, Literature and Sexuality in Spain and Cuba, 1983-93*. Verso: London.

Sontag, S. 1978: *Illness as Metaphor.* 1988: *AIDS and its Metaphors*. (Companion Volumes) New York; Farrar, Straus & Giroux.

Tejada Martín, I. 1996. El SIDA: una enfermedad social, in *Pensar la sida* (Espai d'Art A. Lambert: 19 April – 11 May 1996), edited by P. Miralles. Xábia: Espai d'Art A. Lambert.

Chapter 8

The Role of Local Communities in Developing Unique and Effective Intervention Responses to the AIDS Epidemic: Experiences from Thika, Kenya

Felistus Kinyanjui

Introduction and Background

Since 1984, when the first HIV and AIDS patient was diagnosed in Kenya, the disease has become the country's greatest health challenge akin to what is happening in the global South. The HIV and AIDS pandemic has had a heavy toll, particularly among persons aged between 20 and 49 years. The HIV/AIDS epidemic in Kenya has been tracked through annual sentinel surveillance in antenatal clinics since 1990. Behaviour has been measured through National Demographic and Health Surveys in 1993, 1998, and 2003. The surveillance data indicates AIDS-related deaths have fallen by 29% since 2002 (National AIDS Control Council & National AIDS/STI Control Programme, 2007). The few gains that independent Kenya may have made in regard to reduction in morbidity, mortality and longevity in lifespan are gradually being eroded. Also, the realization of MDGs, 4, 5 and 6 are jeopardized, especially the latter, which targets to combat HIV, malaria and other diseases.

Thus, AIDS has become an urgent developmental issue. Families languish in poverty due to early death of parents, while economies are on the brink of collapsing owing to the loss of its productive human resource. It is against this backdrop that this chapter attempts an analysis of the local initiatives formulated by communities to contain the pandemic. This study is based on the premise that "people can be motivated to practise healthy behavior through information, education, and communication" (IEC). Through billboards, messages over the radio and cinema, lectures in schools and public meetings, people can receive vital health messages. This study was carried out in Thika district (now part of the newly created Kiambu County), which is located 40 kilometres northeast of Nairobi, Kenya's capital. Since 1986, when the first case of HIV and AIDS was diagnosed in Thika, the pandemic has had a heavy toll. Prevalence rates of between 34 and 40 per cent were reported although in the last decade this has nosedived. By 2005 it was estimated that HIV and AIDS prevalence stood at 34 per cent, which was more than double the national rate (RoK 2005), and a prevalence rate of 3.7 per cent – the highest in Central Kenya – was reported in 2012 (*East African Standard*, RoK 2012).

Methodology and Approach of the Study

This study is a socio-historical study that employed both quantitative and qualitative methods of data collection. For qualitative data, this study used participatory approaches where information was gleaned from local people in their own settings. Data was collected through key informants' interviews (KIIs), focus group discussions (FGDs), 'informal' discussions, observations and case studies, which form some of the extracts presented in this chapter. The use of these ethnographic techniques, such as unstructured observations and 'informal' pontaneous discussions – with various categories of informants (among them teenagers, healthcare providers and adults in different social spaces) – proved quite worthwhile given the nature of the topic of study. In particular, participant observation was made as we visited nightclubs and other social places where information related to the study could be obtained. Additionally, life histories in this study were invaluable in representing the case studies of individuals afflicted by the HI-virus. Also, performances – especially songs and dance, skits, poems and aspects of language such as proverbs and sayings – were invaluable for this study. Oral sources therefore formed the major bulk of this set of data for this study. Data from this set of data was corroborated with that obtained from the extant secondary sources and authoritative government records, especially in regard to vital statistics and trends.

Most disciplines and researchers have devised tools for data generation that are used in research, regardless of the cultural context. However, we argue that researching a complex and sensitive issue such as HIV and AIDS, which are (sometimes) directly linked to sex and sexuality (thus they are perceived as taboos and hence cannot be openly discussed), calls for an eclectic and tactful approach in the choice and application of data-generation techniques. Even after selecting a suitable method it becomes necessary to think of ways of engaging participants in the discussions, as there are a number of relations that people associate with personal and private spaces that affect the data collection process.

The cultural norms involving issues of sexuality and taboos poised a great challenge and were manifested when conducting FGDs. The use of FGDs was aimed at gaining deeper insights into the issues of HIV and AIDS. According to Livingstone (2000), the individualistic bias of the researcher can be partially overcome by research methods that either engage with people in the social contexts of their lives (such as participant observation) or by questioning them collectively, as in discussion groups of various kinds. The two approaches, observation and questioning, proved valuable to this study. Discussing matters of sexuality with strangers was not easy and it could also be regarded as socially unacceptable. To make people comfortable, a song related to the HIV and AIDS pandemic was used to relax them before we got into discussion on the topic. The song, for example, contained a message on how the disease was transmitted and its effect on society. From there, people could easily relate to the focus of the discussion and readily contribute to the topic, highlighting what they knew about AIDS and what could be done to contain the pandemic in their cultural contexts. To corroborate primary data, desk research was considered essential, especially for quantitative data – useful to discern the patterns and trends of prevalence. Secondary data sources included UNAIDS reports, government of Kenya reports on HIV and AIDS, policies, plans and strategy documents, district development plans and related documents. Scholarly works in published books, journals and newspapers related to the topic of study were also consulted.

Factors Attributed to High Sero-Prevalence in Thika

Although Thika was far removed from what was initially considered the 'highway' of the epidemic in Kenya and its entre-points, specific conditions prevailed making the Thika unique as a HIV and AIDS study site. In this study, the regional-specific factors that increased Thika's susceptibility to the AIDS pandemic were identified, among others, as: histogeography; persistent denial and inertia; stigma; production and consumption of illicit brews, and transactional and intergenerational sex.

Thika: An Industrial Hub and Locale for Migratory Labour

Dependent industrialisation, which is characteristic of Thika, offers invaluable insights into the understanding of HIV/AIDS in the area. Thika town, which is at the confluence of the Rivers Thika and Chania, traces its origin to the early 1900s, this being the time that white settlers made their way into the area and established coffee, sisal and horticulture farms. Next came the Indian immigrants, who set up *dukas* (Kiswahili for retail shops) and they were followed by African emigrants. With this racial mix attendant segregation became the norm, as was then the case across urban areas in Africa then. The initial development of Thika was accompanied by the establishment of agro-processing, tanneries, textiles, vehicle assemblies and packaging and chemical industries. This led to the christening of the town as the 'Birmingham of Kenya'. Thika's industrial history influenced its socio-economic development and related issues.

From the 1920s through the mid-1980s, Thika was an industrial hub defined by a heavy presence of manufacturing and service industries. Subsequently, it attracted job seeker emigrants from as far afield as Nyanza, Western and Eastern Provinces of Kenya. Women were mainly employed by the textile and food processing plants, partly for their dexterity at work and docility in unionism. The male labour force was absorbed mainly by Metal Box and the automobile industries (Kinyanjui 1987). Both male and female workers were confined to dormitory-type housing, forcing them to leave their families in their rural homes. In 1970 housing was a major problem in the town, whereby an average of 4.2 people shared a tiny room (Kinuthia 1972). Housing would remain a major challenge in future due to increased migration (RoK 1982, 1994). With the influx of newcomers, both rural and urban Thika assumed cosmopolitan status, which has bi-directional positive and negative effects on emigrants and locals. To date, Thika registers high rates of mobile population, some of whom are migrant workers and others daily commuters. In 2002 the migration rate stood at 2 per cent, which outstripped the national rate of 1.5 per cent (UNDP 2002). The commuters are white and blue collar workers who work in the town but return to their rural homes. Akin to what happens in urban settings, migrant workers often form temporary sexual liaisons in their destination, and the same may be said of their spouses back home.

Women from Thika's hinterland who engage in nocturnal activities are not ignorant of the HIV epidemic but they expressed their confidence that, in the town of Thika there were many men who would still be willing to take a woman for the night This confirms findings made by the Kenya Demographic and Health Survey of 2003 (KDHS), conducted by the Ministry of Health (MoH) and the Central Bureau of Statistics, that men who slept away from home more frequently had a HIV prevalence of 9 per cent, compared to 3 per cent for those who did not sleep away from home (RoK 2004). The seemingly 'single' men who are unaccompanied by their spouses fall prey to both resident sex workers and those who oscillate between the rural and urban areas. In most cases, the women who commuted from the hinterland to Thika town maintained other sexual relations in their villages of origin. The cyclic nature of the relationship and high turnover of sexual partners partly fanned the pandemic between the rural and urban areas. The migrant women too contributed to the 'bridge' population that served as a corridor for the high transmission rates of the virus within the rural and urban areas in Thika. Similar findings were made by Mweru (2008) who observed that, among migrant workers in Thika, feelings of isolation, high costs of living, pressure to get married and granting sexual favours to employers increased the likelihood of the women becoming infected.

This implies that men who were isolated from their spouses were at a higher risk of engaging in casual sex or having sexual relations with the commercial sex workers (CSW). Evidence from both informants in the town and rural areas showed that Thika was home to many sex workers who operated in heterogeneous ways; from bars, on the streets and/or in brothels. Many respondents volunteered names of buildings where 'call girls' could be located, suggesting that their operations were less than discreet in as much as prostitution is illegal in Kenya. A proliferation of many social places, frequented by the under-18 youth, was identified as a major factor in the escalation of the pandemic in the area. Commercial sex workers were considered to harbour a great risk due to a high turnover and diverse clientele. Therefore, Thika being a locale for migratory labour with an increased supply and demand for sex trade increases its susceptibility to the spread of the HIV epidemic. This reality in Thika resonates with what Setel et al. (1997) and Lyons (2004) asserted about southern and eastern African migrations that, apart from weakening the stability in the family, it formed an ideal milieu in which sexually transmitted diseases spread.

Thika as a Commercial Agriculture Hub

Closely allied to industrial activities was the commercial agriculture taking place in the tens of coffee, tea and flower farms spread across the district. These plantations presented pockets of high HIV and AIDS prevalence. Since the 1900s, Thika has been home to large coffee, sisal and pineapple estates, which have attracted many job seekers from diverse cultural backgrounds (Cora 1991), many of which are lacking in recreational facilities. This void is taken up by pervasive casual sex, allegedly a preoccupation for most of the under 45-years female workers residing on the estates, particularly on payday (Adagala 1991). One would expect that behavioural change would have been molded positively by the AIDS epidemic but this was not the case until after about two decades of the scourge. One of the coffee estate managers, who had served on different farms in the last two decades or so, was explicit that indulgence in illicit brews and casual sex were the main preoccupations in plantation life (PC 4 May 2010). Casual labourers were at an increased risk of sexual manipulation because of their temporary terms of service. To circumvent possible layoffs, most women extended sexual favours to supervisors who were predominantly male. Although such individuals could be regarded as victims of sexual exploitation they were defensive of their actions, positing that economic deprivation was not comparable to 'sexual exploitation'. Many did not perceive sex trade as a risk, but rather a means to survival or securing a livelihood, *unga*.[1]

Another factor identified as crucial in the spread of the pandemic was the collapse of the agricultural sector, particularly falling returns from coffee. Since the colonial period, coffee had been the 'lifeline' of local people, forcing many to slip into poverty. Hence women from the hinterland were compelled to offer sexual services on a full-time or part-time basis on the estates or in the towns. Previously, casual labour on the coffee farms was a chief contributor of income to rural households. Sex workers who were interviewed in the rural areas were optimistic that, in Thika, it was hard to fail to get a willing customer no matter the circumstances, even in regard to the "AIDS" scare, suggesting that it was not perceived as a health challenge to many. Further, evidence from the Government adduced to the heightening sero-prevalence in the district in 2001, whereby the District Administration expressed an outcry regarding the huge influx of sex workers in the townships of Gatukuyu, Kamwangi, Gakoe, Kanyoni and Kiamwangi, all in the district. These workers had invaded these towns following the release of Sh. 8 million to coffee farmers in the giant Gatukuyu coffee factory. The sooner the money got into the various coffee factories, the CSWs flooded,

---

1   Unga is a Kiswahili word for maize meal, but it is also commonly used to make reference to general livelihood.

calling upon the Provincial Administration to send a wake-up call to the male farmers to be wary of the 'strange visitors' in the area. The extent to which this warning was heeded remains questionable. This begs the question of whether people are aware of the risks they are exposed to or whether they are just ignorant. For instance, the CSWs were well aware of the risks they exposed themselves to, but to a large extent those who were interviewed were categorical that it was better to die ten years down the line than to face instant death due to starvation. Some female respondents in their mid-20s put it thus: '*haribu jina jenga mwili*' (Kiswahili for ruin your reputation, build your body), a cynical reference to the fact that a good name is intangible, but sex-for-money brings home a livelihood. One of these young females opined '*kuishi ni bahati kufa ni lazima*', meaning that to live was a mere chance whereas death was inevitable. From these nuances it was adduced that economic deprivation played a significant role in influencing the decisions that the women had to make as they negotiated for their material survival. Below is a transcript of an interview we carried out with Daisy, which illuminates the dilemma facing young girls in the era of HIV/AIDS:

Daisy, age 19, migrated to Thika immediately after she completed her 'Ordinary Level' of education in a rural school in Kamwangi division. She acquired grade C which was low to secure her university admission. Her peasant parents sent her to stay with her aunt in the neighbouring Ruiru division. Her aunt was well-off and promised to pay her tuition fees in a commercial college where Daisy would pursue a course in Clearing and Forwarding. Daisy was enrolled in college in Nairobi in June 2002. She commuted daily between Ruiru and Nairobi, a distance of 30 kilometres. In the evenings and during the weekends she helped in household chores and sometimes had to undertake tasks on the farm. Her aunt often overloaded her with work, denied her pocket money, making life unbearable for the college girl. When Daisy informed her mother of her aunt's cruelty she advised her to *vumilia* (Kiswahili for bear against all odds) given that her siblings were in school and the familial income was minimal. Daisy managed to get a temporary job as an intern in Nairobi and it was at that time that she took a step in living independent of her aunt. One day she decided not to return to her aunt's house but to take refuge in a church, which she converted into a home. Daisy used to spend her day in Nairobi and wait for night fall, take a snack and finally get into the church to catch her sleep on the wooden benches with no bedding. The wooden church was cold but it was her only home for a period of over one month. She usually left the church compound before dawn, just in time to avoid meeting worshippers who streamed in for morning worship. She was not always lucky because at times she was forced to join worshippers during *kesha* (Kiswahili for night vigil).

During her regular trips to college she interacted and flirted with *matatu* (Kiswahili for taxi) crew who 'showed her love'. One day she sat next to a *matatu* driver who asked her for a date after having noticed her as a regular customer on the Ruiru-Nairobi route. Daisy never left the man's house thereafter. It ended up in 'marriage' and Daisy was happy to have a home that she could call her own. She ended up living with a man she had barely known for a week. Her internship came to an end and she then became a housewife. The marriage was, however, short-lived.

After three months of marriage Daisy fell pregnant and quit college. She developed complications and was bed-ridden throughout her pregnancy. She carried it to term and gave birth to a baby boy. The baby was sickly and needed constant attention but the ailing baby did not give Daisy any clue as to what was happening to her own health. After about six months, she lost her baby to what doctors told her was acute pneumonia. Even before she recovered from the loss, Daisy started ailing and was diagnosed with tuberculosis. This was the first time that she sensed that she may have contracted the deadly virus. At the time of the interview, Daisy was almost certain that she had the virus although she had not taken an AIDS test. She looked emaciated but was optimistic of God's healing power. In the last months of 2004 Daisy was sickly with chest pains, diarrhoea and her once glowing skin was covered with lesions. I visited Daisy in January 2005 only to learn that she had passed away on 23 December 2004. Her mother blamed the union between her late daughter and the driver who was said to have died July 2004.

The tear-jerking story of Daisy resonates with several others in Thika. Financial straits facing many young females put them in a dilemma to make a choice between embracing what appear to be 'promising' opportunities and that of engaging in risky sexual behaviour. Zulu et al. (2004) make a similar observation based on the Nairobi slums whereby transaction sex was not a means for women to obtain luxury items but for basic survival, including rent and food, so that children do not go to bed hungry.

Leisure and Illicit Brews

The normative way for men to spend their leisure time was in consuming liqueur, whether licit or illicit. Due to the high cost of living, bottled beer was out of reach to many. They resorted to the abuse of illicit brew which was cheaper and was purported to 'help them forget' their misery. In the illicit brew dens, HIV and AIDS found a conduit. This was particularly so in the case of indiscriminate sexual relations, which are heightened by substance abuse for which Thika is infamous. Justin Willis (2002), in his book *Potent Brews*, notes that, by the 1950s, there was a very large amount of illicit alcohol production and sale going on across the region. Illicit brew was associated with an escalation in crime. The production and sale was fanned by favouritism, fines and bribes. Without recourse to law, the production continues and its effects can be used to partially explain epidemiology in Thika. In 2001, 50 people died after consuming a local brew in Kiandutu, a slum in Thika. In 2005, Kenya lost 51 lives to an illicit brew that was laced with methanol. This incident took place at Machakos and it was reported that revellers took a brew dubbed *mulika* (Kiswahili for reflect or illuminate). This 'brand' was added to the existing illicit brews that include *muratina* (honey brew), *changaa* gin, *kumi kumi* and *kari kari*.[2] The alcohol content of these *changaa* was rated as high as 98 per cent and at times brewers use methanol to increase potency to give the consumers a 'kick' (*Daily Nation* 14 April 2005). Production of illicit brews was outlawed in Kenya in 1978 but it remains rampant. The local chiefs and their assistants, who are representatives of the Provincial Administration at the grassroots, are accomplices perpetuating this illegality. These Government officers set certain weekly or monthly commissions, which the brewers and traders delivered to them promptly in return for 'protection'. It is well known that whenever producers defaulted in paying 'commissions', swoops and campaigns were vociferously mounted (RoK 1993). According to the people who take these brews, they 'soothe their disturbed nerves and help them forget their troubles'.

Once drunk, HIV/AIDS was of little concern to the patrons and the owners of the *changaa* dens, who were mainly women and who conceded that they frequently engaged in indiscriminate unsafe sex with their 'loyal' clients. To an outsider, the sellers and consumers of these illicit brews can be dismissed as an 'incestuous' community. In Makwa, a village in Kamwangi division, was appropriately christened 'Galilee' because of the proliferation of *changaa* dens, outlets for the liqueur brewed at a riverbank. In one incident, villagers volunteered information on how a mother and her daughter, sellers of illicit brew who also engaged in indiscriminate sex with their clients, both succumbed to the virus within an interval of six months (this information was gleaned from more than one FGD). Many of the adults, both males and females, who were interviewed agreed that there was a close connection between illicit brews and the spread of HIV and AIDS in the district. The dynamics of a combination of *changaa* and sex-trade point to the desperate straits attributable to the marginalization of women in rural Thika. This bears semblance to findings from a study in the 1980s which showed that in Thika town itself, regular 'patrons' of *changaa* dens were also regular sexual partners for the women *changaa* dealers (Kielmann 1997). This also resonates with findings of a study that was conducted in the Kibera slum in Nairobi which revealed that, when a man became a patron and he introduced new customers, he was considered as a reliable person by the owner of the business, who then extended sexual favours to her loyal patrons (Zulu et al. 2004). At the national level, a similar scenario is depicted whereby the KDHS of 2003 revealed that HIV prevalence among women who took alcohol and those who are non-drinkers stood at 19 and 9 per cent respectively (RoK 2003). Therefore the connection between alcoholism and the spread of HIV/AIDS is rather apparent. Although disaggregated statistics to show the link between HIV and illicit brews may not be available, it is safe to argue that

---

2   These terms are used interchangeably to refer to illicit brews; most of the 'brands' cost ten shillings for a mug, which is the unit of measurement, hence the term kumi kumi.

consumption of illicit brew increased chances of engaging in risky sexual behavior that subsequently raised the chance of contracting the dreaded virus. There is need for a medical study to critically examine the relationship between social drinking and the effects of HIV and AIDS.

In focus group discussions people bemoaned unprecedented rates of rape and sexual violence against girls aged between three and nine years. According to official statistics, 185 cases of rape were treated at the district hospital in 2002 (RoK 2003). This figure is conservative when taking into account that most cases went unreported for many reasons which are not covered here. Additionally, sex between members of the same sex – hitherto a little known phenomenon but am not suggesting it did not exist – was on a record increase, particularly for men who visited the illicit brew dens. In Kamwangi and Gatundu divisions, men were reportedly forcefully sodomised.[3] The vice was also traced to the substance abuse that was a major issue in said divisions. According to the Clergy and the Provincial Administration, the district was "experiencing highly unacceptable moral decadence" (Personal Communication).

Lack of proper guidance for the youth increased their vulnerability to contracting HIV. Most of the youth were sexually active, but they relied on peer advice in the absence of proper guidance from parents or teachers. Few knew what family life education (FLE) and reproductive health was, so as to take the necessary precautions to guard against infection. Discussions revolving around sex and death were an abomination among the Kikuyu (quoted in Kiai, Kiuna and Muhoro 2003). It was a taboo topic and so it has remained; even among the educated, sex matters are not discussed openly. Nuances of sex were construed in concealing languages or couched and could not be unsealed to persons younger than the one holding the information. A person was considered of low moral standing if they uttered words related to sexual matters in the public domain. This fact was traced to traditional Kikuyu custom, which considered sexual matters private sphere and, thus, could not be discussed in the public, except probably across age-mates, peers and normally people of the same gender. With this reservation, sexuality matters were left to the realm of imagination, especially for the young, resulting in gross ignorance. In their study on sexuality among the youth in Kenya, Kiai, Kiuna and Muhoro (2003) observed widespread ignorance and doubt among adolescents on sexuality and related matters, which negated the common belief among parents that issues pertaining to reproductive health and sexuality were adequately covered in school through the Family Life Education – FLE – (Kiai, Kiuna and Muhoro 2003). FLE was only introduced in Kenyan schools in 1999, after a protracted battle between parents and the religious fraternity on the one hand, and the Government on the other.

---

3   This information was obtained from individuals, groups and other social gatherings as well as being openly discussed, although the victims of sexual pervasion did not readily admit it until they were taken ill and experts revealed what was ailing them.

The socialisation in silence sharply contrasts with the openness that characterised initiation during the pre-colonial period. In pre-colonial Kikuyuland, circumcision rituals, including *ngwiko* and *kuumithio* rituals, were accompanied by learning sessions or initiation school (Kenyatta 1938). *Ngwiko* entailed controlled sexual activity that allowed newly initiated girls and boys to sleep together, to explore and enjoy each other without penetration. Peer pressure was part of the mechanisms used to maintain the proscribed sexual discipline among girls and boys. Further, taboos, prohibitions and the belief that a breach of conduct would lead to a breakdown of harmony and social balance, leading to disasters and diseases, were extensively used to guide the youth in regard to their sexuality. During *Kuumithio*, which was part of the initiation process, circumcision counsellors, who were selected by the parents of the initiates, guided the novices on their sexuality and expected sexual behaviour.

Presently, and in line with current trends, boys are initiated into manhood with minimal, if any, lessons being taught regarding their newly acquired status. Subsequently, young men engage in indiscriminate sex with several girls (Ahlberg-Maina 1999). Multiple dating and multi-partnerism is embraced by a majority of the youth who are on an "exploration" mission popularly referred to as *Kuhurwo mbiro* (Kikuyu loosely translated to dusting soot from the cooking pot). To the novices this is purported to be a prerequisite to attaining status of a man. This misplaced sexual adventure and machoism exposes youth to risks of contracting the deadly virus. To most youth, the notion 'it cannot happen to me' prevails, assuming that they are not at risk, thus inhibiting modification of sexual behaviour.

Most parents interviewed stated that they felt uneasy discussing the subject. It is in this vacuum that popular theatre has found its place, and appropriately so. Using popular culture, local troupes have contextualised and devised health messages, which are used to mount anti-HIV and AIDS campaigns across Thika.

Towards Effective Intervention Measures

Popular theatre is sometimes referred to as 'theatre for development 'and has been used to convey messages pertaining to health and development in Africa (Colleta and Kidd 1986; Mlama 1991; Godwyll and Ngumbi 2009). It involves the members of a community in their traditional media – dance, music, storytelling, poetry and so on. Popular theatre has played an increasingly important role during the last two decades, not only in Africa but also in Asia and Latin America (Colleta and Kidd 1986). Language as a media of communication is an effective tool for it can be used to shape beliefs and may influence behaviour. Thus, contextualized use of appropriate language has the power to strengthen the global response to the epidemic. Kenya Rugalema (1999) in his study on HIV/AIDS and the Commercial Agriculture Sector posits that the way people talk about the AIDS pandemic reflects how they perceive it and influences how they deal with it.

When AIDS was first diagnosed in Thika it was referred to as *mukingo* (Kikuyu derived word symbolic of emaciation of AIDS victims). This label was stigmatising and value-laden. With time new names have come up as people gradually drop others. The elderly people did not refer to AIDS by any particular name, but commonly make reference to AIDS as 'the big disease' or 'the disease of nowadays'. Whichever term was used, stigma prevailed, and it continues to influence health seeking behaviour for a majority of the people in Thika. It was a double tragedy for HIV-patients seeking treatment from the public health sector, where healthcare providers were insensitive to their conditions, manifested in inhumane treatment, especially by nurses. It was revealed that it was not uncommon to hear a staff callously shout *wapi huyu mwenye kaswende* (Kiswahili for where is the person suffering from syphilis or gonorrhea) (PC with an informant who had previously suffered from an STI). Prior to the advent of HIV and AIDS in both medical and non-medical circles, STDs were often looked upon as self-inflicted problems that were the sole concern of the sufferers (Ngugi and Maggwa 1992). Even with the scourge, People Living With AIDS (PLWAs) were reluctant to seek treatment in public health facilities due to the maltreatment and humiliation they were likely to suffer. This could partly explain why evidence from East and Southern Africa showed that the high prevalence of AIDS was associated with the persistence of ulcerating, untreated and uncured STDs (Caldwell 2000). Stalked with fear of stigmatization, people were reluctant to visit the voluntary counselling centres (VCTs) or seek treatment for opportunistic infections.

AIDS-Support Programmes

In Kenya, akin to most of Africa, the pandemic coincided with Structural Adjustment Programmes (SAPs) that introduced cutbacks on social expenditure. Provision of healthcare in public facilities has dwindled with a reduction in budgets, yet a majority of the poor rely on these facilities. The vacuum left by the exit of the State in the provision of healthcare has been taken up by Non-Governmental Organizations (NGOs), with mixed results that are not addressed here. A variety of interventions have been implemented by NGOs, community and faith-based organizations, funded by the National AIDS Control Council (NACC) under the Community Initiative Account. Their main tasks being: prevention and advocacy; mitigation against socio-economic impact of HIV; treatment; continuum care and support against the socio-economic impact; production and distribution of information; education and communication (IEC) materials; counseling; home-based care; training of trainers; orphan care; support and medical care services. They are 'everything' to those PLWAs. In Thika we find programmes such as Ruiru AIDS Awareness Group, (RAAG); Thika AIDS Awareness Group, (TAAG); Youth Against AIDS Programme, (YAAP); Good Neighbour's Women's Group and Integrated Aids Awareness (IAA). The case study of the Integrated AIDS Programme (IAP) serves as a case example:

The Integrated AIDS Programme

Since 1997, the IAP is one of many community organisations dealing with HIV/AIDS. Its headquarters are located in Kamwangi division, an area with a prevalence rate of 33% in 1998 (RoK 2001). The IAP is funded by the Catholic Agency for Overseas Development (CAFOD). The IAP operates from the Catholic-run Mang'u Dispensary and they accord assistance to the most destitute in the area, selected on a set down criteria. The Community Based Organisation (CBO) works in close liaison with the local communities who present the people affected and infected by the pandemic to its staff. Once the patients are vetted and seen to qualify for assistance they are then registered and they are put on both medical treatment and home care support services. The activities undertaken by the IAP include provision of foods (sorghum, porridge, beans and vegetables) to the patients, counselling and treatment of their clients. The team has some trained counsellors who educate local communities on home-based care (HBC). Patients are treated for opportunistic infections in the dispensary while those who cannot make it there are visited in their homes. Volunteers are committed to providing HBC to patients, particularly in cases where negligence by relatives is evident. In the course of fieldwork, we had the opportunity to participate in some of their activities. Local residents hailed the IAP for its efforts in assisting destitute cases. According to one of the volunteers, "the CBO was based on Christian principles of compassion and care for the less fortunate members of the society. *Theirs is a charity calling to ensure that we express love to these often-neglected people*".

The IAP organised visits to schools where they sensitise the youth on safe sex practices. They emphasised abstinence, a fundamental principle in the Catholic faith, while advising those infected on the need to ensure consistent use of condoms. Through seminars, workshops, theatre, puppet shows and through general advocacy, the IAP raised awareness, especially among the youth. Following the safe sex campaigns, some of the volunteers insisted that there was positive change in people's behaviour. The results from Thika resonate with what has been proven as the potential of theatre, puppetry and indigenous resources in development centres for promoting health care in West Africa. Riley (1990) showed that singing groups, ritual performances and other credible media employ local idiom and are generally accessible and participatory. As such, local media can be adapted to the successful development of messages in particular situations. Available statistics show that in the district, the HIV prevalence rate stood at 33 per cent in 1998 and this had dropped to 18 and 21 per cent in 1999 and 2000 respectively (RoK 2001), while by 2011 the rate stood at 3.7 per cent (RoK 2011).

Creators of health promotion messages should also be cognizant of the social construction of reality that underpins discourses within different cultures, which makes transposing systems or packages from one culture to another problematic. Dutta-Bergman (2004) advocates for development of a culture-centred approach built on a good understanding of the cultural context in which the messages will be consumed. His advice being that communication theorizing ought to locate culture at the centre of the communication process so that the theories are contextually embedded and co-constructed. The troupes in Thika have, in more than one ways, attempted to develop unique performances that are informed by local worldview and culture in order to modify sexual behavior, particularly in men whom, as we have seen, are critical in fanning the pandemic. In the same vein, Christopher Stones contends that in South Africa, "it is men who drive the AIDS pandemic, and if there is to be any major change in the HIV/AIDS infection rate, it is men, rather than women, who need to change their behavior" (2001). This scenario is replicated across Africa, thus there is need to adapt health messages to break this hegemonic masculinity that puts men at the center of the fight against HIV/ AIDS. To shatter this, local media was used to challenge transactional and inter-generational sex, mostly targeting old men who preyed on young females; in local parlance, the 'sugar daddy' phenomenon. Oblivious of the risks those in these relationships were exposed to, some older men dating young females declared *acha iniue ndogo ndogo siachi*, (let it [AIDS] kill me but I will not stop dating young girls). This stance is countered through poems that cautioned against the assumption that all young and beautiful girls who looked healthy could be free of the virus. One such poem warned through the use of the metaphor of a 'beautiful flower that also pricks' – *hiyo maua ina miba* (Kiswahili for that flower has thorns). This message was crucial given the initial perception of local people of those who were infected as being emaciated.

Men, both married and unmarried, who commonly associated with multi-partnerism were warned in more than one way through folk media. In one song the message was delivered *mbembe ni ndoge'* (Kikuyu for maize has been poisoned). It warned men especially that maize, which is a staple food for residents of Thika, was laced with poison and that they would only eat it to their peril. It implied that all maize may look good and edible to the eye, but those who did not heed to caution risked being infected with the virus by the 'poisoned maize'. Thus the message was contextualised in a way that many consumers would not have difficulties in deciphering the intended meanings. Harding (1998) concurs that it is true that indigenous media can be used to further knowledge about HIV and AIDS. This is because it is part and parcel of the culture, it is locally made and contextualised. Similarly, and drawing examples from Uganda, Mushengyezi (2003) argues that communication as a process is hinged on the cultural dialects within a society. Since culture shapes the environment within which a message is decoded, indigenous media continue to present themselves as effective channels for disseminating messages in predominantly rural societies, where population tends to be more orate, that is oral-based rather than literate or written. He illustrates with cases of how both Government and NGOs have utilized indigenous media extensively as a major tool in development programmes. For example, at the inauguration of the anti-AIDS campaign, the radio and TV announcements were preceded by a *ggwanga mujje* drumbeat, which traditionally was sounded to alert people to calamity or danger. This drumbeat resonated a strong message to the people and consequently statistics have shown that response to the AIDS awareness campaign has been positive (Mushengyezi 2003).

In their advocacy for sexual behavior modification, the residents troupes in Thika stressed consistent or 100 per cent use of condoms. For instance, this message was couched in one stanza in a poem titled 'Do not swim in River Chania without a swimming costume' – idiom for condom use whenever one had penetrative sex. Invoking the concept of a river well known to the audience to be infested with crocodiles or 'sharks' – euphemism for danger – the troupes localized the messages in order to make the audience identify with the reality of the scourge. The troupes educate those who are not infected of the life that they will face if they were to contract the disease. They are cautioned that dreams will be shattered, hence the need to seek God's guidance in order to live according to His plan – warning that the life of an infected person is lonely and desolate. In line with the hopeful message, people are encouraged to seek counselling and testing given that contracting HIV and AIDS is no longer synonymous with a death sentence, a paradigm of the late 1980s and much of the 1990s. According to Petty and Cacioppo (1986), an important predictor of the amount of cognitive effort an audience exerts to attend messages is the level of involvement with the topic of the message. Borrowing a cue from this principle, the troupes in Thika did encourage their audience to join them in the dance, and in this participatory way they also become part and parcel of the process. Using music and dance that was contextualized, people easily identified with the reality and messages couched in the various mediums of expression. There are local variations in relation to music and style, dances and songs, but the essence is that it cuts across the various age brackets and implores people to change their sexual behaviour positively. We conclude that the way AIDS information is passed on nowadays contrasts with ways of the mid-1980s, as exemplified by this unequivocal 'AIDS KILLS, WHAT YOU SEE IS NOT WHAT YOU GET!' Such messages were fatalistic and judgmental messages that condemned the initial victims of AIDS to stigma and looming death. Present-day HIV and AIDS education is geared towards influencing people to change their sexual behaviour by attempting to shatter myths and correcting misinformation of yesteryears.

To most youth, AIDS was referred to as *kimiri* or grinder, *kainukia,* or 'that which sends one to an early grave'; *kamdudu,* or 'an insect', and *bumba,* or 'train' (adopted from one of the secular pop songs). The latter implies that it had a heavy toll on people. Seemingly, many of these terms sound less harsh and therefore more readily acceptable compared to those in use in the mid-1980s through the 1990s. Knowingly or otherwise, the youth started fighting the stigma attached to the disease by replacing the judgmental terms with neutral or palatable ones, and without necessarily losing sight of the dangers posed by the pandemic, as its effects are implied in the new terms and other media. Using drama, songs, dance, puppetry, *mashairi* (Kiswahili for poems) and participatory theatre, the communities have been provided with lifesaving information. The groups use vernacular, Kiswahili and English languages to reach their audience. Invariably, health messages were toned down to the specific context: geographical area (river); the maize crop, extra-marital affairs or *mpango was kado* in place of zero-grazing, used to advocate faithfulness to a single sex partner. These were metaphors and analogies embedded within the worldview of Thika residents. People could relate and identify with the health messages. Troupes also fought stigma by enjoining people to desist from apportioning blame – *lawama*, instead focusing on combating the spread of the virus. Commonly, nuances from the poems were neutral, persuasive and apparently seemed to carry a lot of weight, and were more acceptable to the consumers.

Effects of Local Community Interventions: An Evaluation

The success of these community initiatives could be ascertained as the people working with NGOs showed that there was a marked increase in condom distribution and use among the residents of Thika. Condoms were/are now more readily accepted and in use than in the past. They are, for example, dispensed in social places, which was previously uncommon. Regular HIV/AIDS awareness campaigns are mounted, such as those during the World AIDS-week (December 1) and a youth exhibition in the district agricultural show – an event that attracts many farmers from the region, among others. In 2003, a two-day youth exhibition attracted over 5,000 people and 6,000 condoms were distributed to them (RoK 2003). This translates into about one condom each for all in attendance, reflective of a positive behaviour modification towards protective sex previously resisted among the locals. In most open air public meetings/gatherings, or *baraza*, church and local leaders use the forum to talk about the pandemic. Also, workshops for factory and plantation workers are regularly organised, thus reaching more people. We observed first hand that the strategic prevention measures have gained momentum only in the last few years. The divergent approaches synergise each other and have greatly contributed to the containment of the pandemic.

Voluntary Counselling and Testing (VCTs)   Unless people get tested, they can be passing on the virus through sexual intercourse without knowing it. This makes testing a prerequisite in order to mitigate against the spread of the pandemic. The VCT centres have also played a significant role in the drop in prevalence rates. In the early years of this last decade, people were reluctant to consult the few (16) VCTs available. According to a Government report, by 2002 only 14 per cent of the population in the district had been tested (RoK 2002), the majority of whom were the youth. One counsellor in VCT based in a public health facility observed that the youth were attracted by the television set and the lectures delivered at VCTs. Married couples, especially the men, were wary of visiting a VCT centre because they were not assured of confidentiality due to the way STIs and HIV and AIDS victims were initially perceived, as we have already discussed. What happens in Thika is to some extent a microcosm of the Kenyan picture, whereby the majority of the people are reluctant to know their status despite there being many health messages and campaigns stressing the importance of voluntary testing. According to the Ministry of Health (2009), while HIV-testing more than doubled between 2003 and 2007, an estimated 83% of Kenyans living with HIV remained undiagnosed in 2007.

Although more aggressive measures have only recently been embraced to fight the pandemic, the future is bright in as far as HIV and AIDS zero rates is concerned. Our argument is premised on evidence that the decline in infections has been consistent. Evidence to support these declines, for example, comes from behavioural information, including from KDHS and the first national Behavioural Surveillance Survey (BSS). These surveys show an older median age of sexual debut, significant levels of secondary abstinence among youth 3, and fewer people at high risk of HIV due to multiple sexual partnerships and high-risk behavior. Additionally, those engaged in casual sex with non-regular or commercial partners have increased their use of condoms, although condom use is low with regular partners who are trusted. According to the 2012 UNAIDS report, the number of new infections has been reduced from 133,503 in 2005 to 61,691 in 2011. This remarkable decline in the number of new infections in the country is attributed to increased budget to combat the pandemic, as well as concerted effort by communities to fight the pandemic through the local troupes.

Conclusion

The HIV pandemic has ravaged residents of Thika, as well as Kenyans. Thika's history, locale and nature of economic activities provide catalysts that fan the pandemic. Thika's pandemic has defied all theories on location and makes plausible the application of the theory of the concentration of a highly mobile and varied category of vulnerable groups. The fluid population of Thika serves as 'bridge' population, connecting the residents of Thika with a highly susceptible category. Myths and misinformation have been countered by the contextualization of the pandemic through local drama and theatre, which is embedded in the community's culture. Local troupes' plays using localised languages, songs and dance, couch relevant HIV/AIDS information to all, which has partly resulted in sexual-behaviour modification. Respondents reported having reduced the number of sex partners as well as consistent use of condoms. We noted that information alone is not sufficient to motivate behaviour change. In the absence of a vaccine or cure, the main challenge to AIDS prevention is to move people from awareness to behaviour change, such as abstinence and consistent use of condoms, a credit which the local troupes have to some extent registered in Thika. Evidence of the success of local initiatives was partly evidenced in a drop in prevalence rates in the first decade of the century, a trend that has continued to the present. But new infections in the district remain the highest prevalence in Central Kenya. The rise in new infections amplifies the argument that Thika is unique and calls for more intense intervention campaigns for an effective containment of the pandemic. This requires further research and an amplification of local initiatives to situate the pandemic in the appropriate epidemiological and socio-cultural context, away from the conventional text-book panacea. Localised narratives and media carry the key towards containment of the pandemic in the future.

References

Adagala, K. 1991. Households and Historical Change on Plantations in Kenya, in *Women, Households and Change*, edited by Masini E. and Stratigos S. Tokyo: UNUP Press: 206-241.

Ahlberg-Maina, B. 1999. Male Circumcision: Practice and Implication for Transmission and Prevention of STD/HIV in Central Kenya, in *Experiencing and Understanding AIDS in Africa*, edited by Becker C., Dozon J., Obbo C. and Moriba T. Dakar: CODESRIA.

Caldwell, J. (ed.), 2000. *Towards the Containment of the AIDS Epidemic: Social and Behavioural Research*. Canberra: Health Transition Centre: 599-612.

Colleta, V. and Kidd, R. (eds) 1980. *Tradition and Development*. Berlin: German Foundation for International Development.

Cora, P. 1992. *Kikuyu Women: The Mau Mau Rebellion and Social Change in Kenya*. Boulder CO: Westview Press.

Daily Nation 14 April 2005.

East African Standard. 'Thika Maintains Lead in New HIV Cases', 9 July 2012.

Godwyll, F. and Ngumbi, E. 2009 'Problematic Recipe: Alternatives to Public Health Education to Reduce the HIV Pandemic' *Nordic Journal of African Studies* 18 (1): 73-90.

Harding, F. 1998. Neither 'Fixed Masterpiece' nor 'Popular Distraction': voice, transformation and encounter in Theatre for Development, in *African Theatre For Development: art for self determination*, edited by Salhi K. Exeter: Intellect: 5-22.

Kalipeni, E., Craddock, S., Oppong, J. and Ghoshi, J. 2004. *HIV and AIDS in Africa: Beyond Epidemiology.* Malden, MA: Blackwell.

Kenya Ministry of Health. 2009. *Kenya AIDS Indicator Survey 2007.* Nairobi: Kenya Ministry of Health.

Kenyatta, J. 1938. *Facing Mount Kenya.* London: Martin Secker and Warburg.

Kiai, W., Kiuna, S. and Muhoro, N. 2003. The Challenges of Communicating with Female Adolescents: A Case Study of Kenya, in *Gender and HIV and AIDS in Africa*, edited by AAWORD. Dakar: AAWORD.

Kielmann, K. 1997. Prostitution, Risk and Responsibility: Paradigms of AIDS Prevention and Women's Identities in Thika, Kenya, in *The Anthropology of Infectious Disease: International Health Perspectives*, edited by Inhorn, M. and Brown, P. Amsterdam: Gordon and Breach Publishers: 375-411.

Kinyanjui, M. 1987. *The Location and Structure of Manufacturing Industries in Thika*. Nairobi: Kenyatta University M.A. Thesis.

Kinuthia, M. 1972. *Housing Policy in Kenya: The view from the Bottom: A Survey of the Low-Income Residents in Nairobi and Thika.* Nairobi: Urban Praxis.

KNA/AMC/14/20/49: 1982. Thika District Hospital Report.

Mlama, P. 1991, "Women's Participation for Development": The Popular Theater Alternative in Africa", *Research in African Literature,* vol. 22 (3): 41-53.

Mushengyezi, A. 2003. "Rethinking Indigenous Media: Rituals, 'Talking Drums' and Orality as Forms of Public Communication in Uganda", *Journal of African Cultural Studies,* vol. 16, 1: 107-117.

Mweru, M. 2008. Women Migration and HIV/AIDS in Kenya, *International Social Work.* 51 (3): 337-347.

National AIDS/STI Control Programme 2009. *2007 Kenya AIDS Indicator Survey: Final Report.* Nairobi, National AIDS/STI Control Programme.

National AIDS Control Council, National AIDS/STI Control Programme. *Sentinel Surveillance of HIV and AIDS in Kenya 2006.* Nairobi, National AIDS Control Council, National AIDS/STI Control Programme.

Ngugi, E. and Maggwa, A.B.N. 1992. 'Reproductive Tract Infections in Kenya: Insights for Action from Research', in *Reproductive Tract Infections: Global Impact and Priorities for Women's Reproductive Health,* edited by Germain A., et al. New York: Plenum Press: 275-295.

Petty, R.E. and Cacioppo, J.T. 1986. *Communication and Persuasion: Central and Peripheral Routes to Attitude Change.* New York: Springer.

Riley, M. 1990. 'Indigenous Resources in Africa: Unexplored Communication Potential', *Howard Journal of Communication,* vol. 2, 3: 301-314.

RoK. 1993. *Thika Division Monthly Reports from Other Departments.*

RoK. 1994. *Kiambu District Development Plan 1994-96.* Nairobi: Government Printer.

RoK. 1997. *Thika District Development Plan 1997-2000.* Nairobi: Government Printer.

RoK. 2001. *The 1999 Population and Housing Census vol. I,* Nairobi: CBS.

RoK. 2002. *Thika District Plan 2002-2008.* Nairobi: Government Printer.

RoK. 2003. *Kenya Demographic and Health Survey.* Nairobi: Government Printer.

RoK. 2003. *Thika District Hospital Annual Report.*

RoK. 2005. *Thika District Hospital Annual Report.*

RoK. 2005. *AIDS in Kenya: Trends, Interventions and Impact.* Nairobi: NASCOP.

Rugalema, G. 1999. *HIV/AIDS and the Commercial Agricultural Sector of Kenya: Impact, Vulnerability, Susceptibility and Coping Strategies.* New York: FAO/UNDP.

Setel, P., Chirwa, W. and Preston-Whyte, E. (eds) 1997. *Sexual Networking, Knowledge and Risk: Contextual Social Research for Confronting AIDS and STDs in Eastern and Southern Africa.* Canberra: Transition Health Centre.

Stones Christopher, 2001. *Socio-Political and Psychological Perspective on South Africa.* Johannesburg: Nova Publishers.

Thika Times, November 1986.

United Nations Development Programme-UNDP-2002. *Datasheet on Population and Development Indicators from the 1999 Kenya Population and Housing Census Kenya.* New York: UNDP.

Willis, J. 2002. *Potent Brews: A Social History of ALCOHOL in East Africa 1850-1990.* Oxford: James Currey.

Chapter 9

Deconstructing and Reconstructing Cultural Representations to Strengthen HIV/AIDS Interventions in Africa[1]

Arvind Singhal

Whatever one may think about his politics, Ugandan President Yoweri Museveni is hailed globally for leading a highly effective national response to HIV/AIDS. When Museveni became President in 1986, Uganda was ravaged by AIDS with about one in every four adults HIV-positive (Singhal and Rogers, 2003). Within a decade, with concerted political acumen, Museveni helped turned the tide on HIV/AIDS. In a meeting of African Heads of State in 2001, when Museveni was asked how he did so, he responded: "When a lion comes to the village, you don't make a small alarm. You make a very loud one. When I knew of AIDS, I said we must shout and shout" (Mutume, 2001: 21). Museveni emphasized that the 'village chief' had the responsibility to shout the loudest.

The cultural representations of HIV/AIDS (a hungry 'lion') that Museveni invoked for his fellow African Heads of State, emphasizing the role of the leader (a "village chief") to muster urgent political and social mobilization (a 'shout'), is nothing short of brilliant. In many sub-Saharan African countries, tales of heroic valor emphasize the vanquishing of mighty lions with human guile, dexterity, and bravery. By framing HIV/AIDS in highly resonant cultural, linguistic, and colloquial terms, Museveni mobilized Uganda's civil society – the schools, the churches, the mosques, and its mass media – to spread the word on AIDS. So, in Uganda's public schools, student assemblies were the place where headmasters (the educational 'Chiefs') 'shouted' about AIDS. In its mosques, *Imams* (the religious 'Chiefs') 'shouted' about AIDS during congregational prayers, home visits, and community-centered ceremonies such as marriage, birth, and burials (Singhal and Rogers, 2003).

While Museveni orchestrated Uganda's national response to HIV/AIDS, by astutely evoking highly-resonant cultural and linguistic frames, often it is the prevalent cultural representations of HIV/AIDS in societies that impede the implementation of effective HIV/AIDS programs. For instance, in many African countries, including Uganda, masculinity and sexuality go hand-in-hand. The more

---

1 This chapter draws upon some of the author's previous writings: Singhal (2003a; 2003b); Singhal and Rogers (2003); Singhal and Howard (2003).

girlfriends (or 'trophies') a man can boast about, the more virile he is considered (Brown, Sorrell, and Raffaelli, 2005; Campbell, 1997). Other manly pursuits such as serving in the military, getting drunk, and injecting IV drugs further exacerbates the link between masculinity and HIV/AIDS. An extreme and twisted representation of masculinity comes into play when having an STD becomes a marker of manhood.

The purpose of the present chapter is to describe and analyze cultural representations of HIV/AIDS in Africa, mainly focusing on heterosexual (man-woman) experiences. The chapter argues that the dominant biomedical approaches to HIV/AIDS have paid inadequate attention to grasping the socio-cultural representations of the disease, stymieing local, national, and global responses to preventing and controlling AIDS. Through concrete examples from Uganda, Senegal, South Africa, Zambia, and Kenya, we illustrate how cultural representations can be deconstructed and reconstructed in the fight against HIV/AIDS.

Understanding Socio-Cultural Representations of HIV/AIDS

The cultural representations of HIV/AIDS in Uganda (as the 'lion'), and Museveni's (the 'village chief's') ensuing response ('shouting') suggest that cultural, linguistic, and contextual variables can be highly important in inspiring effective HIV/AIDS programs. However, insufficient attention has been paid to understanding cultural factors in the spread of HIV infection and in its prevention and control (Airhihenbuwa, 1995; Basu, 2011; Dutta, 2008; Farmer, 1995; Singhal and Rogers, 2003).

A basic problem with HIV/AIDS prevention and control programs is that the epidemic has been over-defined as a biomedical problem. The biomedical approach looks at the body as diseased, and focuses on 'fixing' the diseased individual. Consequently, adequate attention is not given to the social and cultural factors that fuel the epidemic. This situation seems strange for a disease without a vaccine or a cure. The dominant bio-medical approaches construct HIV/AIDS as a life-threatening disease to be feared, resulting from promiscuous and deviant behaviors of the 'others'. Hence most HIV/AIDS interventions have been anti-sex, anti-pleasure, and fear-inducing (Singhal and Rogers, 2003). While 'sexuality' involves pleasure, bio-medical approaches have rarely constructed sex as play, as adventure, as fun, as fantasy, as giving, as sharing.

The social and cultural context in which HIV infection occurs is important to grasp. The wife of a migrant worker can hardly refuse sex, when her husband, who may have been infected in the city, returns home after a long absence. Nor can she insist on condom use for she may be deemed 'promiscuous'. So, HIV/AIDS prevention programs that routinely advise women to negotiate sexual behavior with a husband/partner fail to adequately grasp the connections between masculinity, sexuality, and patriarchy in a given cultural context. These structural and cultural factors need to be taken into account in designing HIV/AIDS prevention and control programs. Devoid of such cultural considerations, HIV/AIDS programs can easily miss their mark as we illustrate in this chapter.

Certain cultural beliefs in Zambia, for instance, fuelled the epidemic. For instance, "when a married man dies in Zambia, his widow must cleanse herself of his spirit by having sexual intercourse with one of her late husband's brothers or other male relatives" (Singhal and Rogers, 2003: 210). This traditional belief about purification helped spread HIV infection. If the husband died from AIDS and his widow is HIV-positive, she may infect his brother or other male relative, who may in turn infect his wife and future children. A similar cultural belief among the Luo in Kenya led to extremely high rates of HIV/AIDS among this ethnic group.

HIV/AIDS programs that are anchored on the bio-medical approach to 'fixing' the individual's disease "suffer from some certain mistaken assumptions" (Singhal and Rogers, 2003: 211-212).

1. They assume that all individuals are capable of controlling their context. However, whether or not an individual can get an HIV test, use condoms, and be monogamous, s/he is affected by cultural, economic, social, and political factors over which the individual may exercise little control.
2. They assume that all persons are on an 'even playing field'. However, women commercial sex workers (CSWs) are usually most vulnerable to HIV/AIDS. A meta-analysis of HIV/AIDS interventions focusing on commercial sex workers noted that a majority of them simply focused on imparting education about HIV and promoted condom negotiation and use (Shahmanesh, Patel, Mabey, and Cowan, 2008). None of the interventions focused on altering the deep-seated socio-cultural structures that perpetuate inequality and vulnerability of CSWs (Basu and Dutta, 2009; Dutta, 2008).
3. They assume that all individuals make decisions of their own free will. However, whether a woman is protected from HIV is often determined by her male partner (Bujra, 2002).
4. They assume that all individuals make preventive health decisions rationally. Why would one logically put one's life in danger by engaging in unsafe behaviors? In Kenya, a popular Kiswahili saying is "*Aliyetota hajui kutota*", which means "The one who is wet does not mind getting wetter" (Singhal and Rogers, 2003: 212).

Anthropologist Richard Parker's work in Brazil demonstrates why understanding socio-cultural representations of HIV and sexuality is important (Parker, 1991; Daniel and Parker, 1993). Parker notes that the "erotic experience" is often situated in acts of "sexual transgression", understood as the deliberate undermining in private of public norms. Common Brazilian expressions such as "*Entre quarto paredes, tudo pode acontecer*" ("Within four walls, everything can happen") or "*Por de baixo do pano, tudo pode acontecer*" ("Beneath the sheets, everything can happen") signify how the erotic experience lies in the freedom of such hidden moments (Daniel and Parker, 1993 cited in Singhal and Roger:

213). This social and cultural construction of eroticism may explain why a married man, with a home life and children, visits CSWs. Within four walls, a CSW may perform a range of sexual acts that a 'proper' wife would not.

Parker's (1991) work in deconstructing "sexuality" provides social and cultural explanations for why the act of anal sex is perceived as relatively more routine in Brazil than in most Asian or African country contexts. Parker explains that anal sex is widely practiced in Brazil both between men-men and men-women, and that such sexual scripts are learned early. In the game of *troca-troca* ("exchange-exchange"), adolescent boys take turns inserting their penises in each other's anus (Daniel and Parker, 1993). Sexual encounters between adolescent boys and girls routinely involve anal intercourse to avoid pregnancy.

HIV/AIDS interventions rarely take into account such contextually-bound cultural and social constructions of sexuality. Understanding such social and cultural constructions of masculinity, sexuality, and vulnerability in a society, is a crucial ingredient in launching more effective HIV/AIDS prevention and control programs (Jana et al., 2004).

Toward Culture and Context-Centered Approaches

Many culture-centered scholars and practitioners have called for moving away from individual-centered biomedical approaches to preventing and controlling HIV/AIDS to more multi-level, cultural, and contextual interventions (McMichael, 1995; McKinlay and Marceau, 1999; 2000). Others have called for viewing culture not just as a hindrance or barrier but also for its strengths (Airhihenbuwa, 1995; 2007; Parker, 1991). Culture-centered scholars have called for exposing, deconstructing, and reconstructing the coupling of culture and barriers in HIV/AIDS interventions, so that new, positive cultural linkages can be forged (Airhihenbuwa and Obregon, 2000). For instance, smoking cessation programs among Latinos identified the cultural strength of the value of *familismo* ("family ties"), harnessing it to reduce smoking (Airhihenbuwa, 1995; 1999; Diaz, 1997). Similarly, close family ties are valued in Indian society, where the definition of the family includes neighbors and colleagues. Understanding and harnessing these strong family bonds can lead to more effective HIV/AIDS prevention, care, and support interventions (Mane and Maitra, 1992).

Senegal is one country that has done a noteworthy job of strengthening its national response to HIV/AIDS by strategically tapping into several socio-cultural and spiritual aspects of Senegalese society. For instance, the cultural norms in Senegal value the universality of marriage and the rapid remarriage of widow(er)s and divorced persons. These practices uphold the sanctity of both marriage and partner fidelity. Senegalese culture also morally condemns all forms of sexual cohabitation not sanctioned by religious beliefs, curbing irresponsible sexuality (Lom, 2001). The fear of dishonoring one's family provides a strong motivation for acting responsibly (Diop, 2000). Such cultural "entry points" for HIV/AIDS interventions exist in every other society or country; however, few programs have strategically explored or actively pursued this cultural path.

HIV/AIDS intervention programs can fare better if scientific explanations of the disease are couched in local, cultural contexts of understanding (Harris, 1991). Such context-based explanations are called syncretic explanations (Barnett and Blaikie, 1992). A diarrhea prevention campaign in northern Nigeria illustrates the importance of providing syncretic explanations. When missionaries in Nigeria were alarmed by the number of infant deaths due to diarrhea, they tried to teach mothers about water-boiling. The mothers were told that their children died because of little animals in the water, and that these animals could be killed by boiling the water. Talk of invisible animals in water was met with scepticism. Babies kept on dying. Finally, a visiting anthropologist suggested a solution. There were, he said, "evil spirits in the water; boil the water and you could see them going away, bubbling out to escape the heat" (Okri, 1991: 134-135). This message had the desired effect, and infant mortality due to diarrhea dropped sharply.

So, how can HIV/AIDS intervention programs more strategically harness peoples' local, context-centered cultural understandings? We illustrate with some examples from the African context: The cultural attributes of the Nguni people in Southern Africa, for instance, reveal points of entry for implementing HIV/AIDS interventions (Airhihenbuwa, 1995). Among the Nguni, responsibility for providing sex education to the young is usually delegated to an aunt or an uncle, at the onset of a youth's puberty. Cultural emphasis is placed on sexual abstinence. Further, "a strong taboo exists against bringing one's family name to disrepute. Members of an extended family take turns in caring for the sick, to avoid burdening one person. No orphans exist, as extended family members take care of children without parents" (Singhal and Rogers: 219).

Among the Zulus of Southern Africa, the practice of *ukusoma* (or non-penetrative sex) is commonly practiced, both to preserve virginity and to prevent pregnancy (Airhihenbuwa and Obregon, 2000). The woman keeps her thighs closely together, while the man finds sexual release. Other groups use a bent elbow for a similar purpose. Similar non-penetrative sex practices exist among certain groups in Ethiopia (commonly referred to as "brushing") and the Kikuyu in Kenya.

The Ngunis, Zulus, and Kikuyu cultures in Africa are not unique when it comes to non-penetrative safe sex practices. A range of "outercourse" (in contrast to "intercourse") practices manifest themselves in all countries and cultural contexts: From kissing, to fondling, to masturbation, to rubbing and stroking. Compared to penetrative sex, these outercourse practices significantly reduce the risk of pregnancy and sexually-transmitted diseases. While no substitute for sexual abstinence, non-penetrative sexual practices do expand the range of behavioral options to prevent and control HIV/AIDS.

Deep cultural understandings can lead to the identification of alternatives to existing harmful practices. Consider the case of HIV entering Nyanza Province, the heartland of the Luo people in Western Kenya, in the mid-1980s, where it spread rapidly. Like many other East African cultures, the Luo practise widow inheritance. When a husband dies, one of his brothers or cousins marries the widow. This tradition guarantees that the children remain in the late husband's family, and that the widow and her children are provided for. Sexual intercourse with the late husband's relative cements the bond between the widow and her new family (Blair et al., 1997). However, this cultural practice led to disastrous consequences in an era of AIDS.

Focus group discussions in Nyanza showed that the widow-cleansing practice is important for the Luo to "avoid *chira*, a curse that befalls a person who does not perform traditional rites" (Singhal and Rogers, 2003: 221). However, focus group discussions with community elders also suggested possibilities for replacing the rite of "intercourse" with alternative rites, such as the male relative placing his leg on the widow's thigh, or hanging his coat in her home (Blair et al., 1997). Elders noted that such alternative rites were quite acceptable, as the Luo used to practice them decades ago. Such culture-specific understandings are critical in designing effective HIV/AIDS interventions.

Cultural insights from Nyanza Province suggest that HIV/AIDS program managers should go beyond the identification of harmful cultural practices (such as 'wife-cleansing') in order to implement culturally-acceptable alternative rites. PATH (Program for Alternative Technology in Health) and WGEB (Women's Global Education Project) have worked with local NGOs in Kenya, such as Ntanira Na Mugambo Tharaka Women's Welfare Project, to create an alternative ceremony for young girls in Kenya called 'Circumcision with Words'. In this alternative rite of passage, young girls (12 to 17 years) are "secluded" (as is common with the traditional ceremony) for one week. During this time they undergo empowerment training with their mothers and other female leaders. After one week, "community members gather to celebrate the girls' passage into adulthood. The girls perform uplifting songs and dances, and local leaders, especially women, give speeches. And, instead of genital cutting, a cake is cut to celebrate the girls entering womanhood" (www.womensglobal.org). Several thousand Kenyan girls participate in these ceremonies, thus avoiding the risk of HIV infection during cutting ceremonies.

In Yoweri Museveni's Uganda (referenced at the beginning of the chapter), *Imams* (Muslim religious leaders) incorporate accurate information about HIV/AIDS in Islamic teachings, promoting messages of mutual fidelity and moral responsibility in congregational prayers. When participating in sacred family birth and death rituals, they advise community members about the risks of contracting HIV through male circumcision (when an unsterilized razor may be used for several infants), and in the ablution of the dead (when body orifices may be cleaned without wearing protective gloves).

In Uganda and in Kenya, several HIV/AIDS interventions have replaced the biomedical metaphor of safe sex as "negotiation" with the metaphor of safe-sex as "play" (Adelman, 1992). Negotiating safe sex is a sterile, rational, and non-emotional strategy, devoid of sensuality and sexuality (Metts and Fitzpatrick, 1992). It denotes "time out," an abrupt pausing of a sexual script. Instead, playful approaches focus on "healthy passions" i.e. teaching people how to have "good sex" that is "safe sex", as opposed to prevention messages promoting sexual abstinence (Singhal and Rogers, 2003).

Consistent with the sentiment of "healthy passions", Bolton (1995) asked whether HIV prevention programs with gay communities can recruit attractive gay men to educate their partner about the joys of safer sex. Bolton's question is relevant at many levels. First, it extends the discussion of cultural representations beyond heterosexual relationships to also include same sex relationships. Second, Bolton is asking if, contrary to present-day biomedical approaches, is it possible to liberate sexuality (as opposed to denying or repressing it), increase the sum of sexual gratification (as opposed to reducing it), and adopt healthy sexualities (as opposed to continuing with unhealthy ones)?

Conclusions

At a UNAIDS meeting in Geneva (in which the present author participated), a representative from Kenya talked about how young schoolgirls in Kenya rendered sexual favors to urban middle-class and affluent men, commonly known as 'Sugar Daddies', in exchange for the 3Cs: cash, cell phones, and cars. Sugar Daddies seduce by asking young girls: "Can I buy you chicken and chips?" or "Can I give you a lift in my car?" Such seductive offers put these schoolgirls at risk of contracting HIV. Ethnographic research with schoolgirls in Kenya showed that they were well aware of the high risks of their liaison with Sugar Daddies, but they were willing to take their chances (Singhal and Rogers, 2003). Why say no to such glamorous offers, when the alternative is to struggle through school and college, find a job, get married, and then to attend to one's husband, domestic chores, and raising children.

In Kenya as elsewhere, strong cultural undercurrents about masculine sexuality – beliefs in virility associated with bedding young girls, and power and prestige associated with such symbols of modernity as cash, cell phones, and cars – complicate the design of HIV interventions directed at young girls and Sugar Daddies. Messages directed at individuals such as "Stay away from Sugar Daddies" or "Stay away from schoolgirls" miss their point (Singhal and Rogers, 2003: 214) for they mistakenly believe that individuals make preventive health decisions rationally, irrespective of power and prestige considerations.

While an understanding of cultural factors is highly important in effectively responding to the AIDS epidemic, insufficient attention has been paid to them. Because they are focused on biomedical concerns, most HIV/AIDS intervention programs rarely take into account how sexuality is socially and culturally constructed in a society. Invariably, expert-driven knowledge trumps localized, culture-specific potentialities, and as long as the epidemic is represented as a biomedical problem, cultural factors will be shortchanged.

Behavioral interventions will continue to be the mainstay of HIV prevention programs, and for them to succeed, interventions must ultimately respond to the nuances of cultural representations, particularity, and detail (Parker, 1991). They must be based on an understanding of sexual experience as rooted in cultural meanings and social systems (Parker, 1989). Otherwise, HIV/AIDS intervention programs for the most part will be flying blind and be culturally rudderless.

References

Adelman, M.B. 1992. Healthy passions: Safer sex as play, in *AIDS: A communication perspective*, edited by T. Edgar et al. Mahwah, NJ: Lawrence Erlbaum Associates, 69-89.

Airhihenbuwa, C.O. 1995. *Health and Culture: Beyond the Western Paradigm*. Thousand Oaks, CA: Sage.

Airhihenbuwa, C.O. 1999. Of culture and multiverse: Renouncing "the universal truth" in health. *Journal of Health Education*, 30(5), 267-273.

Airhihenbuwa, C.O. 2007. *Healing Our Differences: The Crisis of Global Health and the Politics of Identity*. Lanham, MD: Rowman and Littlefield.

Airhihenbuwa, C.O. and Obregon, R. 2000. A critical assessment of theories/ models used in health communication for HIV/AIDS. *Journal of Health Communication*, 5, 5-15.

Barnett, T., and Blaikie, P. 1992. *AIDS in Africa: Its present and future impact.* New York: Guildorm Press.

Basu, A. 2011. HIV/AIDS and subaltern autonomous rationality: A call to re-center health communication in marginalized sex worker spaces. *Communication Monographs*, 78, 391-408.

Basu, A. and Dutta, M. 2009. Sex workers and HIV/AIDS: Analyzing participatory culture-centered health communication strategies. *Human Communication Research*, 35, 86-114.

Blair, C., Ojakaa, D., Ochola, S.A. and Gogi, D. 1997. Barriers to behavior change: Results of focus group discussions conducted in high HIV/AIDS incidence areas of Kenya, in *Confronting the AIDS epidemic: Cross-cultural perspectives on HIV/AIDS education*, edited by D.C. Umeh. Trenton, NJ: Africa World Press, 47-57.

Bolton, R. 1995. Rethinking anthropology: The study of AIDS, in *Culture and Sexual Risk: Anthropological Perspectives on AIDS*, edited by H. Brummelheis and G. Herdt. Amsterdam: Gordon and Breach, 285-314.

Brown, J., Sorrell, J., and Raffaelli, M. 2005. An exploratory study of constructions of masculinity, sexuality and HIV/AIDS in Namibia, Southern Africa. Available at http://digitalcommons.unl.edu/psychfacpub/54 [accessed: 23 August 2012].

Bujra, J. 2002. Targeting men for a change: AIDS discourse and activism in Africa, in *Masculinities Matter*, edited by F. Cleaver. London: Zed Books, 209-234.

Campbell, C. 1997. Migrancy, masculine identities and AIDS: The psychosocial context of HIV transmission on the South African gold mines. *Social Science and Medicine*, 45, 273–281.

Daniel, H. and Parker, R.G. 1993. *Sexuality, Politics, and AIDS in Brazil*. London: Falmer Press.

Diaz, R.M. 1997. Latino gay men and psycho-cultural barriers to AIDS prevention, in *In Changing Times: Gay Men and Lesbians Encounter HIV/AIDS*, edited by M. Levine et al. Chicago: University of Chicago Press, 221-244.

Diop, W. 2000. From government policy to community-based communication strategies in Africa: Lessons from Senegal and Uganda. *Journal of Health Communication*, 5, 113-118.

Dutta, M. 2008. *Communicating Health: A Culture-centered Approach.* Cambridge: Polity.

Farmer, P. 1995. Culture, poverty, and dynamics of HIV transmission in rural Haiti, in *Culture and Sexual Risk: Anthropological Perspectives on AIDS*, edited by H. Brummelheis and G. Herdt. Amsterdam: Gordon and Breach, 3-28.

Harris, D. 1991. AIDS and theory. *Linguafranca*, 1(5), 16-19.

Jana, S., Basu, I., Rotheram-Borus, M.J. and Newman, P.A. 2004. The Sonagachi project: A sustainable community intervention program. *AIDS Education and Prevention*, 16, 405-414.

Lom, M.M. 2001. Senegal's recipe for success. *Africa Recovery*, 15(1-2), 24-25.

Mane, P. and Maitra, S.A. 1992. *AIDS Prevention: The Socio-cultural Context in India.* Mumbai: Tata Institute of Social Sciences.

McKinlay, J.B. and Marceau, L.D. 1999. A tale of three tails. *American Journal of Public Health*, 89, 295-298.

McKinlay, J.B. and Marceau, L.D. 2000. Public health matters. To boldly go. *American Journal of Public Health*, 90(1), 25-33.

McMichael, A.J. 1995. The health of persons, populations, and planets: Epidemiology comes full circle. *Epidemiology*, 6, 663-636.

Metts, S. and Fitzpatrick, M.A. 1992. Thinking about safer sex: The risky business of 'know your partner' advice, in *AIDS: A Communication Perspective*, edited by T. Edgar et al. Mahwah, NJ: Lawrence Erlbaum Associates, 1-19.

Mutume, G. 2001. African leaders declare war on AIDS. *Africa Recovery*, 14(4), 1, 20-23.

Okri, B. 1991. *The Famished Road.* New York: Oxford University Press.

Parker, R.G. 1989. Bodies and pleasures: on the construction of erotic meanings in contemporary Brazil. *Anthropology and Humanism Quarterly*, 14, 58–64.

Parker, R.G. 1991. *Bodies, Pleasures, and Passions: Sexual Culture in Contemporary Brazil.* Boston: Beacon.

Singhal, A. 2003a. Overcoming AIDS stigma: Creating safe communicative spaces. *Journal of Communication Studies*, 2(3): 33-42.

Singhal, A. 2003b. Focusing on the forest, not just the tree: Cultural strategies for combating AIDS. *MICA Communications Review*, 1(1): 21-28.

Singhal, A. and Rogers, E.M. 2003. *Combating AIDS: Communication Strategies in Action.* Thousand Oaks, CA: Sage Publications.

Singhal, A., and Howard, W.S. (eds) 2003. *The children of Africa confront AIDS: From Vulnerability to Possibility.* Athens, OH: Ohio University Press.

Shahmanesh, M., Patel, V., Mabey, D. and Cowan, F. 2008. Effectiveness of interventions for the prevention of HIV and other sexually transmitted infections in female sex workers in resource poor setting: A systematic review. *Tropical Medicine and International Health,* 13(5), 1-21.

Chapter 10

Representing HIV/AIDS in Africa: Pluralist Photography and Local Empowerment[1]

Roland Bleiker and Amy Kay[2]

The difficulties of stemming the spread of HIV/AIDS are in part due to the fact that the disease is not only a medical problem but also a social, cultural, and political challenge. Perhaps more so than any other disease in history, HIV/AIDS has generated countless political debates, scientific publications, donor appeals, public protests, education campaigns, and artistic engagements (see Miller 1992, McNeill 1998, Elwood 1999, Ogdon 2001, Crimp 2002). Paula Treichler (1999: 1) thus speaks of an "epidemic of signification", which is to say that the nature and political impact of HIV/AIDS is intrinsically linked to how the disease is represented, and how these representations influence key issues, such as the production of stigma and discrimination.

The purpose of this chapter is to examine the nature and political consequences of representing HIV/AIDS. We do so by focusing on how different methods of photography embody different ways of understanding and dealing with HIV/AIDS in Africa, the continent where the disease has taken its greatest toll. Since the early 1980s, some 16.7 million Africans have died from AIDS-related illnesses. In South Africa alone there are 1,600 new infections every day (Freedman and Poku 2005: 665–667). Africa is, of course, far too diverse a continent to be represented in homogeneous ways. That is, in fact, one of the stereotypical representations we critique in this chapter. HIV infection rates for people between the ages of 15 and 49, for instance, range from 1 per cent in Mauritania to almost 40 per

1   This chapter appeared first published in *International Studies Quarterly* (2007) 51, 139–163.

2   Authors's note: Thanks are due to John Ballard, Thomas Bernauer, Gerard Holden, Emma Hutchison, Subhash Jaireth, and Hanspeter Kriesi as well as the ISQ editorial team and their anonymous referees for insightful comments on earlier drafts of this chapter. We would also like to acknowledge the generous help of Eric Gottesman, who repeatedly took the time and care to respond to our inquiries. Much of the background information about our case study on pluralist photography is based on these interviews, which took place either by phone or e-mail between June 2004 and July 2006. Rather than citing the interviews individually throughout the text, we acknowledge them here collectively.

cent in Botswana and Swaziland. Major differences also exist with regard to key factors influencing HIV/AIDS, such as gender disparity, poverty, mobility, and intravenous drug use. Sub- Saharan Africa is the most affected region, containing 25.8 of the estimated 40.3 million people living with HIV/AIDS worldwide in 2005 (UNAIDS 2005).

We focus on photographs in our chapter because they play an important role in shaping private and public understandings of HIV/AIDS. The political dimensions of photographic representations become particularly acute when they enter the realm of mass media. Popular perceptions, policy frameworks, and development priorities are all influenced by the visions that mass media create with respect to a particular issue. Photographs are central to this process. The likelihood of a story making it to print, especially on the cover of a publication, increasingly depends on the quality of the pictures that accompany it. At a time when we are saturated with information stemming from multiple media sources, images are well suited to capture issues in succinct and mesmerizing ways. They serve as visual quotations (Sontag 2003: 22, 85; 2004: 22). Some of the most influential means of representing HIV/AIDS in Africa have thus been through photography. From iconic photographs in mass media to local artistic engagements, photographic portrayals of HIV/AIDS have created a range of powerful effects, from apathy and fear to empathy and engagement.

We distinguish among three photographic methods of representing HIV/AIDS: naturalist, humanist, and pluralist. Each embodies different forms of representation through which we give meaning to political phenomena. Exploring such sites of representation, we argue, reveals how different ideological assumptions generate different public understandings of – and thus reactions to – the HIV/AIDS pandemic.

Naturalist approaches portray photographs as neutral and value free, as reflecting an objective reality captured through the lens (see Hall 1997: 98). Photographs are seen as having a truth value, allowing the viewer realistic insight into the events and people they depict. In its pure form, such a position is, we believe, not tenable. Photographs cannot portray the world as it is. A photograph is no different from any other form of representation, even though the seemingly naturalistic reproduction of external realities may deceive us initially. A photograph is taken at a certain time of the day, with a certain focus, and from a certain angle. These choices make up the very essence of the photograph: its esthetic quality. But they result from artistic and inevitably subjective decisions taken by the photographer – 140 Representing HIV/AIDS in Africa decisions that have nothing to do with the actual object that is photographed. As there is relatively widespread scholarly consensus about these limits to naturalist photography, we do not engage the respective practices – and their underlying assumptions – in detail. Instead, we focus our attention primarily on two alternatives to naturalism: humanism and pluralism.

Humanist photography is the first of two non-naturalist approaches we examine systematically. We do so by focusing on a meanwhile iconic "AIDS photograph" taken by photojournalist Ed Hooper. It depicts a Ugandan mother and her baby, both in the last stages of fatal, AIDS-related illness. We examine the Hooper photograph as a particular type of image that symbolizes broader western practices of representing HIV/AIDS in Africa. Taken in 1986, during the relatively early years of western recognition of the HIV/AIDS epidemic as a major crisis, the Hooper photograph reveals how HIV/AIDS was first visualized in the press, and how such early visualizations of suffering and victimization have had implications that still shape the HIV/AIDS discourse today (Bhattacharya et al. 2005: 8). It also symbolizes how very specific, humanist forms of representations continue to influence our understanding of HIV/AIDS in Africa (for a recent example, see Annan, Gordimer and Kennedy 2003). The political assumption behind such humanist approaches is that images of suffering can invoke compassion in viewers, and that this compassion can become a catalyst for positive change. Although accepting the basic premise underlying this position, we inquire further into the values involved in these practices, and the form of change that issues forth from them. We show that humanist photographic engagements, well meant as they are, contain residues of colonial values. They are more likely to invoke pity, rather than compassion. They reflect how western – and thus very often universalized – accounts of HIV/AIDS in Africa are based on very specific assumptions, even stigma, revolving around the portrayal of people affected by HIV/AIDS as passive victims, removed from the everyday realities of the western world.

We then juxtapose humanist practices of photography prevalent in western media sources with different, more local, and more diverse photographic engagements. We term them pluralist photography. They differ from both naturalist and humanist approaches. They share with the latter the belief that photographs can become important catalysts for social change, but actively oppose the humanist focus on iconic photographs and their implicit association with western and often universalized positions. Pluralist photography, by contrast, seeks to validate local photographic practices in an attempt to create multiple sites for representing and understanding the psychological, social, and political issues at stake. To illustrate this form of engagement, we focus on the recent work of photographer Eric Gottesman and the Addis Ababa community of *kebele* (neighborhood) 15. Gottesman worked with local children affected by HIV/AIDS, teaching them how to use photography to represent for themselves what it means to live with HIV/AIDS in a community that has both high-infection rates and high levels of related stigma. We examine the potential – and limits – of such local photography to overcome the stereotypical image of the passive victim. While we advocate the use of pluralist photography, we fully recognize that this tradition is not void of bias either. It cannot give us authentic local knowledge. But by generating multiple and creative ways of representing HIV/AIDS, it helps viewers recognize that the process of representation is inherently incomplete, and thus inevitably political. Such engagements with representation can offer more effective ways of addressing the spread and sociopolitical effects of the disease. This is why, we argue, pluralist photography should be used more widely in attempts to understand and contain the spread of HIV/AIDS.

Before we begin our inquiry, a few words on methodology are in order. The photographs we have chosen for our case studies are obviously not meant to provide a comprehensive account of how the issue of HIV/AIDS in Africa is being represented. Doing so is not – and cannot be – the purpose of a short chapter. Our main empirical focus rests with an iconographic photograph portraying HIV/AIDS in Uganda during the mid-1980s and a series of photographs taken more recently by Ethiopian children affected by AIDS. These photographs are taken two decades apart, at times when HIV/AIDS occupied a very different place in public discourse.

They deal with two completely different parts of Africa. We have chosen the photographs in question because they symbolize, in an ideal way, specific kinds of photography. Studying them allows us to understand the sociopolitical dimensions entailed in different representations of HIV/AIDS, which is the main objective of our chapter.

A similar disclaimer is in order with regard to the three categorizations we use: naturalist, humanist, and pluralist. These concepts are meant to differentiate between ideal types of photography. We are fully aware that in reality, a photograph and its public use may simultaneously contain elements of multiple approaches – say a combination of humanist and pluralist traits. But by focusing on ideal types of photographs – archetypes, so to speak – we are able to identify more precisely what is at stake in the process of representation. We use our own, relatively ad hoc terms, in part because we wanted to use everyday language, rather than jargon, in part because there are comparatively few relevant conceptual discussions, at least in the literature on international relations. Among the similar studies that do exist, Francois Debrix and Cynthia Weber distinguish between practices of representation, transformation, and pluralization (Debrix 2003: xxi–xxii). While our approach is influenced by their typology we nevertheless retain our own, slightly different concepts. We do so because Debrix and Weber focus on how an image is being mediated in the process of creating social meaning while our own task is mostly limited to understanding practices of representation themselves.

Beyond Naturalism: Representation and Western Media Constructions of Stereotypes

Photographs deceive. They seem to give us a glimpse of the real. They provide us with the seductive belief that what we see in a photograph is an authentic representation of the world: a slice of life that reveals exactly what was happening at a particular moment. This is the case because a photograph is, as Roland Barthes (1977: 17) stresses, "a message without a code". As opposed to a linguistic representation, or a painting, a photograph is "a perfect analogon". Indeed, its very nature, as Barthes continues, is defined by this analogical perfection. In the realm of documentary photography, for instance, it was for long commonly assumed that a photographer, observing the world from a distance, is an "objective witness" to political phenomena, providing authentic representations of, say, war or poverty (see Strauss 2003: 45). Theoretically, such naturalistic positions hinge on the belief that a photograph can represent its object in a neutral and value-free way, transferring meaning from one site to another without affecting the object's nature and signification in the process. Debrix (2003: xxiv, xxvii–xxx) stresses that this belief is part of a long western search for transcendental knowledge, be it of a spiritual or secular nature.

While most scholars who work on photography acknowledge that photographs mimic vision in one way or another, few if any claim that such representations, even if they are pictorial simulacra, are authentic representations of the world as it is (see Friday 2000: 356–75). We agree. But rather than critiquing naturalist understandings of photography in detail we find it more productive to explore how alternative approaches recognize that photographs are practices of representations and thus of an inherently political nature. Two aspects make such alternatives to naturalism convincing.

First, and as already mentioned, a photographic representation reflects certain esthetic choices. It cannot be neutral because it always is an image chosen and composed by a particular person. It is taken from a particular angle, and then produced and reproduced in a certain manner, thereby excluding a range of alternative ways of capturing the object in question (see, for instance, Barthes 1977: 19, Sontag 2003: 46).

Second, and more importantly, a photograph cannot speak for itself. It needs to be viewed and interpreted. This is why Barthes (1977: 17–19) stresses that there are always two aspects to a photograph. There is the "denoted message", which is the above-mentioned analogically perfect representation of a visual image. But there is also a "connoted message", which includes how a photograph is read and interpreted, how it fits into existing practices of knowledge and communication. Some refer to this process more specifically as "secondary image construction", which takes place when photographs are "selected out from their original ordering and narrative context, to be placed alongside textual information and reports in a publication" (Hall 1997: 86). It is not our intention here to engage the complex and rather diverse literature on photography, visual culture, and media representation. Doing so would go far beyond the scope of this chapter. But we would like to point out briefly that there is widespread scholarly agreement that a connoted message cannot take the form of an unmediated representation of reality. John Berger (1980: 55), for instance, points out that photographs "…only preserve instant appearances". When we look at a photograph we never just look at a photograph alone. We actually look at a complex relationship between a photograph and ourselves (Berger 1977: 9). Our viewing experience is thus intertwined not only with previous experiences, such as our memory of other photographs we have seen in the past, but also with the values and visual traditions that are accepted as common sense by established societal norms. Guy Debord (1992: 4), likewise, stresses how everything directly lived becomes distanced through representation. It becomes part of a "spectacle", which he defines as a "social relationship between people that is mediated by images". For David Levi Strauss (2003: 45), the important aspect of this process is that there are always relations of power at stake, that there is always an attempt to tell a story, and that this story is always told from a particular, politically charged angle.

What makes photographs unusually powerful – and at times problematic – is that their analogically perfect representation of a visual image masks the political values that such representations embody. The assumption that photographs are neutral, value free, and evidential is reinforced because photography captures faces and events in memorable ways. For instance, if one looks at an image of a person affected by AIDS-related illnesses, one could easily believe that one actually sees that person as he or she was at that moment. Michael Shapiro (1988: 124, 134) writes of a "grammar of face-to-face encounters". And he stresses that the analogical nature of this encounter makes photographic representations particularly vulnerable to being appropriated by discourses professing authentic knowledge and truth. We may succumb to such a "seductiveness of the real" to the point that we forget, as photojournalist David Pearlmutter (1998: 28) warns us, that "the lens is focused by a hand directed by a human eye". Add to this that the public rarely sees the news media as purveyors of commercially profitable stories and images. Instead, the news is perceived as a reflection of the actual, as a neutral mediator between a subject, and, in the case of most international news, an object usually located in another part of the world.

The fusion of information and entertainment, and the commercial need for recognizable headlines and simple stories, inevitably favors stereotypical representations over more complex ways of representing sociopolitical issues, such as HIV/AIDS. Barthes (1977: 22) even goes as far as arguing that a photograph only achieves meaning "because of the existence of a store of stereotyped attitudes which form ready-made elements of signification". This tendency is exacerbated when a news item refers to events in the developing world. In such cases, western media sources tend to fall back on the scripts of global news agencies circulated in wire services. Once the parameters of a news story have been set, coverage can lapse into a standard formula. Photography may thus give a pandemic such as HIV/AIDS the meaning of familiar crisis by cueing an audience to formulaic events via particular images. Such practices can, for instance, revolve around a micrograph picture of the virus or an image of a person dying of AIDS-related illnesses. They reinforce static pictures of HIV/AIDS and make it difficult to generate change (Watney 1990). Photographs can thus strengthen the perception that the disease is not part of daily life, but something less real and more remote, something that may resemble what Edith Wyschogrod (1973) once called a "death event" (Wyschogrod 1973).

HIV/AIDS and Colonial Perceptions of Africa

Portrayals of Africa epitomize how western media sources produce and reproduce stereotypes. Since the early years of the HIV/AIDS epidemic, western science and modern media have constructed a concept of "African HIV/AIDS" that is closely linked to the colonial heritage and its mystifications of Africa (see Watts and Boal 1995: 105). Part of this Eurocentric perception is the tendency to view Africa as a homogenous continent seen through a "prism of misery" (Kean 1998: 2). The Kenyan author and playwright Binyavanga Wainaina (2006) writes of the western tendency to write as if Africa were one country, a place that "is hot and dusty with rolling grasslands and huge herds of animals and tall, thin people who are starving". Methods of photography that use standardized representational practices reinforce such colonial stereotypes, creating what David Campbell, in a series of innovative and convincing essays, calls an "iconography of anonymous victimhood" (see Campbell 2003a: 69, 70–71, 84; 2003b: 67; 2004: 62, 69).

The result is a fatalistic apathy in the western viewer, leading to the impression that each crisis is simply part of a larger pattern of misery and gloom that is so deeply entrenched that it cannot possibly be reversed. Cindy Patton (1990: 83) points out how images of Africans suffering and dying from AIDS-related illnesses perfectly fit into such stereotypical images of "a wasting continent peopled by victimbodies of illness, poverty, famine". Patton stresses how this pre-conceived image neglects to recognize the many instances where development has actually taken place: moments, for instance, when local communities managed to thrive, when personal and societal achievements prevailed over doom and gloom.

Practices of representation are among the most influential elements in encounters between the North and the South (see Doty 1996: 2). This is particularly the case with western representations of Africa, which correspond to what Edward Said (1979: 2–3) termed orientalism: a style of thought – and a corresponding mode of governance- that is based not on geographical, political, or cultural facts, but on a series of stereotypical assumptions about the values and behavior of people who inhabit far off and "exotic" places. Central here is a stark division between the orient and the occident. This division is characterized by the juxtaposition of fundamental opposites, which are presented as essential cultural traits. The West is characterized by values such as reason, progress, activity, optimism, and order, while Africa is associated with emotion, stagnation, passivity, pessimism, and chaos (see Mitchell 1998: 293; Bancroft 2001: 96). The practices of authority and domination that issue from such representations have insinuated themselves into all domains of life, from philosophy, science, history, and tourism to governmental regulations, economic structures, artistic traditions, and scientific methods. Early practices of photography are as much part of these colonial power relations (see Higgins 2001: 22–36) as are contemporary perceptions of HIV/AIDS.

Representations of HIV/AIDS do, indeed, fit into established patterns of orientalism. Consider, for instance, how some of the first media accounts of HIV/AIDS revolved around theories that traced the origin of the disease in Africa. One particular theory was based on the assumption that the HIV virus had actually been present in Africans for years but simply remained undiagnosed. That is, until they "passed it out to the world as civilization reached them" (Hilts 1988: 2). Another theory stipulated that HIV evolved from a parent virus discovered in wild African green monkeys. The disease was then said to have crossed species barriers and found a human host in Africans, who later passed it on to the rest of the unknowing world. Although debated by the medical community (see McNeill 1998: 11–17; Smith 1998: 330–333; Bancroft 2001: 92–4), theories based on the origins of HIV/AIDS can often lead to problematic practices of blaming others and generating racist stereotypes (Sabatier 1988). In this particular case, HIV/AIDS is represented as emerging in faraway places, from bodies of "others" that then "contaminate" the rest of the world. The result is an emphasis on questions of origins, rather than an engagement with the underlying causes of infection. It would be far more productive to emphasize how certain behaviors and practices put all people at increased risk for HIV infection. Equally important are efforts to understand factors that contribute to a person's vulnerability, such as power relations and societal norms that limit women's choices to protect themselves against infection (see Sarin 2002, DeSantis 2003, Roudi-Fahimi 2003, UNDP 2007).

Stereotypical portrayals of Africa are epitomized by assumptions surrounding the sexual transmission of HIV. Rather than relying on scientific data or pragmatic policy deliberations, western perceptions of HIV/AIDS in Africa have been dominated by moral judgments and prejudices (see Sabatier 1988: 1). This is, as Susan Sontag (1988: 27) stresses, not necessarily new or surprising. She points out that many diseases that are said to be linked to sexual fault (such as syphilis) tend to "inspire fears of easy contagion and bizarre fantasies of transmission by nonvenereal means in public places". But such tendencies have been particularly pronounced with regard to representations of HIV/AIDS in Africa. Sexual practices have been moralized and demonized by western doctors and other experts. As with previous epidemics such as cholera, the disease is being interpreted "...as a sign of moral laxity or political decline" (Sontag 1988: 142). Representative of this practice is an American doctor, who stressed in a press interview that "there is a profound promiscuity in Uganda, and a virus which takes advantage of it" (cited in Hooper 1990: 28). The ensuing HIV/AIDS discourse mingles medical and moral assumptions, making it difficult to prevent the production and diffusion of stigmatizing ideas (Patton 1990: 105). The result is a public discourse based on an entrenched suspicion about the disease and, more importantly, about the people who live with it.

Prevalent journalistic styles of reporting further reinforce stereotypical images of HIV/AIDS in Africa. This is particularly the case of so-called "parachute reporters", who are flown into a crisis zone for a short time and then report back to the "rest of the world". One of many examples: in the years immediately following recognition of the epidemic in Uganda, President Museveni announced an "open door policy", designed to draw the world's attention to the impact of the epidemic in Africa (Sabatier 1988: 91). In the wake of this policy announcement, western journalists entered the country, flooding hospitals in an attempt to visualize the pandemic though images of African AIDS victims. But such parachute reporters often lack knowledge of the political and cultural context that surround the issues they seek to cover. They are given only limited time and resources to do their work. The ensuing coverage almost inevitably leads to a reinforcement of existing stereotypes. The reaction of some local African governments to the crisis often exacerbated the effect of the stereotypical images that prevail in the western public discourse. Particularly fateful, Treichler (1999: 109) believes, is the combination of "doomsday predictions" by western media sources and categorical denials by governments in developing countries. The latter not only increases fear, stigmatization, and the spread of the disease, but paradoxically reinforces stereotypes. When western reporters seek to deal with HIV/AIDS in Africa, their representations often clash with the institutionalization of silence imposed by local public policies. Ministries in some African countries have often banned researchers and physicians from talking to the press. Various arguments are presented for such silencing, including fears that representations of HIV/ AIDS could damage thriving industries, such as tourism, on which many African countries depend (Sabatier 1988: 96, Fleury 2004: 1). The result is an entrenchment of the problematic practices described above: foreign reporters rely more heavily on available foreign sources, thus reinforcing preexisting narratives of Africa and silencing the far more complex and intertwined local stories that characterize the epidemic's spread and sociopolitical consequences. The so-produced dehumanizing images of Africa are not just reflective of media representations, but permeate most western engagements with the continent. Raymond Apthorpe (2001: 112), drawing on decades of experience with humanitarian work, emphasizes the deeply entrenched tendency of western development workers and aid agencies to rely on stereotypical, reproducible, recognizable, and self-affirming views of Africa, thus reproducing a virtual reality that contains only "token roots in the actual, domestic reality of the land beneath".

The fact that HIV/AIDS is increasingly seen as a security issue may further add to these stereotypical attitudes. While many commentators welcome new ways of conceptualizing global health issues (see Singer 2002: 145–8), others are growing concerned that framing HIV/AIDS through the language and practices of security may further extend monitoring and surveillance traditions that go back to eighteenth-century Europe. This is why Stefan Elbe (2005: 403–19) fears that unless the securitization of HIV/AIDS is approached with great caution, the ensuing modes of governance could easily generate new forms of orientalism and racism. Extending the logic of security to health could, for instance, legitimize numerous, rather problematic practices designed to control, and contain parts of the population deemed "unhealthy" and seen as a risk to the vital and thriving core of global society.

Confronting Suffering: Humanist Representations of HIV/AIDS

So far, we have portrayed a fairly grim picture, one that highlights how western stereotypes about Africa render the problem of HIV/AIDS more difficult than it already is. Photography plays an integral part in these neocolonial practices of domination. But this is not the end of the story. Photography can also play an important role in overcoming stereotypes, creating alternative images of HIV/AIDS, and thus new ways of understanding, discussing, and addressing the spread and impact of the disease. We begin our inquiry into these alternatives by focusing on humanist photography.

Humanist photography has a mission: it aims to use photography in the service of a human cause. Such photographic engagements emerged as a direct reaction against early naturalist tendencies to consider photographs as pieces of evidence, as authentic records that reflected a true image of the world. Humanist approaches, by contrast, stress that documentary photography can provide access to both facts and feelings. Lewis Hine (quoted in Beloff 1983: 171), one of the early proponents of this position, stressed that he "wanted to show things that had to be corrected". Photography can thus be used as a specific political tool, as a way of rallying public opinion in favor of a particular issue. We term this approach humanist because it contains key traits associated with humanism as it is broadly understood: a modern attempt to "replace God with man", that is, to reject the notion of a divine will in favor of a world where people take charge (Caroll 1993: 2). But humanism also created a specific understanding of agency and order, one that revolves around the search for certitude, one that sees humanity in absolute and often universal terms (see Doty 1996: 24, 125, Edkins 2005: 379).

Humanist photography is able to live up to many of humanism's key goals, most notably to the idea that human beings are able to shape their social and political environment. Few commentators would question that the reaction of the western world to human suffering in other countries is linked to the influence of key photographs on the formation of public opinion. Pictures of impoverished children, of villages devastated by natural disaster, or of people dying of AIDS-related illnesses are often circulated with the hope that an outpouring of humanitarian support will help those who are in need (Schwartz and Murray 1996: 1, Sankore 2005). Humanist photography has become an important aspect of what Michael Ignatieff (1998: 10) calls the new "internationalization of conscience". While the impact of photographs on public discourses is beyond doubt, the exact nature of this influence is far more difficult to assess. We now address this challenge by examining a widely circulated iconic HIV/AIDS photograph, taken in 1986 by Ed Hooper. Reprinted as Figure 10.1, this picture epitomizes the key ideas behind humanist photography. It depicts a Ugandan woman named Florence and her child, Ssengabi, sitting outside their home in Gwanda, Uganda.

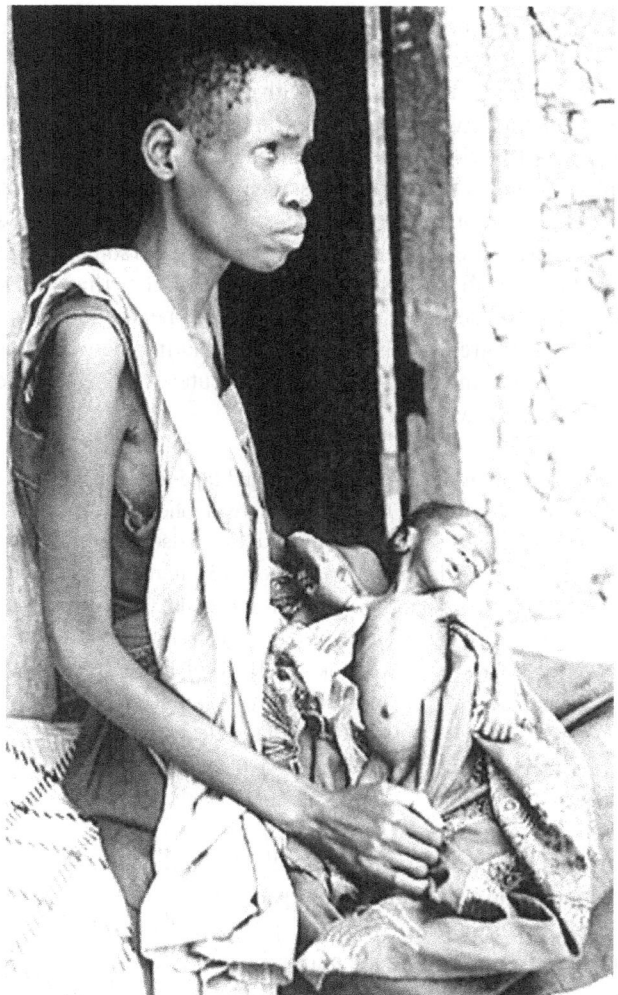

Figure 10.1 Florence and Ssengabi
Source: Hooper (1990).

Both Florence and Ssengabi were visibly ill. Taken during the early period of western public awareness about HIV/AIDS, the Hooper photograph provided a "face" that could symbolize the AIDS crisis in Africa. It was published widely in the international media, including Newsweek and the Washington Post. Florence died four weeks after the photograph was taken. Her baby Ssengabi died four months later. The photograph is very confronting in its direct visualization of illness, suffering, and death. It is part of a long tradition, deeply rooted in Christian art, of depicting the human body in pain. Some label this practice "demonic curiosity" (Friday 2000: 363). Some even compare it with pornography, for images of suffering and death expose in public a person's most intimate and vulnerable features (Dean 2003: 91–3, see also Scarry 1985, Sontag 2003: 41–42).

One of the most obvious problems associated with the Hooper photograph is the unequal power relationship between the photographer and his object. Any western photographer, no matter how well meant and sensitive his or her artistic and political engagement is, operates at a certain distance from poverty, conflict, and disaster. And there is, of course, an even greater distance between the viewers of the photographs and the content they convey. Making public a person's private suffering may well draw attention to the issue of HIV/AIDS, but perhaps only by compromising the dignity of those being photographed. Hooper's subsequent reflections reveal that he was aware of this dilemma, oscillating between his humanist desire to draw attention to the AIDS crisis and an acute awareness of the privileged position he occupied as a western photographer:

> I feel that we were right, that day in Kyebe, to use film and tape to record the brutal realities of Slim [HIV/AIDS]; for Florence had agreed, and in the end permission was surely hers to grant or withhold. Nevertheless, I also know that I participated in something of a media rape. For the next 15 minutes, barely containing... excitement... I photographed the mother and child from every angle, with every lens. Cameras clicked and whirred, pausing only for the changing of films... Some minutes later, we took our leave of Florence and her family... and I gave some money... On one level it was a simple gesture of assistance to people whom we had met... who were in a hopeless situation. On another... it was payment for taking the photographs... payment to help ease our consciences (Hooper 1990: 48–9).

Hooper's moral agonizing touches upon a range of political and ethical dilemmas. But above all, it underlines one key point: the privileged position of the photographer and the consequences that issue from this position. The photographer controls the action, from staging and framing the photograph to deciding about the appropriate compensation for the so-captured object. Hooper depicts HIV/AIDS not unlike Baudelaire's famous *flaneur* observed the contradictions and undersides of urban life in the late nineteenth century. Peeking out of his secure bourgeois existence, the *flaneur* voyeuristically strolls through the city's darker parts, thereby discovering its neglected and suffering population (see Sontag 1977: 55–6, Debrix 2003: xxxii–xxxvi). And just as the disturbed *flaneur* uses his gaze in the hope that it might engender social change, Hooper's photograph too was taken and reproduced largely in the context of a humanist engagement for positive change. But this does not deflect from the fact that the ensuing practices of representation are unequal, perhaps even exploitative. This is the case because the photographer, and the western press in general, have the privilege to frame, and thus politicize, another person's suffering.

Two main interrelated critiques have been raised against such forms of humanist photography: that it estheticizes suffering and that it leads to compassion fatigue. The former critique is epitomized through a prominent essay by Ingrid Sischy (1991: 92) about Sabastiaõ Salgado's beautiful and politically engaging photographs.

She found them problematic insofar as they "anesthetize" the viewer. "The beautification of tragedy", she stresses "results in pictures that ultimately reinforce our passivity toward the experiences they reveal". This passivity, some commentators assert, is reinforced by the very confronting nature of photographs like those by Hooper. Shock can only work for a limited period of time before its mesmerizing capacity loses sway. Even the most horrific image becomes banal when it is repeated ad infinitum. It may end up normalizing suffering, and thus rending the viewer numb and indifferent (Sontag 1977: 19–20, Dean 2003: 88). The result, some stress, is what Susan Moeller (1999) termed "compassion fatigue" or, as it might be called in the case of our specific topic, "AIDS fatigue".

We believe that both critiques are not warranted, at least not in an unqualified manner. But as the issues at stake are rather complex, and as they touch only marginally upon our main objective, we only draw brief attention here to some of the scholars who have provided counter-arguments. David Campbell (2004: 62), for instance, stresses that the compassion fatigue position cannot be sustained in an unqualified manner, not least because there is widespread evidence that the public often reacts generously when charity organizations appeal for help (see also Cohen and Seu 2002: 200). At a theoretical level, debates about the effects of estheticized suffering go back at least to Walter Benjamin's (1977: 168) concern that all attempts to "render politics esthetic" end up in war, or Theodor Adorno's (1955: 31) controversial remarks that it is impossible to write poetry after Auschwitz, that even the attempt to do so would be barbaric. But these remarks emerged in a very specific political context, that of fascist Germany. As general statements, they are, we believe, neither tenable nor, for that matter, compatible with Benjamin and Adorno's overall scholarly positions. Various authors, such as David Levi Strauss (2003: 9), have thus questioned the idea that an estheticized image is somehow politically less relevant or that beauty cannot be a call to action. Rather than dismissing esthetics as politically problematic per se, one should try to understand the nature and political consequences that are entailed in particular types of esthetic representations. Doing so is our task here, and we engage it now through a closer reading of the Hooper photograph.

The Political Consequences of Decontextualizing Suffering

The Hooper photograph gives us a very particular image of suffering. It depicts a dying mother and child, sitting alone in an open doorway somewhere in Africa. No other people are visible, nor are there any features that can be recognized as part of a particular society or culture. Hooper displays Florence and Ssengabi passively, as if they were unable to do anything but wait for death. They are seen in one function only, as sufferers. Indeed, Florence and Ssengabi are entirely defined by their suffering. But this was, of course, not their only identity, even though they were facing immanent death. One could have just as well presented them in different ways, as being integrated in their surroundings, or as pursuing an activity. But the Hooper photograph is an attempt to capture the universal nature of death, stripped free of culture and context. As a result, it shows an image of passive victims, void of agency, history, belonging, or social attachment.

The decontextualized and universalized nature of Hooper's humanist photograph becomes, not surprisingly, further reinforced by its subsequent usage in western media sources. The photograph was published in leading western media outlets, including Newsweek and the Washington Post Journal of Health. The former used the picture with a generic caption that read: "Two Victims: Ugandan Barmaid and Son" (Nordland, Wilkinson and Marshall 1986: 44). The names of the victims are already lost, having been replaced with more generic terms of "victim" and "Ugandan". Florence is, furthermore, framed pejoratively as an anonymous barmaid.

The Washington Post story does mention the names and ages of Florence and Ssengabi. It does so in the caption accompanying the photograph. Given its shocking nature, the photograph stays in the reader's mind, but the corresponding article never mentions Florence and Ssengabi again. We never hear what Florence has to say about her situation. We only see a snapshot of her suffering and that of her baby, and even this picture is framed by someone, as Hooper (1990: 47–50) himself acknowledges, who barely knows her and her family. Further, the Washington Post story appeared two years after the Newsweek story but used the same photograph, rendering its use even more generic and universal.

As reproduced in the western press, the Hooper photograph was meant to shock readers and draw their attention to the urgency of an issue. It was meant to "hook" them, not only to shocking AIDS images but also to a particular consumer product: a newspaper or magazine that operates according to profit-seeking principles of market economics. That in itself would not necessarily hinder representational sensitivity, but due to the lack of context provided by Newsweek and other media sources, the Hooper photograph soon turned into a symbol, an archetype used years after it was first taken. And from there, it is only a short step to stereotypes. This is, we believe, the most characteristic and also the most problematic aspect of Hooper's humanist photograph: its attempt to capture a generic image of AIDS, a universalized and decontextualized notion of human suffering. We are left with an increasingly fixed image, frozen in time and place, inevitably feeding into stereotypical images of Africa we have already identified in detail earlier in the chapter: a dark and homogenous continent, populated by passive victims stripped of either voice or agency. Although the Hooper photograph is meant precisely to escape from this doomsday scenario, its generic nature paradoxically feeds into the same problematic tradition. It also evokes a long photographic tradition, epitomized by National Geographic, which has represented Africa through typical orientalist images of "dark-skinned, bare-breasted women, in their customary dress, looking at the camera without awareness of their impending status as spectacles of adolescent Western eyes" (Grundberg 1990: 173). Although corresponding reporting practices have become more sensitive, many of its key features remain intact, as demonstrated by recent issues of National Geographic on "Living with AIDS" (September 2005) and Time on "Global Health" (November 2005). Even the shocking nature of an AIDS photograph is not enough to break through such stereotypes. Sontag (2004: 23) even believes that the opposite may be the case, for "the image as shock and the image as cliché are two aspects of the same presence".

Several consequences emerge from the decontextualized nature of humanist photography. The basic idea behind this approach, as already stressed, is to generate compassion in viewers, which, in turn, ought to engender social change. But the universal nature of humanist photography is unlikely to generate compassion, at least if we define compassion as Hanna Arendt (1990) does: as sentiments that are directed toward particular individuals. Humanist photography is more likely to inspire what Arendt calls pity, a more abstract and generalized form of politics.

In a compelling application of Arendt's typology, Luc Boltanski (1999: 4) stresses how a politics of pity views the unfortunate collectively, even though it relies on singling out particular misfortunes to inspire pity in the first place. It is evident that the ensuing dynamics entail a fundamental dilemma, one that perhaps cannot be solved. A generalized portrayal of HIV/AIDS as a political problem is unlikely to inspire pity. Statistical data, for instance, cannot do this, no matter how much evidence it provides of the devastating impact of the disease. To arouse pity, Boltanski (1999: 11) stresses, "suffering and wretched bodies must be conveyed in such a way as to affect the sensibility of those more fortunate". That is the function of the Hooper photograph. But problems arise as soon as this image is used to establish and defend a more generic political stance. This is the case, for instance, when the Hooper photograph is being used to draw public awareness in the West about the general problem of HIV/AIDS in Africa. The image of suffering then inevitably becomes detached from both the sufferer and local circumstances.

Manifestations of pity often mask unequal power relations. It was precisely in the seemingly selfless Christian practices of pity that Nietzsche (1991: 947) detected a will to power, a thirst for triumph, a desire to subjugate. Pity then becomes linked to several features that fundamentally contradict the original humanist desire for social change. Images of suffering in Africa subconsciously contain a range of moral judgments and sentiments, including resentment and fear (see Sontag 2003: 75). They may also remind western audiences of what they are free from. Paradoxically, the very disturbing nature of the Hooper photograph thus provides a certain feeling of safety and security to some of those viewing it. Death in a distant and dangerous elsewhere can then become a way of affirming life in the safe here and now, giving people a sense of belonging to a particular group that is distinct from others (Biehl 2001: 139, Radley 2002: 2, see also Nussbaum 2001: 297–454 for a more general discussion of pity and its distinctiveness from compassion, sympathy, and empathy).

Local Representation through Pluralist Photography

Despite the humanist aspiration to change the world for the better, we are, then, back to a more pessimistic interpretation of photography and its ability to engage political dilemmas. Or are we? Not necessarily, for photography has the potential to break through stereotypes. It may even be able to engender compassion, rather than mere pity.

To scrutinize this potential, we now examine what we call pluralist photography. Just as humanist approaches do, pluralist ones oppose the naturalist belief that photographs are authentic and value-free representations of the world. Photography is seen in the context of sociopolitical practices. And it is endowed with the explicit mission to shape these practices actively. But as opposed to humanist photography, pluralist approaches do not aim to capture a generic and universal notion of suffering. Photography is, instead, seen as a method to validate multiple local knowledge and practices, thereby disrupting existing hierarchies and power relationships – as for instance the ability of western photographers and media representations to frame the suffering of others. The basic idea behind this approach is to provide people affected by HIV/AIDS with the power to decide for themselves what kind of information and representation is most appropriate to capture the social, political, ethical, and psychological challenges they face. The ideal result of this practice is a form of dialog that opens up spaces for communities to work through the problems that confront them. Photography would then facilitate what Debrix and Weber (Debrix 2003: ix) called a ritual of pluralization: a practice of mediation whereby the represented person takes an active role in the process of inscribing social meaning, but does so without attaching to it an exclusive claim that silences other positions and experiences. Our engagement with such pluralist photographic practices is strongly shaped by and indebted to the work of William Connolly (1995, 2005), even though we refrain from drawing specific linkages to his conceptual elaborations on pluralism.

We examine the potential and limits of pluralist photography by focusing on a project initiated by documentary photographer Eric Gottesman. Between November 2003 and March 2004, Gottesman (2003) worked on a photography project in Ethiopia, collaborating with HIV/AIDS-affected children in a particular neighborhood of Addis Ababa, in kebele 15. Participation in the project, which has continued since then in different forms, was voluntary. It was coordinated through a local NGO, Hope for Children. It took place in a country with the second highest population of HIV/AIDS orphans in the world. Some 720,000 children have been orphaned as a result of HIV/AIDS-related deaths or stigma. About 200,000 of them live with HIV/AIDS, many of them in the streets of Addis Ababa (USAID 2003: 19–23; UNICEF 2004: 26).

The objective of the Addis Ababa project was, in part, to place cameras in the hands of children affected by HIV/AIDS, giving them a tool to represent what it means to live with the disease in a community where HIV infection rates and HIV/AIDS-related stigma are high. This practice includes providing a medium and space to share stories and visions, rather than giving this authority away to a professional photographer whose products are then reproduced to fit media priorities and pre-existing narratives of Africa. Gottesman's project is based on a method pioneered by photographer Wendy Ewald, who worked with children in different contexts, from inner cities in the United States to small towns in Columbia and rural areas in India and Mexico. Ewald's understanding of photography evolved as she worked with students in different places. It began with the idea of sharing the camera with children but then moved into situations where children took charge and created images themselves (Ewald 1998: 1–3). These approaches are part of a larger set of development communication methods designed to promote multidimensional and dialogic ways of representing and engaging communities. They are meant to replace centralized, professionalized, and consumer-oriented communication practices, which tend to silence many people, particularly those who live at the margins of society. Pluralist photography is part of an alternative, more democratizing means of representation that seeks to create space for diverse and localized ways of communicating meaning (see Servaes 1986: 211–215).

Children involved in the Addis Ababa program were taught how to use the cameras themselves. On some occasions digital cameras were used, but in most cases the technology was as simple as possible, consisting of Polaroid Propack cameras that automatically produced a black and white photograph with negatives attached. Some of the so-taken photographs deteriorated relatively quickly, as is evident with some of the pictures represented here. But the method also has several advantages, including providing the young photographers with control over what was destroyed or kept for further use.

Pluralist local photography begins before any photograph is actually taken. It seeks to facilitate understanding of photographic representations and the type of values and power relations embedded in them. The children who participated in the project met each week with Gottesman, either on a one-to-one basis, or in a group. They were encouraged to develop their own methods of photography, so that they could tell their unique stories from their own, unique angle. Crucial to this process were preliminary discussions about the methods that would be used to represent their lives and those they loved and also lost. This included using photography to document not only the present but also the past. In one class, students were asked to reconstruct the history of their own parents who had died of AIDS – parents who often died before the children could get to know them. Thus, this process required using methods of photography to merge fact, fiction, and feeling into a composition that recovered and represented what had been lost in a parent's untimely death. Gottesman stresses that everyone involved was aware that they took decisions, and that these decisions affected the ways in which photographs represented them and their surroundings. This form of collaboration, he believes, is rather different from traditional photographic portrayals of developing countries as seen in National Geographic and other magazines. Both Gottesman and Ewald learned from their work that photographs taken by children are often more complex than the reality that professional representations usually assign to their experiences.

We now focus on the work of Tenanesh Kifyalew, a 12-year-old girl who was living with HIV/AIDS and participated in the Addis Ababa project. Tenanesh means "she is health" in Amharic. She was named by her grandmother who, after her daughter had died of AIDS, refused to believe the doctor when he diagnosed her granddaughter with HIV. Tenanesh agreed to work with Gottesman while living with AIDS-related illnesses that often drained her energy. Like Florence and Ssengabi, Tenanesh died shortly after the photographs by and of her were created.

Tenanesh took over 100 photographs, mostly in her home, where she spent much of her time confined by her illness. She either took the photographs herself or asked others to take photographs of her in particular situations. The impressions that these photographs convey are very different from the ones evoked by Hooper's picture of Florence and Ssengabi. Tenanesh's self-portrayal of what it means to live with HIV/AIDS is not nearly as dramatic, not nearly as shocking as Hooper's representation. When analyzing Tenanesh's photographs, we found two types of pictures, each of them differing markedly from humanist photography. In the first type Tenanesh represented her illness; in the second she portrayed her daily life. Images of the first type, are represented by Figures 10.2 and 10.3.

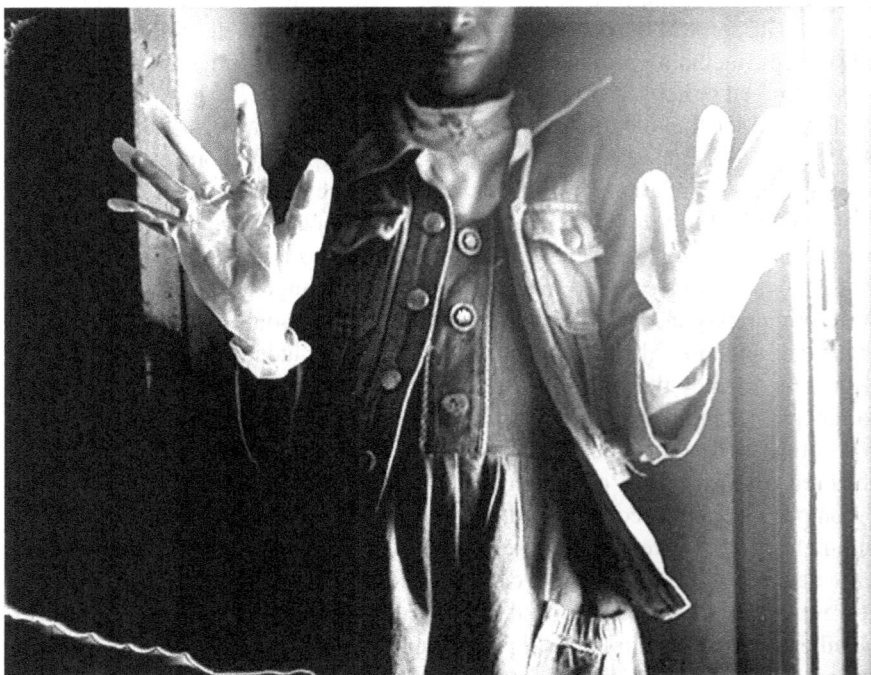

Figure 10.2 Tenanesh Kifyalew, "Untitled"

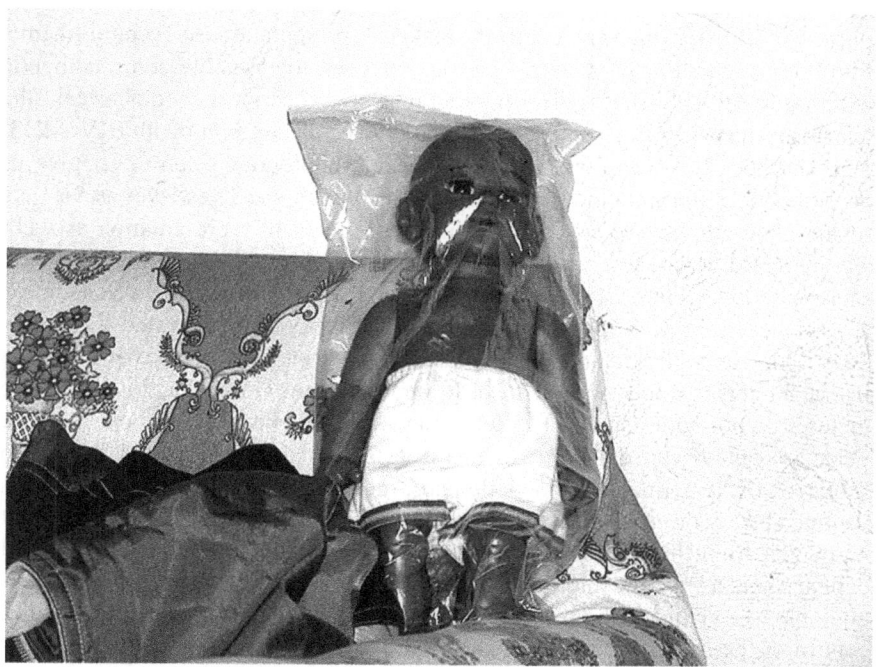

Figure 10.3 Tenanesh Kifyalew, "Untitled"

We consciously resist the temptation to over-interpret Tenanesh's photographs. We do so in order to offer a form of commentary that illuminates the issues at stake but then refers authority back to the photographs themselves (see Heidegger 1981: 194). It would have been tempting indeed to speculate what the rubber-gloved hands exactly signify, or how the quasi-cling-wrapped doll may express a sense of suffocation or fear of the outside world. But the death of the photographer – in this case unfortunately not only metaphorical but also real – is as paramount a phenomenon as the much-discussed death of the author. We cannot know what Tenanesh intended to represent when she took the photographs, nor does it matter. She does not retain any control over how viewers subsequently see the photographs.

In order to leave the process of interpretation open to the reader and viewer, we only highlight how Tenanesh captures the nature of living with HIV/AIDS through a conscious process of abstraction. But the nature of Tenanesh's abstraction is fundamentally different from that of Hooper's. The humanist photographs of the latter contained elements of naturalism insofar as they sought to depict an authentic external reality: the "real" face HIV/AIDS as epitomized by a representative single person living with HIV/AIDS. A very particular image is frozen to then produce generalities from it. The process of representation and abstraction is masked by the shocking "reality" of the image. Tenanesh's portrayal of suffering, by contrast, makes representation its central theme. She does not take a photograph that is supposed to resemble some authentic external image of suffering. Her photographs are much more metaphorical. She addresses the psychological and emotional dimensions of living with HIV/AIDS. And she does so by explicitly recognizing that photographs can never give us an authentic representation of the realities in which she lives. We, as viewers of the photographs, are confronted with the process of representation as well: we are asked to imagine what it means for her to face HIV/AIDS. As a result, representation becomes a site of politics, open to interpretation and debate.

The second type of photograph that Tenanesh took is illustrated in Figures 10.4–10.6. Here, her pictures do not represent suffering. They place her existence in a larger personal and social context. As opposed to the Hooper photograph, these pictures do not portray a decontextualized world of darkness and gloom. Instead, Tenanesh captures the dailyness of her life, its ups and downs, her determination to lead a relatively normal childhood. Perhaps, she does so precisely because she was confined by her disease, unable to attend school, or go outside for long. We cannot know that from the photographs alone. But we see a certain defiance, a playful defiance, and a way of demonstrating that she has not lost her agency. Tenanesh is not a passive victim in the way Hooper portrays Florence and Ssengabi. She has control of the camera, and with it she shows that she has some control over her

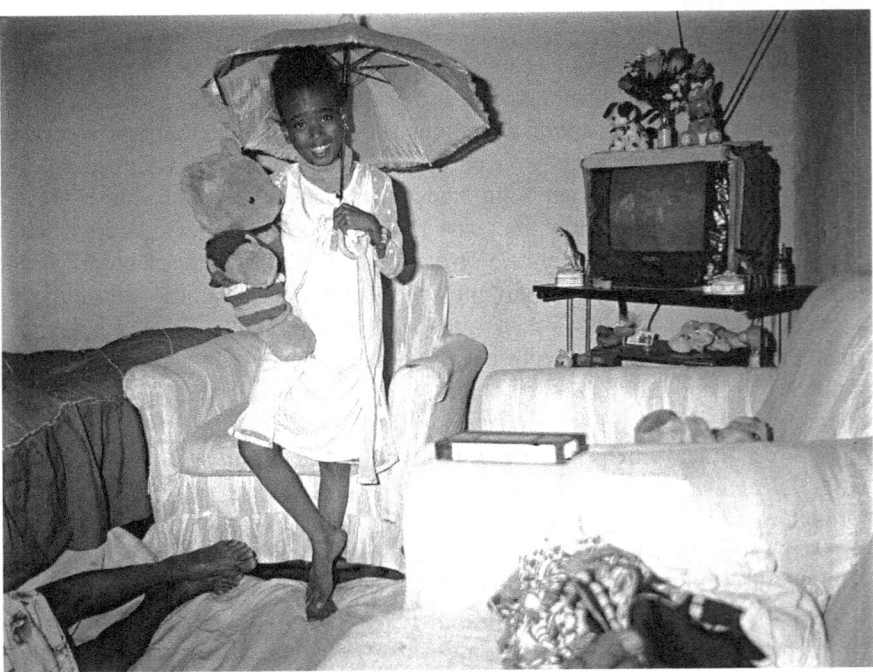

Figure 10.4 "My Favorite Things"

surroundings too. As opposed to Florence and Ssengabi, Tenanesh's identity is not reduced to that of a sufferer alone. She is also a child, a Christian, a member of a family, part of a social community. We are inevitably confronted with the life of a single person, rather than an abstract image of a disease.

If Tenanesh's photographs shock, then it is not because we are graphically confronted with the agony of dying from AIDS-related illnesses. The pictures surprise because they portray Tenanesh living a seemingly normal, even vibrant childhood in the face of death. In a sense, her photographs symbolize a shift away from portrayals of people "dying of AIDS", which were particularly dominant in the early days of the pandemic (see Watney 1990: 173–192, Nixon and Nixon 1991) toward an attempt to show people "living with AIDS" (see Mendel 2006: 42–51). Figures 10.4 and 10.5, for instance, depict Tenanesh in her surroundings. In Figure 10.6, she photographs some of her family members. These pictures do not fit into a preconceived image of what it means to be living with and dying of AIDS in Africa. Western viewers cannot easily create a safe distance from these pictures by reassuring themselves that the life portrayed in them takes place in some far off, dangerous continent. The daily objects Tenanesh chooses as symbols to represent her life are uniquely personal and universal at the same time. From the teddy bear and the television set to pictures of Jesus, they suggest her attachment to "favorite things". They also capture her faith in the divine. Although such images can evoke shared experiences around the world, they do so without generating a generic picture of "AIDS in Africa". Tenanesh's unique environment is presented as an essential element of who she is and what it means to be affected by HIV/AIDS. It is thus much less likely that such context-specific pictures can feed into a pre-existing neo-colonial image of Africa as a dark continent, caught in a web of gloom and doom, populated entirely by helpless victims.

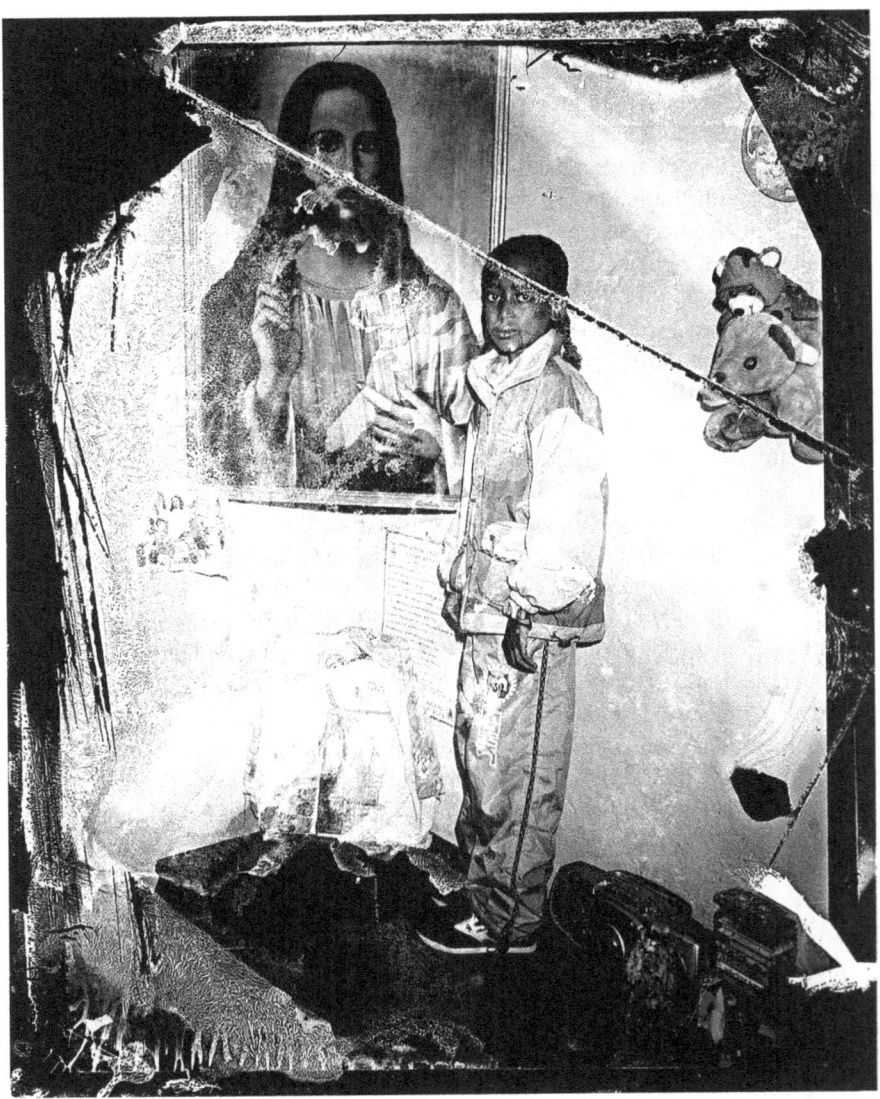

Figure 10.5 Tenanesh Kifyalew, "Untitled"

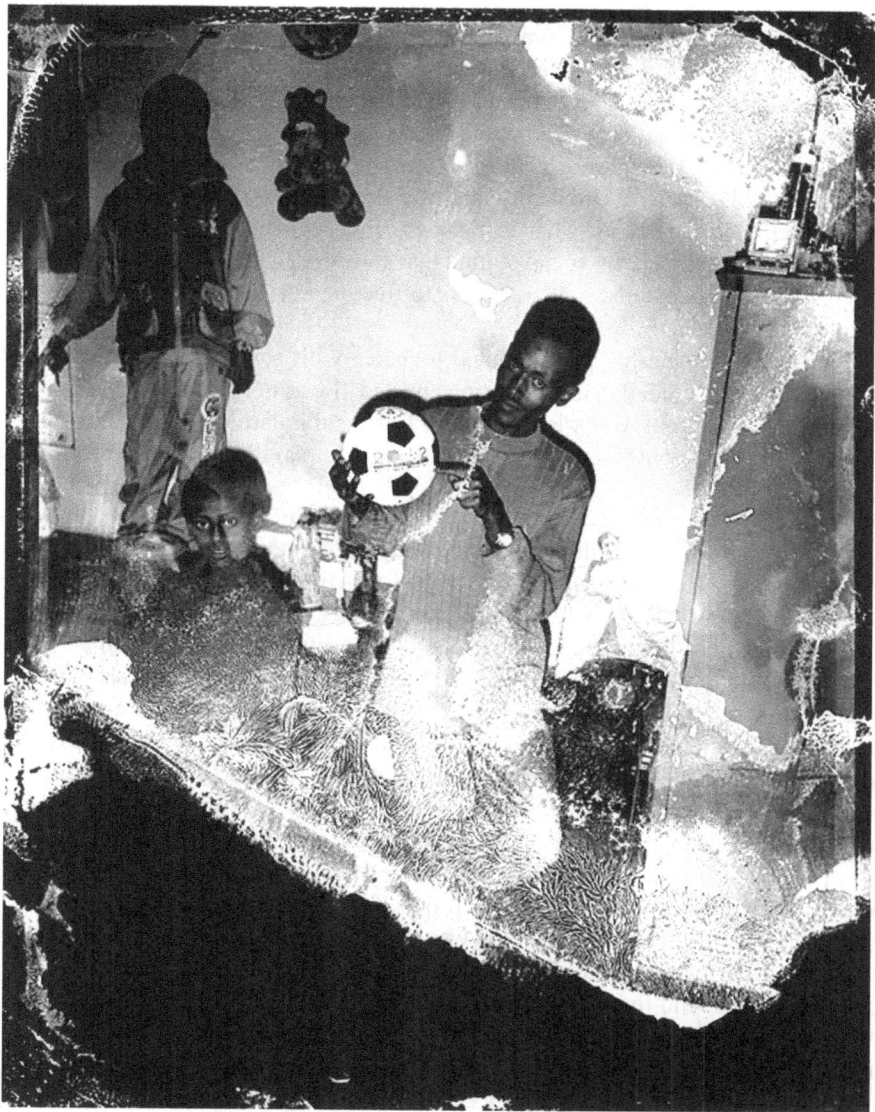

Figure 10.6 Tenanesh Kifyalew, "Untitled"

Pluralist Photography and Community Dialog

The practices of displaying pluralist photography are as novel as their composition. Tenanesh's photographs were an integral element of her activism. She used her remaining life to become an outspoken advocate for a movement called People Living with HIV (PLWHA). She advocated the use of life-prolonging drugs, such as antiretrovirals, which were available only to a very small minority of people living with HIV in Ethiopia. Tenanesh spoke to thousands of people at public gatherings and eventually became an Ambassador for UNESCO on behalf of HIV/AIDS affected children. She wrote letters and postcards in which she made her claims public. They were addressed, among others, to Ethiopians abroad, students at Addis Ababa University, and the President of the United States. In these letters, she described what it meant to live with HIV/AIDS, telling, for instance, how she faced the social stigma that surrounded her. She also advanced specific political demands, such as access to free medical assistance for children affected by HIV/AIDS.

Sixteen of Tenanesh's photographs, together with some of her letters and postcards, were included in an exhibition entitled "I was not a child when I was a child" (translated from Amharic). Tenanesh's original Polaroid photographs were scanned and then printed at a local advertising company that had a large-scale printer.

During the month of March 2004, the exhibition, which also featured photographs by 14 other children, traveled to 21 different kebeles in Kifle Ketema Subcity, as well 156 Representing HIV/AIDS in Africa as to City Hall in Addis Ababa (Figure 10.7). Just as Tenanesh's photographs were created as a result of a dialog, the exhibition too made dialog one of its central themes. As members of a community, viewers were asked to add letters and pictures to Tenanesh's work, thus creating a verbal and visual dialog that became an essential and constantly changing part of the exhibition. The idea that spectators are not just passive consumers but active contributors to the work of art is, of course, not new. It goes back at least to Marcel Duchamp and is practiced today by a range of prominent artists, such as Rirkrit Tiravanija (see Tomkins 2005: 82–95). By embracing such an approach, the Addis Ababa exhibition promoted new forms of discussion about what it means to live with HIV/AIDS. It thus provided a creative and safe space for dialog. The idea behind this dialog was to break through some of the silences, taboos, and stigma that characterize HIV/AIDS in a city where almost everyone knows someone who lives with or has died of the illness. The objective was thus very practical: to influence the conditions under which people live with HIV/AIDS and to find more appropriate ways of stemming the spread of the disease and related stigma. This is why, for instance, the Addis Ababa exhibition also provided information about local organizations that are engaged in dealing with the increase in HIV infections and the impact of HIV/AIDS.

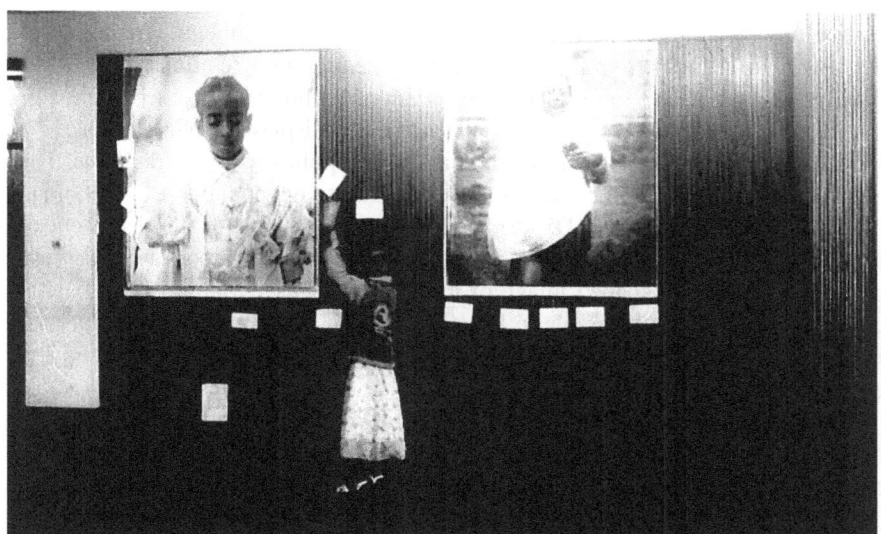

Figure 10.7 Tenanesh Kifyalew, Preparing the Exhibition

The Addis Ababa exhibition told multiple stories about HIV/AIDS in the context of a unique local environment. By refusing to uphold one correct way of portraying the issues at stake, the exhibition drew attention to the political nature of representation. Such communication practices are, of course, rather different from those represented through the iconic images of humanist photography, where the flow of information is controlled, hierarchical, and works in only one direction.

While we believe that pluralist photography has the potential to challenge some of the taboos and stigmas that shroud HIV/AIDS, it is important not to idealize this form of representation. Two particular limitations stand out.

First: just as any other photographic approach, the type of image that pluralist photography projects is neither authentic nor, for that matter, void of power relations. From Tenanesh's photographs alone, we do not know what her life is like, at least not entirely. We still have only snapshots of particular moments and situations. Add to this that she was integrated in a photography project that was shaped by western assumptions about representation. Gottesman provided not only the cameras needed for the project but also the know-how. He instructed the children involved in the project about the use of cameras and the different possibilities of capturing images with them. Although Gottesman was careful to teach the children how to make their own representational choices, his esthetic influence cannot be extricated from the project. The same is the case with the subsequent exhibition, which was only possible as a result of Gottesman's know-how and funding from a variety of sources, including UNICEF and the Ethiopian HIV/AIDS Prevention and Control Office. Funding does, of course, always come with constraints, either explicit or implicit ones. Gottesman retained some editing authority about the display at the exhibition, even though Tenanesh was actively involved in it from the beginning to the end. Power relations would have been present even had the project been organized without western influence or participation. For better or for worse, taking and displaying photographs is a form of representation, and thus open to a range of political uses and abuses. The Addis Ababa exhibition, for instance, focused exclusively on the fate of Ethiopian children affected by HIV/AIDS. It did so, some would say, to the detriment of drawing attention to the affected adult population, thereby portraying a very particular, politically shaped image of the issues at stake. Many of the societal groups that are most vulnerable to HIV/AIDS, such as commercial sex workers, intravenous drug users or men who have sex with men, remain marginalized and even criminalized.

Human relations cannot exist outside power. But the nature of pluralist photography minimizes the oppressive effects of these relations by consciously problematizing representation. The collaborative and dialogical nature of pluralist photography can provide ways through which multiple perspectives may be seen and validated. By undermining the authority of professional photographers and commercialized organizations to tell the truth about HIV/AIDS, pluralist photography retains the ability to step out of pre-existing narratives and to surprise the expectation of the viewer/reader.

Second: the sociopolitical impact of pluralist photography can only be partial and gradual. As opposed to iconic humanist photographs, pluralist versions are less likely to be used by global media networks as symbols representing a particular issue. They cannot appeal to the same mass audience. But this does not mean that pluralist photography is void of social impact. The Addis Ababa exhibition may not on its own have transformed the situation in Ethiopia, where stigma, myths, misinformation and silence continue to surround HIV/AIDS and related issues of sexuality and health behavior. But the exhibition is part of a larger, ongoing effort to change the way people think about themselves and their surroundings. It reached some viewers who, in turn, may influence others through their experience. The exhibition was also part of an effort to convince the Ethiopian government of the need to make antiretrovirals available to the population. This has already started to happen, with the introduction of a first, although limited program aimed at supporting some 30,000 affected people (Thibodeaux 2005).

At times pluralist photographs may even have an impact beyond their local setting. The Addis Ababa project, for instance, reached an audience wider than the *kebele*, even though the mechanisms of diffusion were neither instant nor global. Ethiopian national television covered the exhibition in what were the country's first televised pictures of people living with HIV. In a society where one in six people are infected with HIV, this was an important and long-overdue step (see Hope for Children 2003: 2). The actual video images were provided by the children who participated in the exhibition. Versions of the exhibition also traveled to the United States and Australia. The exhibit changed as it traveled on, engaging new audiences and retaining its interactive and dialogical nature in an attempt to bring the children of *kebele* 15 in contact with western audiences. Even more opportunities would 158 Representing HIV/AIDS in Africa and will exist through the Internet, which is not only global, but pluralist itself. It may thus be particularly suited to diffuse pluralist photography.

Conclusion

In the 20 years since the recognition of HIV/AIDS as a pandemic, the disease has become a global challenge. This challenge is not only of a medical nature but also involves various political, social, and psychological factors. The lives of those who are infected or affected by HIV/AIDS have come to be decisively shaped by how we represent what it means to live with the disease. This is particularly the case in acutely affected African communities, where HIV/AIDS has taken its greatest toll. As in many parts of the world, people here live with a condition that is shrouded in silence, taboos, and stigma. The resulting practices of representation not only marginalize and oppress people affected, but also fuel the spread of the disease.

In this chapter, we have examined how photographic representations either contribute to or break with stereotypical portrayals of HIV/AIDS. We began by discussing naturalist positions, which view photographs as authentic representations of external realities. Various problems emerge from such assumptions. When photographs are accepted as unquestioned factual representations, our eyes become passive instruments, rather than tools for broadening vision and understanding. We forget that the photograph was framed by a particular person, who made a range of esthetic and inherently subjective choices in this process. We have thus explored two approaches that use photography as an active catalyst for social change. Both acknowledge that photographs cannot portray the world as it is, that they always involve both facts and feelings. Humanist engagements seek to use iconic photographs as a way of visualizing the devastating aspects that can be a part of the reality of HIV/AIDS, hoping that the so-generated feeling of shock in western viewers would serve as a catalyst for social and political change. Pluralist photography, by contrast, is more concerned with finding ways through which people can express the multiple and often local manifestations of what it means to live with HIV/AIDS. Such forms of representation can open up possibilities for a democratic and constructive public dialog.

We examined humanist photography by interpreting one of the most influential iconic HIV/AIDS photographs; Ed Hooper's portrayal of a dying Ugandan woman and her child. The process here revolves around a western photographer being in control of virtually all esthetic and political choices involved in the process of representation. The object of the photograph, in this case Florence and her child, Ssengabi, are objects indeed. They are deprived of voice and agency – a loss that is further exacerbated by the manner in which iconic photographs are then used in global mass media. The result is a symbolic representation of HIV/AIDS, one that may shock western viewers and evoke pity in them. But this shock comes at the expense of understanding the complexities of the local and personal situation. A symbolic representation of a person dying of AIDS-related illnesses can easily turn into an archetype, which feeds into deeply entrenched stereotypical images of Africa as a dark and homogenous continent, populated by nameless victims who are helplessly exposed to a never-ending series of crises. Suffering, then, becomes idealized and stigmatized at the same time – a combination that is particularly fateful with regard to a disease like HIV/AIDS, which is already surrounded by a range of prejudices and taboos. Gazing at the suffering of others in far off places may also become no more than a way of affirming the safety of the here and now, thus undermining the very humanist aspirations for social change that have inspired the respective photographic engagements in the first place. There are alternatives to iconic humanist photography. These alternatives are of a more pluralist nature, consisting of attempts to open up spaces for people living with HIV/AIDS to decide for themselves how they would like to be represented, and how these representations should be used. Trying to understand the potential and limits of such approaches, we have examined Eric Gottesman's collaborative approach with HIV/AIDS-affected children in a community of Addis Ababa. Here, we see very different images of what it means to live with HIV/AIDS. We do not see victims stripped of voice and representational authority. Instead, each child finds her or his own way of representing life with a stigmatized disease. In the photographs we analyzed, for instance, we saw a 12-year-old girl, Tenanesh, trying to capture her unique struggle and her normal daily routine of living with HIV/AIDS. The Addis Ababa project alone will not change the global image of HIV/AIDS, but it has empowered those who participated in it, giving them the opportunity to express their own visions of what HIV/AIDS means, using collaborative and dialogical means to do so. And, perhaps more importantly, it is part of a broader, long-term, and much-needed process of finding more diverse and appropriate ways of representing what it means to live with HIV/AIDS.

Pluralist approaches offer a viable alternative to naturalist and humanist photography. This is not to say that they are without problems. As any other form of photographic representation, pluralist approaches too are always open to political interpretation and appropriation, for better or worse. But because pluralist photography refuses to universalize suffering it is less likely to lead to stereotypical representations. Particularly when embedded in community projects that promote dialog, pluralist photography – perhaps more so than any other photographic practice – has the potential to challenge some of the deeply entrenched and highly problematic taboos and stigmas that are associated with HIV/AIDS. Or so suggests the type of interpretative research and analysis we have conducted for this chapter. Whether or not our results can be confirmed by empirical evidence remains to be seen. Doing so is no easy task, for, as Stanley Cohen and Bruna Seu (2002: 188) stress, "far more is known about the space between the pristine object – the tortured body, the massacred corpses, the homeless refugee – and its public representation than the space between the resultant image and its public perception". The exact impact of pluralist photography on sociopolitical practices remains to be investigated, and it can be done only through carefully designed case studies. But such studies are only possible once we have more systematic insight into the representative practices that characterize our knowledge of and political attitudes toward HIV/AIDS. Contributing to this process has been the main objective of our chapter, and we hope that by doing so we have taken a modest step toward dismantling some of the stigma and discrimination that continues to shape the impact of HIV/AIDS.

References

Adorno, T.W. 1955. *Prismen: Kulturkritik und Gesellschaft*. Frankfurt: Suhrkamp.

Annan, K, Gordimer, N. and Kennedy. R. 2003. *Pandemic: Facing AIDS*. New York: Umbrage.

Apthorpe, R. 2001. Mission Possible: Six Years of WFP Emergency Food Aid in West Africa, in *Evaluating International Humanitarian Action: Reflections from Practitioners*, edited by A. Wood, R. Apthorpe and J. Borton. London: Zed Books, 102–121.

Arendt, H. 1990. *On Revolution*. Harmondsworth: Penguin Books.

Bancroft, A. 2001. Globalisation and HIV/AIDS: Inequality and the Boundaries of a Symbolic Epidemic. *Health, Risk and Society* 3(1): 89–98.

Barthes, R. 1977. The Photographic Message, in *Image, Music, Text*, edited by S. Heath. London: Fontana Press.

Beloff, H. 1983. Social Interaction in Photographing. *Leonardo* 16(3): 165–171.

Benjamin, W. 1977. Das Kunstwerk im Zeitalter seiner technischen Reproduzierbarkeit, in *Illuminationen: Ausgewa"hlte Schriften 1*, edited by S. Unseld. Frankfurt: Suhrkamp, 136–169.

Berger, J. 1977. *Ways of Seeing*. London: Penguin.

Berger, J. 1980. Uses Of Photography, in *About Looking*, edited by J. Berger. New York: Vintage.

Bhattacharya, S., Gulan, K., Pramod, K., and Sharma, M. 2005. Arts and Media Transforming the Response to HIV/AIDS Strategy Note and Implementation Guide. New York: UNDP.

Biehl, J. 2001. Life in a Zone of Social Abandonment. *Social Text* 68 19(3): 131–149.

Boltanski, L. 1999. *Distant Suffering, Morality, Media and Politics*, trans. by Graham Burchell. Cambridge: Cambridge University Press.

Campbell, D. 2003a. Salgado and the Sahel: Documentary Photography and the Imaging of Famine, in *Rituals of Mediation: International Politics and Social Meaning*, edited by F. Debrix and C. Weber. Minneapolis: University of Minnesota Press, 69–96.

Campbell, D. 2003b. Cultural Governance and Pictorial Resistance: Reflections on the Imaging of War. *Review of International Studies* 29: 57–73.

Campbell, D. 2004. Horrific Blindness: Images of Death in Contemporary Media. *Journal of Cultural Research* 8(1): 55–74.

Caroll, J. 1993. *Humanism: The Wreck of Western Culture*. London: Fontana Press.

Cohen, S. and Seu, B. 2002. Knowing Enough Not to Feel Too Much: Emotional Thinking about Human Rights Appeals, in *Truth Claims: Representation and Human Rights*, edited by M.P. Bradley and P. Petro. New Brunswick: Rutgers University Press, 187–203.

Connolly, W.E. 1995. *The Ethos of Pluralization*. Minneapolis: University of Minnesota Press.

Connolly, W.E. 2005. *Pluralism*. Durham: Duke University Press.

Crimp, D. 2002. *Melancholia and Moralism: Essays on HIV/AIDS and Queer Politics*. Cambridge: MIT Press.

Dean, C.J. 2003. Empathy, Pornography and Suffering. *Differences: A Journal of Feminist Cultural Studies* 14(1): 88–124.

Debord, G. 1992. *La Société du Spectacle*. Paris: Gallimard.

Debrix, F. 2003. Rituals of Mediation, in *Rituals of Mediation: International Politics and Social Meaning*, edited by F. Debrix and C. Weber. Minneapolis: University of Minnesota Press, xxi-xvii.

Desantis, D. 2003. HIV Prevention and Protection Efforts Are Failing Women and Girls. UNAIDS: The Global Coalition on Women and AIDS. Available at: www.unaids.org [accessed May 2004].

Doty, R.L. 1996. *Imperial Encounters: The Politics of Representation in North-South Relations*. Minneapolis: University of Minnesota Press.

Edkins, J. 2005. Exposed Singularity. *Journal for Cultural Research* 9(4): 359–386.

Elbe, S. 2005. AIDS, Security, Biopolitics. *International Relations* 19(4): 403–419.

Elwood, W.N. (ed.) 1999. *Power in the Blood: A Handbook on AIDS, Politics, and Communication*. London: Lawrence Erlbaum Associates.

Ewald, W. 1998. Innocent Eye, Conversation with Wendy Ewald. Available at: http://globetrotter.berkeley.edu/Ewald/ewald-con4.html [accessed February 2004].

Fleury, J. 2004. Development Journalism or Just Good Journalism. Available at: www.bbcworldservice.com [accessed 1 May 2005].

Freedman, J., and Poku, N. 2005. The Socioeconomic Context of Africa's Vulnerability to HIV/AIDS. *Review of International Studies* 31(4): 665–686.

Friday, J. 2000. Demonic Curiosity and the Aesthetics of Documentary Photography. *British Journal of Aesthetics* 40(5): 356–375.

Gottesman, E. 2003. Project Proposal, Hope for Children [E-mail document from Eric Gottesman, July 2003].

Grundberg, A. 1990. *Crisis of the Real: Writings on Photography*. New York: Aperture.

Hall, S. 1997. *Representation: Cultural Representations and Signifying Practices*. London: SAGE Publications.

Heidegger, M. 1981. *Erla"uterungen zu Ho"lderlins Dichtung.* Frankfurt: Klostermann.

Higgins, N. 2001. Image and Identity: Mexican Indians and Photographic Art. *Social Alternatives* 20(4): 22–36.

Hilts, P.J. 1988. Out of Africa: Dispelling Myths about AIDS: Origins, Values, Politics. *Washington Post*, May 24.

Hope For Children. (2003) Annual Report 2003. Addis Ababa: HFC.

Hooper, E. 1990. *Slim: A Reporter's Own Story of HIV/AIDS in East Africa.* London: The Bodley Head.

Ignatieff, M. 1998. *The Warrior's Honor: Ethnic War and the Modern Conscience.* London: Chatto & Windus.

Kean, F. 1998. Another Picture of Starving Africa: It Could Have Been Taken in 1984, or 1998. *Guardian Media Supplement*, June 8.

McNeill, W. 1998. *Plagues and Peoples.* New York: Anchor Books.

Mendel, G. 2006. Looking AIDS in the Face: An Activist Photographic Project from South Africa and Mozambique. *The Virginia Quarterly Review* 82(1): 42–51.

Miller, J. 1992. *Fluid Exchanges: Artists and Critics in the HIV/AIDS Crisis.* Toronto: University of Toronto Press.

Mitchell, T. 1998. Orientalism and the Exhibitionary Order, in *The Visual Culture Reader*, edited by N. Mirzoeff. New York: Routledge.

Moeller, S.D. 1999. *Compassion Fatigue: How the Media Sell Disease, Famine, War and Death.* New York: Routledge.

Nietzsche, F. 1991. *Zur Genealogie der Moral.* Frankfurt: Insel Taschenbuch.

Nixon, N. and Nixon, B. (1991) *People with AIDS.* Boston: David R. Godine Publisher.

Nordland, R., Wilkinson, R., and Marshall, R. 1986. Africa in the Plague Years. Newsweek, November 24.

Nussbaum, M. 2001. *Upheavals of Thought: The Intelligence of Emotions.* Cambridge: Cambridge University Press.

Ogdon, B. 2001. Through the Image: Nicholas Nixon's 'People with HIV/AIDS'. *Discourse* 23(3): 75–105.

Patton, C. 1990. *Inventing HIV/AIDS.* New York: Routledge.

Pearlmutter, D. 1998. *Photojournalism and Foreign Policy: Icons of Outrage in International Crisis.* London: Praeger.

Radley, A. 2002. Portrayals of Suffering: On Looking Away, Looking At, and the Comprehension of Illness Experience. *Body & Society* 8(3): 1–23.

Roudi-Fahimi, F. 2003. Women's Reproductive Health in the Middle East and North Africa. Population Reference Bureau, MENA Policy Brief. Washington, DC: PRB.

Sabatier, R. 1988. *Blaming Others: Prejudice, Race and Worldwide HIV/AIDS.* Philadelphia: New Society Publishers.

Said, E. 1979. *Orientalism.* New York: Vintage Books.

Sankore, R. 2005. Behind the Image: Poverty and Development Pornography. Pambazuka News: Weekly Forum for Social Justice in Africa. Available at: www.pambazuka.org [accessed 1 May 2005].

Sarin, R. 2002. The Feminization of AIDS, in *Worldwatch Paper 161*, edited by D. Nierenberg. Washington, DC: Worldwatch Institute.

Scarry, E. 1985. *The Body in Pain: The Making and Unmaking of the World*. New York: Oxford University Press.

Schwartz, J., and Murray, D. 1996. AIDS and the Media. *Public Interest* 125: 57–71.

Servaes, J. 1986. Development Theory and Communication Policy: Power to the People! *European Journal of Communication* 1(2): 203–229.

Shapiro, M.J. 1988. *The Politics of Representation: Writing Practices in Biography, Photography and Policy Analysis*. Madison: University of Wisconsin Press.

Singer, P. 2002. AIDS and International Security. *Survival* 44(1): 145–158.

Sischy, I. 1991. Good Intentions. *The New Yorker*, September 9.

Smith, R.A. 1998. *Encyclopedia of AIDS: A Social, Political, Cultural, and Scientific Record of the HIV Epidemic*. New York: Penguin.

Sontag, S. 1977. *On Photography*. New York: Picador.

Sontag, S. 1988. *HIV/AIDS and Its Metaphors*. New York: Farrar, Straus and Giroux.

Sontag, S. 2003. *Regarding the Pain of Others*. New York: Farrar, Strauss and Giroux.

Sontag, S. 2004. Regarding the Torture of Others. *The New York Times*, May 23. Available at: www.nytimes.com [accessed May 2004].

Strauss, D.L. 2003. *Between the Eyes: Essays on Photography and Politics*. New York: Aperture.

Thibodeaux, R. 2005. Women, Children Hardest Hit by Ethiopia's Deepening AIDS Crisis. Voice of America, February 11. Available at: www.aegis.com/news/voa/2005 [accessed 20 February 2006].

Tomkins, C. 2005. Shall We Dance? The Spectator as Artist. *The New Yorker*, October 17, 81(32): 82–95.

Treichler, P.A. 1999. *How to Have Theory in an Epidemic*. Durham: Duke University Press.

UNAIDS. 2003. AIDS Epidemic Update, December 2003. Available at: www.unaids.org [accessed February 2004].

UNAIDS. 2004a. AIDS Epidemic Update, December 2004. Geneva: UNAIDS/WHO.

UNAIDS. 2004b. 2004 Report on the Global HIV/AIDS Epidemic. Geneva: UNAIDS.

UNAIDS. 2005. AIDS Epidemic Update, December 2005. Geneva: UNAIDS/WHO.

UNICEF. 2004. Children on the Brink 2004. Available at: www.unicef.org [accessed 1 May 2005].

UNDP. 2007. Women's Rights Initiative. Available at: www.harpas.org/womanright.asp [accessed 4 January 2007].

USAID. 2003. *USAID Project Profiles: Children Affected by HIV/AIDS. Third Edition.* Washington DC: USAID.

Wainaina, B. 2006. How to Write about Africa. Granta 92. Available at: http://www.granta.com/extracts/2615 [accessed February 2006].

Watney, S. 1990. Photography and HIV/AIDS, in *The Critical Image: Essays on Contemporary Photography*, edited by C. Squiers. Seattle: Bay Press, 173-192.

Watts, M., and Boal, I. 1995. Working-Class Heroes: E.P. Thompson and Sebastiao Salgado. *Transition* 68: 90–115.

Wyschogrod, E. 1973. *The Phenomenon of Death: Faces of Mortality*. New York: Harper & Row.

Chapter 11

AIDS Phobia (*aizibing kongjuzheng*) and the People who Panic about AIDS (*kong'ai zu*): The Consequences of HIV Representations in China

Johanna Hood

Introduction

All across the globe, stories of HIV are not simply about illness. Frequently, they speak of structural violence, suffering and inequality, but they may also show how individuals and communities transform adversity and pain into narratives of resilience and strength. Stories of HIV are often fraught with the ideological struggles that unfold when global health and disease research priorities and governmental aid dollars are pitted against—and usually prioritized over—local knowledge and approaches. The general triumph of biomedicine and Western development practice in managing and understanding HIV has placed great importance on both quantification (numbers of people tested, HIV positive, NGOs, and activists), investigation (program transparency and efficacy), and democratic processes (civil society). In this process, the individual voices and experiences of the people who have HIV are sometimes lost or misrepresented. Additionally, as funds earmarked for particular interventions have not always been delivered in ways that satisfy donors, reports on the successes and failures of HIV interventions or evaluations of increasing rates of HIV infection may also tell of perceived inadequacies in the developing world. Such judgments may be underwritten by racist and sexist beliefs, intolerance and Western-centric governance and research strategies. These tensions shape understandings of the virus and those who carry it, and interventions into its spread. Their outcomes frequently have deep and unintended consequences for local communities.

In many ways, China's stories of HIV and its political and civic engagement with the virus share similarities with those of many other countries. China is a diverse nation made up of over fifty recognized ethnic groups. However, the Han Chinese represent over 90 per cent of the population and are generally wealthier, more powerful, and better educated than those from minority groups. Western biomedical knowledge, combined with urban Han Chinese ideologies and interpretations of it impact HIV prevention strategies, conceptions of HIV transmission risk, and the communication of HIV in China's media and public health campaigns. This often occurs with unintended yet far reaching consequences. Over time, communication strategies for HIV have enabled the virus to become largely understood as a problem that only affects non-urban, non-heteronormative, and frequently non-Han people. I call this trend "imagined immunity" (Hood 2011). The virus is also highly stigmatized (UNAIDS, Marie Stopes International China office, and Institute of Social Development Research of the China Central Party School 2009, Sullivan et al. 2010).

In this chapter, I approach representations of AIDS in China through the recent emergence of a phenomenon known as *kong'ai* (恐艾) or *aizibing kongjuzheng* (艾滋病恐惧症)—literally, "AIDS fear or panic" and "AIDS phobia"—which has recently been classified as a psychological disorder (F. Wang, Li, and Yue 2006, J. Fu et al. 2008, C. Wu 2009, Y. Xiao 2009, Y. Liu and Shao 2010). Those people suffering from panic are known as *kong'ai zu* (恐艾族) or *kong'ai min* (恐艾民), which I translate loosely as "people who panic about AIDS." To my knowledge, the condition is reported mainly in urban areas in media and on forums. It varies from the discrimination and marginalization that many with HIV experience from the stigmatization of the virus (Zhou 2007). AIDS panic presents itself through combinations of the following symptoms: repeat hospital visits to test for HIV when exposure is suspected (but not confirmed); irrational fear of HIV; irrational fear of the HIV positive; and irrational fear of the moral qualities of those suspected of having HIV or increased susceptibility to it, such as ethnic minorities, sex workers, or drug users (Jinling Hotline [金陵热线] 2009, 99 Healthnet [99 健康网] 2010, Qilu.net [齐鲁网] 2012, Z. Xia 2012, X. Zhang 2012). Although it could be deemed as lacking academic validity, the contributors to the Chinese equivalent of Wikipedia define AIDS panic as follows, "the panic can be accompanied by anxiety, depression, hypochondria, etc., a variety of symptoms of abnormal psychological conditions and behavior. Sufferers suspect themselves to be infected by HIV, and are especially paranoid of infection to the point that they develop an obsessive preoccupation with cleanliness (so as to avoid HIV)" (Baidu Encyclopedia [百度百科] 2012). The relatively recent diagnosis of AIDS panic means that the latest accessible information on it circulates most readily within mainstream culture. This general fear of HIV has also led to members of the public using HIV as a threat in robbery, extortion, and to flee public security forces (Dong 2006, Qilu.net [齐鲁网] 2012).

Here I aim to contextualize this pathological fear of HIV within the State's management of its public health and media, and the ways in which representations of HIV-positive people are authored and then read by the urban Han public. To do so, I first provide an overview of China's experiences with HIV infection. I explain the ways in which HIV and HIV prevention are generally managed, transmission paths and trends, and the dominant attitudes about HIV among urban Han Chinese. Next, I focus on representations of HIV, particularly the changing embodiment of HIV and AIDS sufferers in urban China's media and public health campaigns over three decades. Following this, I explain the role played by the frequently drastic and shocking stories contained in China's media in encouraging the spread of HIV-related *kong'ai* reported among urbanites. In conclusion, I highlight the importance of representations of disease to the public health and well-being of the population. I suggest that the emergence of the so-called people who panic about AIDS is a result of the combination of media representations of HIV, state management of public health, and pre-existing local ideology and understandings of those who typically are shown as having HIV (usually disadvantaged rural and minority people). To reduce the spread of this new fear, these representations, China's public health, and the discriminatory attitudes toward non-urbanites need further attention from those who are attempting to address the stigmatization of HIV/AIDS in China. Such representations should also be taken into account by any media strategies used in society and by public health bodies.

Responses to rates of HIV transmission in China

Governing geopolitical complexity and diversity

China is a large, complex, and diverse country of almost 1.3 billion people. Today, it has also become one of the world's most unequal societies, and is home to some of the richest and poorest people in the world (Central Intelligence Agency 2012, Hodgson 2012, Sun and Guo 2012). Contemporary China's Gini coefficient, which lies approximately between 50 and 60, is controversial and sensitive enough for the central government to refuse to release it to the Chinese people (Fang and Yu 2012, Cai 2012). The inequality that has characterized China's social and economic development over the last three decades has directly shaped the way HIV and AIDS have affected the nation and the ways in which the virus has become a problem of governance for China's political leaders.

Although the country has just one political party, the development and implementation of governance policies—from healthcare to economic development—in its many geographic regions is a challenge. The implementation of central policies is, in particular, shaped by the ways in which these are administered and adhered to (or not) by local leaders. Other factors that shape this process are human and financial resource availability, political will and corruption, and investment plans and strategies. For example, regional leaders were slow or reluctant to admit HIV infection rates. This was frequently due to fear that portraying socioeconomically depressed areas as having anything but robust climates and populations would have a negative impact on potential investment in their region. HIV has also impacted upon the central government and continues to do so. One of the possible contenders for the post of president in 2012, Li Keqiang was the Provincial Governor of Henan while HIV was ravaging its citizens, some of China's most marginalized. Allegations have been made that he and Propaganda Minister Li Changchun were involved in covering up this situation (The Economist 2012, B. Chen 2010). Due to this controversy, it is only through the mentorship and support of current President Hu Jintao that Li Keqiang remained a candidate for the Premiership, a post he assumed in November 2012 (Ballentine and Sofer 2012: 3).

Social and geographic distributions of inequality in China

China's current and extreme inequality has its roots in the late 1970s. After decades of effective isolation from the non-socialist world, the Chinese government under Deng Xiaoping commenced a series of economic development and modernization reforms. Over a short period, these reforms privileged the "opening up" (*kaifang* 开放) of China's coastal regions, provinces, and large cities along water routes to trade and neoliberal development. Areas such as Guangdong, Jiangsu, and Chongqing municipalities flourished. However, these choices led to widened geographic and ethnic inequalities that further disadvantaged inland provinces with large minority populations like Sichuan, Gansu, and Ningxia. Huge numbers of people flooded from these places into developing urban areas in search of factory work, in what has become one of the largest migrations in human history.

Around the same time, the government also attempted two major reforms to its healthcare system. The first occurred in the 1980s under the philosophy of "using economic measures to govern healthcare" (*yunyong jingji shouduan guanli weisheng shiye* 运用经济手段管理卫生事业), which was a disastrous attempt to marketize what was then an impressive social medical system (Y. Liu, Rao, and Hsiao 2003). As a result, the majority of China's population was left without healthcare coverage, and many ended up in medical debt when they fell ill (Hossain 1998, Ma et al. 2011). For example, one World Bank survey showed that 37 percent of tuberculosis (TB) patients were unable to seek care because of financial difficulties, and many became poor because of treatment costs (The World Bank News 2010). The second medical reform, the *xin yiliao gaige* (新医 疗改革 usually known simply as *yigai*), commenced in the mid-2000s and is an ongoing attempt to recapture the social coverage that was lost in the first reform. Its aims include addressing the widening gap between rural and urban health systems, addressing medical corruption and improving coverage and access to care and prescription medicine (Lin 2012).

HIV and inequality

In China HIV is a problem of inequality. Although great gains in the past decade have been made in policies governing the treatment and care for those with HIV, the HIV positive in many places are unable to access medications and care, in spite of their new entitlements (*The Economist* 2012, B. Chen 2010). This problem, particularly where HIV is concerned, is shaped by the country's sharp ethnic and class divisions and the inequality between these groups (Huan 2010). Assumptions about the value and character of peasants and minority cultures, and the places they live, have also had a direct impact on policy and responses, as well as on the representations of HIV in public health and consumer media (Hood 2012).

As mentioned above, China is ethnically diverse. However, socioeconomic power and resource access and acquisition have become monopolized by the Han—who make up the vast majority of its population—and in particular Han urbanites. As with the differences between incomes and living standards in urban and rural areas, the massive disparities between Han and non-Han fuel social discontent and form challenges to social stability.

These disparities lie at the root of many class and inter-ethnic conflicts today, such as those in Tibet and Xinjiang, but the trend stretches back for centuries. Particularly since the Ming Dynasty, which saw the expansion of industrial development and trade, those identifying or identified as Han have generally occupied better land and have largely dominated trade patterns (Siu and Faure 1995: 2, 12). This has given rise to widespread prejudice: urban Han believe rural Han and non-Han minorities to be of lower moral caliber and quality, as is well documented in current—predominantly anthropological—research (Blum 2001, Jacka 2009, Schein 2002). Additionally, the dominant role networking (*guanxi* 关系) plays in contemporary Chinese society has enabled particular individuals, families, and clans—frequently those who had connections to resource distribution and power in Maoist China—to prosper disproportionately (Chan, Madsen, and Unger 1984, Unger and Chung 2012). As a result, corruption is endemic in government–business linkages.

These dominant Han ways of seeing rural Chinese and ethnic 'others' have direct and unintended consequences on policies (be they health-related or otherwise) and the way they are communicated (Huan 2010, Y. Wan and Beijing Aizhixing Institute 2011, Zhuang and Hua 2002). This is certainly true with regards to the country's experience of HIV/AIDS (Hyde 2007, S. Liu 2011). As Hyde (2007: 7) states, the focus of interventions in the late 1980s and early 1990s was in minority-rich areas. When an epidemic began to brew among poor Han farming communities in central China, "the underlying assumption was that the Tai [an ethnic minority in Yunnan Province] are a loose and sexually uninhibited people (*luanjiao* 乱交) and that their sexual practices were leading to high rates of STIs, and now, HIV/AIDS." These beliefs, in combination with the greed of cadres and corporations and the lack of value placed on farmers and their livelihoods in contemporary China (G. Chen and Tao 2004), meant that an HIV epidemic exploded on China's central plains area, spread through unsterilized equipment and blood pooling practices (Shao 2006), which I explore in the next section. Those directly involved in blood selling and in diagnostics and treatment predict that up to and over one million farmers died undiagnosed (*The epic of central plains* 2007, Gao, Shang, and Guo 2003, K. Zhang 2005). Although it was these people who were first overlooked and then ignored by the State's mismanagement of blood collection facilities and later HIV testing centres, they were later represented in China's public health and media as an underclass of poor HIV-positive peasants. They came to symbolize HIV for urban Chinese audiences, and thus to distance them from it, regardless of what was actually happening in the country's epidemiological landscape (Hood 2012).

A history of HIV in China

The Chinese government confirmed the first official case of HIV in China in 1984, but official statistics reported very few infections outside of Yunnan province until the 2000s. Then, in 2002, the United Nation (UN) report *China's Titanic Peril* predicted that national rates of infection stood at 1.2 million and had the potential to reach 10 million if no steps were taken to curb it. Like other international evaluations of China's HIV problem, this estimate differed wildly from local statistics and accounts. However, ten years later, the figure quoted by most organizations is of an estimated 740,000 to 780,000 sufferers in the country (Carter 2012, Jinghua Li et al. 2012). Of these, only approximately 200,000 are confirmed.

In the mid-1980s, HIV was detected in China among those who had consumed imported plasma products for the treatment of conditions such as haemophilia. It was also later detected in sex workers, in communities with high rates of intravenous drug use, and in minority groups, such as those along the borders of southern China, notably Yunnan province (Hyde 2007, S. Liu 2011). Its detection among China's then invisible MSM community was late. Following these first infections, China banned imports of blood in the mid-1980s. As most Chinese were—and continue to be—unwilling to donate blood voluntarily, a blood shortage arose. This led to the rapid establishment of a massive blood-selling industry in areas characterized by exceptionally poor-quality soil and high drought and flood risks, which were generally excluded from the benefits of China's modernization and development policies. The only saleable resource for residents of such areas was their "liquid gold" or "red oil" (Anagnost 2006, Erwin 2006, Gao, Shang, and Guo 2003, Su 2010, Zhou 2007). Blood-selling also occurred in urban and modernizing areas to which inland people migrated in search of work, but instead found themselves easily exploited by the unscrupulous henchmen of the blood economy. The unsanitary practices prevalent at blood collection stands (such as shared needles and the pooling and reinjection of red blood cells following plasma extraction, or plasmapheresis) favored the rapid spread of HIV through entire communities. China's most populous province, Henan, became the epicenter of this tragedy, and others such as Anhui, Shaanxi, and Sichuan were also affected.

Since the early 2000s, HIV has also become a major concern in Xinjiang and some areas of Sichuan province among IDU populations. Mother-to-child transmission has also been detected nationwide, but not in large numbers. HIV has also begun to be reported among particular populations in urban China. For example, considerable HIV-related panic was directed toward the internal migrant population mentioned above (see Chinese celebrity Pu Cunxin's Public Service Announcement *Migrant Workers*, 2006). This group is made up of young people who are largely single or separated from their spouses and are thus popularly perceived to be 'at risk' from HIV. In this sense, the discourse in China seems to be informed by international experiences of HIV spreading along transport routes and through male-dominated migrant communities in developing nations (UNAIDS 2011). However, this preoccupation with migrant workers was deemed unjustified by many Chinese social scientists involved in detection projects that I spoke to during my fieldwork in the mid-2000s. All the same, transport was a contributing factor to Henan's infections, with the worst affected areas being those which lay close to newly resurfaced roads (Jing and Worth 2010: 19).

Since 2008, sexual transmission has overtaken injection drug use and blood commodification as the primary transmission path of HIV in China. The groups most affected by this transmission path are sex workers and the gay (MSM) community, although the growing infection rates in the latter may reflect concerted efforts to popularize voluntary counselling and testing (VCT) among gay men (Jacobs 2009). HIV infection in non-urban areas is now reported to be concentrated primarily in marginalized communities in poorer inland provinces, such as Xinjiang and Guangxi. These areas have populations with large proportions of ethnic minorities and are home to China's poorest and most vulnerable people. This seems to indicate that although HIV has transitioned away from the rural communities who sought to better their lot in the 1990s through large-scale blood-selling, marginalization remains a key factor for risk of HIV infection in China.

Structural inequalities and demographies of HIV infection

The social problems arising in such a diverse and unequal society continue to shape China's experiences of HIV, as do the country's patterns of public health investment and education, its diagnostic technologies and capabilities, and government-business corruption, among other factors. Although nationwide HIV prevention and treatment policies and plans exist, their implementation varies from region to region, as do the resources assigned to them and patient access to diagnostic technologies and support (Y. Shao 2001). For example, although ARVs in China can be received for free under the Four Frees and One Care policy, currently only a quarter of registered HIV positive in China actually have access to them (Carter 2012).

China's HIV problem has been exacerbated by many interrelated structural and ideological factors. The first was the reform of social medicine described above. When China marketized its health sector in the 1980s, its ability to detect and report new infectious diseases diminished and only began to recover after SARS and the reinvigorated commitment to health on the part of the central leadership that followed. Lack of financing in the 1980s and 1990s meant that many rural hospitals closed. Furthermore, doctors and hospital staff were not able to stay apace of changing epidemiological trends and thus became undertrained. The few who did specialize in HIV were practicing and researching far from areas where the virus was actually spreading (K. Zhang 2005). Private healthcare in urban areas was effectively the only option available for HIV diagnosis and treatment, but those who carried the virus and those most at risk from HIV usually could not afford such care.

A second factor to have negatively affected China's experience with HIV has been its choices about where and how to implement modernization reforms. China's modernization followed a general pattern that prioritized the advancement of urban over rural and of coastal over inland. As outlined above, people from areas and classes that failed to benefit from these reforms quickly fell prey to the so-called plasma economy (*xiejiang jingji* 血浆经济) (Guo 1997, Qi 1997, Zhu 2001, X. Zhao, Yao, and Kang 2005) as blood-selling became an easily accessible source of income for them. As both blood-sellers and blood collection workers lacked education, and were driven to profit from the blood trade, most did not know what HIV was (and those that did considered it a disease that only affected Africans or EuroAmericans), nor were they aware of safe procedures for donation. In modernizing China, commercial sex work once again became a viable source of income for many women who were earning meager wages in factories or could not find other sources of income, and as such, it is an important path through which HIV is spread. Although many CFSW understand how HIV is transmitted, clients are often reluctant to wear condoms. This is particularly problematic among older sex workers (Huang 2010, Jing and Worth 2010, G. Xia and Yang 2005). Finally, the massive changes that China's society has undergone in the past decade have meant rising levels of unemployment, inflation, and social and economic stress for those who do not have the education and skills to navigate and succeed in the new society. Drug use is an increasing problem and also a key path for the spread of HIV (Jing 2010). The link between the spread of HIV, modernization, rising unemployment and ethnicity has been well established (Hou 2009, Huan 2010, Zhuang 2005). In a time of HIV, those who are left behind (for whatever reasons) are the worst affected. As Jing and Worth assert regarding China's social geography of infection:

> HIV is not indiscriminate in its choice of victim, and this applies to China as well. The routes for HIV transmission are behaviourally based, but there is a definite socioeconomic gradient in the ways in which it affects people. The behaviours rendering certain populations susceptible to HIV very much hinge on that population's social standing, economic status and everyday experiences of struggling against various adversities [...] the majority of those who have borne the brunt of the HIV epidemic in China live at the bottom of Chinese society. (2010: 14)

The lack of appreciation for local disease economies forms a third factor informing China's HIV experience. Dominant international understandings of at-risk populations guided health personnel regarding where to look for HIV and whom to target their prevention efforts at. Many key local and international personnel involved in HIV prevention, treatment, and policy were trained in Western epidemiology and public health, and worked in urban areas. They maintained ties to international networks and to international ways of doing and seeing. This exposure reinforced understandings about who was believed to be at risk from HIV. As such, over the past three decades, HIV could be said to have become a problem of looking, rather than of detection per se. For example, as the phenomenon of blood-selling was unheard of internationally, much less connected with standard risk groups, commercial plasma donors were not identified as a risk group in a timely fashion. This problem was further exacerbated by local governments' resistance to reporting health problems and the under-valuation of peasants' lives (Yun et al. 2005). Similar understandings about local populations' risky behavior, and in particular ethnic behavioral norms, also played a role in policy development in ways such as those identified by Hyde (2007), as discussed above.

Finally, as in other countries, the way HIV spreads and the length of time it takes to express itself further hindered detection, as healthy adults often live for years without experiencing strong symptoms or secondary infections. Although Chinese people were becoming HIV positive from contact with the virus through sex or tainted equipment when selling blood and using drugs, the delayed appearance of symptoms meant that HIV became removed from the practices that caused transmission. This situation was exacerbated by the lack of up-to-date medical technology, the resistance to blood donation, the unscrupulous and unhygienic use of the machinery used to extract human plasma from whole blood (plasmapheresis), and inconsistent access to care.

The multiple factors that impact HIV transmission in Chinese society, combined with the delayed expression of the virus, have posed difficulties in understanding and controlling its spread. In spite of the gains that the *yigai* has brought since 2009, there are outstanding problems that are of public and mental health concern. These include Chinese citizens' problematic access to medical care and the chronic underfunding of public health and prevention plans (Y. Liu, Rao, and Hsiao 2003, Ye and Yao 2012, Y. Zhang 2012). In order to understand how HIV has been represented and discussed in public, how it has attracted social interest and donor funding, and how its stories have evolved in China, the dynamics of the global political economy of HIV must be understood, along with the dominant role HIV has assumed in research and country-to-country aid in China. In the next section I explore how the international sphere has impacted upon China's experiences. I show how international investment is a key incentive for keeping HIV a focus of China's public health and media reports, and thus as a key illness in the public sphere.

The glamorous social life of HIV: uneven economies of disease

HIV in China attracts a disproportionate amount of resources and funding in comparison with the amount of people it affects. HIV draws attention from the general public through sensational media stories and celebrity advocacy, and from educated audiences through research grants and employment in HIV-related programs. These are important given the context of increasing consumerism, rising unemployment—notably China's "ant army" (*yi zu* 蚁族), or unemployed university graduates—and the growth in state funding for research projects. For example, the early involvement of the British government in HIV-related projects in China through its China-UK AIDS Program has produced a generation of social scientists specializing in HIV program evaluations and monitoring (Carter 2012).

Other governments, corporations, and business organizations followed suit and the popularity of donating for HIV research and social organization support broadened. Many NGOs and similar grassroots and civil society organizations have been formed that deal solely with HIV. Their activities and relationships to the academic community have informed and improved anti-discrimination laws and policies enabling access to medication and social services such as schooling for the children of low-income families with HIV. The latter was part of the 2004 four frees and one care (*si mian yi guan'ai* 四免一关爱) policy. Yet in spite of these gains, these organizations have failed to address other issues, such as the disproportionate pattern of HIV infection in China according to income, ethnicity, geographic origin, and social status. Although they have paved the way for other organizations to learn from their struggles and avoid their pitfalls and unpleasant encounters with state public security bodies, non-HIV-based organizations have been slower to develop and funding windfalls on a scale similar to those sustained for HIV are absent.

Viral comparisons

Although the prevalence rates of HIV in China are low in comparison to TB or hepatitis, HIV attracts a disproportionate amount of resources and attention. According to international and domestic studies on TB released between 2010 and 2012, China has the second largest TB epidemic in the world and the highest annual number of cases of multidrug-resistant TB infections. These amount to 25 per cent of the world total (People's Daily Online [人民网] 2011, The World Bank 2011, Y. Zhao et al. 2012, 2165, The World Bank News 2010). Some 1.5 million in China are currently infected with active TB (Floyd et al. 2011: 12, table 2.1) while 500 million are suspected to carry the virus without knowledge of this (Ministry of Health 2010, People's Daily Online [人民网] 2011). When China's AIDS 'problem' was coming to light in the early 2000s, TB infection rates were even higher than they currently are, as there have been considerable improvements in TB control in China over the past decade (Levine 2007, Floyd et al. 2011: 1, 7). TB nonetheless remains one of the contributing factors to deaths from AIDS in contemporary China.

Hepatitis is an even graver problem; approximately one in ten Chinese people carry it, putting the total number of estimated sufferers at 120 million (China Ministry of Health 2010). Discrimination against those with hepatitis is widespread (Fan 2007, Beijing Yirenping Center 2008, Jiang and Wang 2009, China Daily [中

国日报网] 2012). As a result of its hepatitis problem, China also has an elevated incidence of liver cancers.

Despite these high prevalence rates for hepatitis and TB, few celebrities publicly support the causes of either TB or hepatitis (J. Wang 2012). Popular pop singer and actor Andy Lau and folk singer and civilian Major General Peng Liyuan are two exceptions, although their engagement with HIV and other causes is arranged by public relations companies and the World Health Organization. Both celebrities also endorse and support campaigns around HIV and other social issues (World Health Organization 2011, International Public Relations Network 2012). Few organizations in existence solely support TB or hepatitis sufferers. One internationally well-known exception is Yirenping. This situation forms a stark contrast to that of HIV, for which there are over 600 organizations (Couzin 2007). In spite of this, many local forms of advocacy around hepatitis have evolved without the major injection of funding that shapes HIV. For example, liver hospitals maintain websites with information about hepatitis transmission and treatment, and there are sites with topical (*shequ* 社区) chatrooms and information on hepatitis, such as Dr51, HBV39, Utter Devotion, Liver Treasure, Club Sohu, and HBVHBV, the largest support site.[1] This seems to indicate that there are differing modes of activism, marketing, and representation at stake within each disease economy, and that HIV is an exception.

Although HIV affects approximately 1 in every 1,000 people in China—in other words, it is a hundred times less prevalent than hepatitis—HIV prevention, treatment and research have been the focus of funding from many overseas governments and organizations, including the Red Cross, various organizations affiliated with the UN, the Gates and Clinton Foundations, as well as corporate social responsibility (CSR) initiatives from companies such as Bayer and Durex. As the exact amount of funding HIV/AIDS receives is difficult to ascertain, direct comparisons to funding figures for hepatitis and TB are impossible, but interest in the latter two is limited outside organizations that engage multiple diseases (i.e. the Global Fund to Fight AIDS, TB and Malaria, or the Global Health Initiative of the World Economic Forum's foci on AIDS and TB). The number of Chinese celebrities (from Jackie Chan to Pu Cunxin) who offer public support for HIV campaigns overwhelms those concerned with hepatitis and TB. The same is true of the number of creative artists (from Yan Lianke to Yu Hua) and documentarians and filmmakers (from Ai Xiaomin to Zhao Liang) whose work focuses on HIV, and of the governmental and non-governmental charities and corporations that target it. This disproportionate attention reinforces HIV's dominant status within the unequal disease economy.

---

1   The urls and/or forum links are as follows: Dr51 [http://hbv.d.51daifu.com], HBV39 [http://hbv.39.net/], Utter Devotion [http://www.gandanxiangzhao.com/forum.php], Liver Treasure [http://jibing.ganbaobao.com.cn/], Club Sohu [http://club.health.sohu.com/l-zfj000-0-0-0.html], HBVHBV [http://www.hbvhbv.com/forum/forum.php].

The media life of HIV: Reporting and representing HIV

The media have played a seminal role in educating the Chinese public about HIV and drawing attention to it; over 90 per cent of people in China learn about HIV through media sources, be they audiovisual, text, or virtual (UNAIDS et al. 2008). Considerable academic attention has also been paid to the importance of the Chinese media in public health messaging. Academic research by Li Xiguang and Zhou Mei (X. Li and Zhou 2005) has carefully documented trends in Chinese HIV reporting, such as the specific topics covered or the places where the Chinese press reports HIV and HIV-related problems to exist. Yet more needs to be said about the choices behind these particular messages and representations, the rapid changes that have occurred in the embodiment of HIV, the multiple media that HIV information is communicated through, and the effects this visual culture has on readers. Additionally, according to Nathan Serlin, it is of critical importance to acknowledge the "hybridizing" of public health media in contemporary society and the differing variables, from institutional to virtual, that shape health communication practices and media (2012: xiv, xviii). In China, media censorship—be it official or self-imposed (for fear of losing one's job or being demoted)—and market forces have played a key role in shaping public discourses and government responses to HIV. The privatization of state media in the 1980s threw the media open to market forces, leading to an increased presence of the sensational stories that attract larger audiences (M. M. Yang 2002). For HIV, this meant that stories of suffering sold well; images accompanying HIV coverage were often graphic, contrasting with the previous era's reporting style, which had focused on robust figures embodying good socialist governance. These practices established a culture of reporting on HIV characterized by the following pattern: initially, the media was prevented from broadcasting China's HIV stories; next, only limited information was conveyed about the virus, mainly through non-local HIV reports, reports on HIV in minority areas and sensational coverage of China's blood-selling epidemic. This practice had a significant impact on the way that both the general public and China's leadership understood HIV. These understandings, in turn, affected the policy and public health responses, or lack thereof, to the virus.

From the Chinese media's complex and diverse narrative of HIV, three main paradigms have emerged to explain the virus's origins, and with them, dominant ways of embodying HIV. In the mid-1980s, HIV was portrayed as an international problem that impacted upon a very small amount of Chinese through imported blood products (*AIDS: The Super Epidemic* 1990, *AIDS: Threatening the Chinese* 1996). In the late 1980s and early-to mid-1990s, HIV became portrayed as a problem affecting EuroAmerican gay men and poor black Africans and Haitians (J. Shi, Zhi, and Li 1991, Cui 1992, Bai 1995), but not the Chinese. Both of these characterizations of the virus reflect biomedical explanatory and detection models, and indeed there was no available media on local infection trends beyond the connection with haemophilia. The third paradigm differed however. In the mid-to late-1990s, a major shift occurred in how the demography of China's infection was explained to the general public. HIV gradually became a local problem that was reported, albeit infrequently, among specific populations—mainly drug users and sex workers—living in China. These groups usually inhabited locations that were hard to access, including urban slums such as those described around Guangzhou railway station, and villages of ethnic minority populations in mountainous rural parts of Yunnan that required days of travel and a four-wheel drive to reach. Only in the very late 1990s was HIV infrequently reported on in "AIDS villages" in Henan, Shaanxi, and Anhui. Areas with high HIV prevalence were typically described using language that emphasized the unfamiliar and rural nature of these locations. In one of the earliest reports by *Southern Weekend* (*Nanfang Zhoumo* 南方周末), the journalist, Shen, describes a long journey to a "remote" AIDS village in Yunnan. Shen travels along narrow, winding dirt roads that challenge his/her luxury car, and through thick forests, and paddy and sugar cane fields. This lush physical environment contrasts with Shen's description of the village as dilapidated, poor, and eerie (1997: 2).

Coverage in the late 1990s and early 2000s of HIV in China also diversified the geography of infection greatly. As the media began to focus on local cases of HIV, the numbers of Chinese risk groups and the range of places where HIV could be found multiplied. These groups and places ranged from the blood-selling agrarian populations who inhabited impoverished areas of Central China such as Henan, Shaanxi, and Anhui, through to the floating and migrant populations (although this was mainly in public health campaigns and not popular media. For example PSAs, see those directed and produced by Ruby Yang and Thomas Lennon, available on http://www.campfilms.org/projects/aids/psas.html) to groups of petty criminals formed by ethnic minorities in urban areas. For example, in a 2003 article by Li Qingchuan, the author describes a trip to Anhui Province to interview an HIV sufferer who contracted the virus through tainted blood. Li provides details of an epic journey involving multiple buses, old borrowed motorcycles, impassable winding rural roads, and walking into an AIDS village, Linlou, on foot. The language of such articles continued to stress non-urbanity and distance in this period, but the process of embodying HIV as a Chinese problem associated it firmly with poverty, greed, backwardness, social waywardness and rural livelihoods. Rarely was it portrayed as an urban concern, except in connection with the presence of underclasses in urban areas.

One of the main features of HIV coverage is its attention to the visible impact the virus has on the body. Regardless of whether they were intended for lay or specialist audiences, most programs, texts and articles on HIV were accompanied by drastic images of the HIV positive. These usually showed people suffering emotionally and physically from the advanced stages of HIV or full-blown AIDS. The most renowned and well circulated are Lu Guang's and Gao Yaojie's photos. The former is an internationally celebrated photojournalist and the latter is a retired gynecologist now living in self-imposed exile in New York where she is writing about Henan's blood scandal from Columbia University. These images present emaciated sufferers with naked limbs or bodies, rashes, and other visually affronting secondary infections typically associated with HIV. In others, rural poor show their scars from selling blood. In almost all, the HIV positive are portrayed as destitute and suffering, and through the repetition of this narrative, they began to form a marginalized underclass of their own.

At the same time, the narratives on each particular risk group diversified and the coverage of the virus became more complicated. No longer was HIV illustrated exclusively as a terrifying disease causing corporeal decay and social exclusion. Instead, the narrative shifted to include tales of resilience, state concern and the social rehabilitation of those who had been stigmatized for being HIV positive. This is most clearly identifiable in the coverage of China's AIDS orphans (*aizi gu'er* 艾滋孤儿), the children of blood-sellers, and HIV-oriented celebrity-endorsed philanthropy in urban areas. This may also have been influenced by the role of journalist training center programs, such as the joint initiative between Beyer-Schering pharmaceuticals and Tsinghua University that opened in 2004 to train the next generation of journalists using different techniques and reporting strategies.

Transmission numbers also fluctuated greatly in local media coverage. For example, the infection rate was reported as being relatively low until 2002, when, as described above, it escalated rapidly following the publication of the UN report *China's Titanic Peril*, which detailed the government action required to stem infections in China's various at-risk communities (United Nations Theme Group on HIV/AIDS 2002). This and other reports associated panic with what had, up to then, been perceived as a threat affecting primarily rural, lower class populations, which further marginalized those with HIV. HIV statistics have been—and continue to be—unreliable. The reported numbers of predicted infections dropped from 1.2 million in 2002 to 600,000 several years later. Numbers then rose to 840,000, and now sit at approximately 740,000. The variance in these numbers from year to year has incited great panic and drawn funds and social, political, and industrial attention to HIV. These shifts have been used to show that China is making national strides in HIV prevention and treatment. However, the actual situation is much more complex—for example only 200,000 of the 740,000 are registered—and varies regionally.

Although reports and representations did not always reflect actual demographies of infection, with the media focus being typically on rural underclasses, the shifting ways of explaining HIV infection that characterized the 1990s and 2000s have continued into the present. Now, HIV is also shown to be more widespread and problematic in urban areas through reports identifying HIV in non-normative populations, such as among sex workers, drug users, and, increasingly, gay men. Men over 50 years old are also a newly identified risk group (Stan 2012, J. Shan 2012, W. Xu 2012).

Despite the occasional publication ban and the levels of self-censorship that plague China's media generally, HIV has remained a well-reported concern since the mid-1980s, particularly around World AIDS Day, December 1. Regardless of this, HIV continues to be a moralized subject in non-academic public discussion.

Particular research findings on it remain sensitive, such as the relationship between ethnicity and HIV infection (Huan 2010, Jing and Worth 2010: 28), in that non-Han have significantly higher infection rates in provinces such as Yunnan, Xinjiang, and Gansu, and increased difficulties in accessing ARVs (Y. Wan and Beijing Aizhixing Institute 2011, Y. Wan et al. 2009). Despite this, HIV research in China is well developed and well reported. The sheer numbers of publications and media on the social aspects of the virus and on living positively with it suggest there are other benefits to be gained from keeping stories about a problem that only one in 1,000 have in focus in the media today.

The afterlife of HIV

Over the past three decades, images of both Chinese and international HIV sufferers and related topics have been used indiscriminately in China's media.[2] While researching HIV discourses and representations, I attempted to republish images of black Africans used in China's early HIV media. During my struggle to gain copyright permissions for these, I found that publishers of the Chinese materials in question often could not trace the origin of the images or that they had been used without copyright permission. In one case, a popular weekly publication kindly gave me permission to republish images that they did not actually own. According to one journalist who was helping me at the time, the use of images without copyright permission was standard practice (confidential conversation with author, 2009). I later discovered that images published in the Chinese media about HIV and Africa may have been drawn—unacknowledged— from online image repositories such as those run by Corbis, Getty, World Press Photo, and UNAIDS.

When images are removed from their original context and transplanted like this to new contexts without reference to this process, the new context informs the ways the images are interpreted. They often acquire new meanings, which Larissa Heinrich has called their "afterlife." Heinrich's work on this issue is driven by the question "what happens when ideas about illness and identity meet ideological imperatives?" (2008: 17). Although she analyzes the meanings ascribed to images of amputation and smallpox, a corresponding trend can be identified in the images and stories circulating within China's HIV media, which also have a fascinating afterlife.

Heinrich describes how the image of a Chinese child was initially used in Asia to "signify China's invention of the practice of inoculation [against small pox] as a technological achievement in advance of the West" (2008: 2). However, when transplanted to France, the decontextualized image came to mean something different. "Far from symbolizing technological prowess…in the context of their

---

2 The EuroAmerican notion of copyright is not indigenous to China, although adherence to international conventions is growing and increasingly enforced.

representation these images in fact stood for a kind of backwardness, a kind of vulnerability to disease coded implicitly as Chinese" (2008: 2).

A similar process occurs during the borrowing, reusing and recycling of representations of HIV/AIDS within China's public health and popular media. In this way, images are given new meanings that affect popular imagining of illness and transmission risk. Given the major role that the media plays in public health in China, the afterlife of these stories can be linked to widespread misunderstandings about HIV, serious levels of discrimination against HIV positive, stigmatization of the virus and those who have it, social panics, and the extreme cases of *kong'ai*. I turn to these in the following section.

Representations of HIV and social and public health problems

Fear, stigma, discrimination, and social suffering

In addition to being unique for the disproportionate amounts of attention and resources it receives, HIV is also unique for the levels of discrimination (*qishi* 歧视) and consequent suffering (*chiru* 耻辱, *shouku* 受苦, *qinhai* 侵害, and *wuming* 污名) endured by those carrying the virus. Although there is discrimination toward hepatitis and TB carriers, the stigma around these is, as one sufferer put it, "not as serious" (*Together* 2010).

The discrimination and suffering endured by HIV-positive Chinese originate in dominant social understandings of HIV and in political responses to the virus. The social science research of Shao Jing (2006) Shao Jing and Mary Scoggin (2009), Jing Jun (2006, 2007, 2010), Yun et al. (2005) Liu Yuehua (2010) and the work of activists like Wan Yanhai (2009, 2011), documentary makers like Zhao Liang (*Together* 2010) and Ai Xiaomin (*Epic of Central Plains* 2007), and authors like Yan Lianke (2006) show that levels of suicide and depression are high among Chinese HIV sufferers. In scientific research, suicide and depression are also included in discussions of non-medical factors impacting the success of anti-retroviral therapy (Lai et al. 2011).

Theories about social suffering by Kleinmann, Lock, and Vas (1996, 1997) and Farmer (1996) help to understand the experiences of China's HIV positive, and the particular role of the state and society within them. Social suffering results from, "what political, economic, and institutional power does to people, and, reciprocally, from how these forms of power themselves influence responses to social problems" (Kleinman, Das, and Lock 1996: xi). For carriers of HIV in China, being HIV positive has become a serious "marker of disadvantage, relative powerlessness, and devastating effects of social change, and in this sense is a moral indicator of cultural or societal disorder" (Kleinman 1999: 391). Portrayals of suffering in both urban and rural areas are frequent and widespread in public media. Since the late 1990s, and particularly since the 2000s, much attention has been given to the graphic and disproportionate suffering the HIV positive endure by China's more open media, such as the *Southern Weekend* (Guo 1997, Qi 1997, Shen 1997), Southern People Weekly (*Nanfang Renwu Zhoukan* 南方任务周刊) (L. Chen et al. 2004, Q. Wan 2004), Newsweek (*Xinwen Zhoukan* 新闻周刊) (Chenguang Wu 2001, Z. Liu 2003, Yingli Liu 2004) and Xinmin Weekly (*Xinmin Zhoukan* 新民周刊) (Jin 2002, Q. Li 2003, J. Yang and Huang 2004). Many of these include images to illustrate the suffering of the HIV positive in China, which are sometimes recirculated in discussions on China's micro-blogging (*weibo* 微波) community, and uploaded to *Youku* (忧酷), China's YouTube (For examples, see: Chris 2006, Q. Fu 2007: image numbers. 7, 8, 10, 14, 15, 16, 18, Gao 2007, M. Xiao 2007, M. Shan and Xu 2012).

In blogs and online diaries about HIV that are readily available to the public, HIV-positive Chinese describe how high levels of public anxiety about the virus affect their lives. They frequently face discrimination, rejection at hospitals and anguish over disclosing their seropositivity status to their families for fear of abandonment (UNAIDS, Marie Stopes International China, and Institute of Social Development Research of the China Central Party School 2009: 8). As the HIV-positive author of *Diary of an AIDS Girl*, Zhu Liya, recalled in a documentary about her experience of stigma and discrimination directed and produced by Ruby Yang and Thomas Lennon:

> When I found out I was HIV positive I was given two choices by the University Principal. One was to leave school the other was to take leave (*Julia's Story Trailer* 2005: 00:46). From that evening I couldn't live together with my classmates. I wasn't allowed to dine with them. I couldn't enter the classroom (*Julia's Story* 2005: 2:30). I was numb to everything. At that time it was like I wrapped myself in a dark cloth. I also didn't know when it was light and when it was dark. I went and bought sleeping pills. I didn't take enough and the next day at 4 pm I was resuscitated. (*Julia's Story* 2005: 4:00–4:50)

In China's 2009 *Stigma Index Report*, which was based on interviews with over 2000 HIV positive, only 5 per cent of females and 10 per cent of males said they were able to tell their closest family members and friends about their HIV status (2009: 6). Many had lost their houses, jobs, friends and family (2009: 8). These findings are echoed in the latest report by Asia Catalyst and Korekata AIDS Law Center (2012). Accordingly, stigma and its consequences—from violence to job loss—represent "an indication of the gravity of stigma surrounding HIV" (UNAIDS, Marie Stopes International China office, and Institute of Social Development Research of the China Central Party School 2009: 6), as do the high levels of suffering endured by HIV-positive Chinese. However, there is little research that explains HIV-based suffering as being a consequence of media coverage and of structural factors such as the initial state censorship of HIV stories, its endorsement of commercial blood donation, and the avoidance and underfunding of public health campaigns.

Imagined immunity

Another consequence of media representations of HIV is what I call "imagined immunity" (Hood 2011). Urbanites with some secondary, tertiary, or university education generally feel 'distance' and a lack of risk association with HIV. Many I have spoken to about the virus feel that it is a disease of the 'immoral' and is therefore a problem of others. They thus believe themselves to be 'immune' to catching the virus through their actions, whether these are risky or not (Long 2005, Medical Doctor Net [医药医生网] 2011, China Medical Tribune (医学论坛网) 2012). During my fieldwork in China from 2003 to 2008, audiences at HIV-related events were frequently polled about their understandings and impressions of HIV. At Peking University, Renmin University, Minzu University, and Tsinghua University, students consistently subscribed to the misunderstanding (*wujie* 误解) that HIV was a problem of others (*taren* 他人, *waidiren* 外地人) and not something that could affect them (Jing 2007).

These feelings of distance dominate understandings of personal risk even when those in question understand the transmission paths of the virus and behave in ways they can identify as risky. Others choose to take risks that may lead to contact with the virus, for example commercial female sex workers who decide to not wear condoms because many clients will pay a higher rate for unprotected sex (Huang 2010: 46–7, Zheng 2007). Other factors—fear, for example—inform decisions about whether or not to engage in discriminatory behavior toward HIV-positive people and whether to get tested repeatedly for HIV when contact with the virus is suspected, which I discuss in the next section.

Social panic, AIDS panic, and the kong'ai zu

In addition to the sense of imagined immunity described above, HIV also inspires considerable fear among the general public (Medical Doctor Net [医药医生网] 2011, C. Xu 2012). Such fear is aroused and maintained through local media coverage of HIV, through which stories of the virus are quickly sold and circulated regardless of their accuracy. The country's public health campaigns are often underfunded and ineffective in combating this trend, and although there are exceptions, they have not been effective in creating more effective communication platforms.

Media coverage of the everyday life struggles of HIV positive people and incidents involving HIV-based stigma and discrimination typically characterizes them as having low moral caliber. Coverage also reinforces existing urban Chinese understandings of ethnic minorities such as the Yi and the Uighurs, migrants and residents of inland provinces such as Henan, all of which are seen as vulnerable target groups and vectors of infection in the literature, that is, as more prone to disease.

One widespread fear is of the intentional transmission of HIV via blood, mainly through needle pricking. In 2002, Tianjin newspapers reported a needle pricking in a popular market (Jiaming Li 2002: 193–196). The circulation of this news caused thousands of people to present in hospital emergency rooms with similar claims. In the decade that followed, needle prickings have also been alleged in Beijing, Shanghai, Hangzhou, Tianjin, Xi'an, and Urumqi, although to my knowledge none of the needles in question were confirmed to have been infected with HIV. Like the Tianjin incident, these reports resulted in surges of hospital visits by other people who believe they have been pricked. In the particular case of Urumqi, the story united Han Chinese racism toward ethnic Uighurs with popular fears of HIV. In August 2012, China Central Television reported that a male taxi passenger had sat on a syringe suspected to contain HIV (CCTV 13 News [CCTV 13 新闻] 2012). Unlike the incidents mentioned above, in this case the syringe actually contained the virus. Within days, the story had been cross-posted online and rebroadcasted on many other stations, evidence of the social currency that HIV-related reporting has in China (Jiarui Li 2012, M. Xu 2012). The man's girlfriend was then reported as having requested they terminate their relationship out of fear that she too would be infected (M. Shi 2012), despite the scientific community's repeated statements that the virulence of the virus is significantly diminished when stored outside the body, and that the risk of becoming infected with HIV in such circumstances was minimal (G. Yang 2012).

Also common is the fear of behavior that could not possibly lead to infection, such as working with HIV-positive colleagues or consuming agricultural produce from regions rumored to have high HIV prevalence. For example, in the summer of 2001, many Beijing residents would not buy watermelon from Henan for fear that they would catch HIV from eating it (People's Daily [人民日报] 2001, Y. Li 2001, Medical Doctor Net [医药医生网] 2011). In a 2012 post on HIV infection, *Lucky in Love, [unlucky] in AIDS!* blogger lanbh21 admits in how difficult people find it not to treat someone with HIV differently:

> Everyone understands the logic, but if I put myself in such a position I know perfectly well that I would really struggle to treat someone with AIDS the same as I treat everyone else, you can say that I'm selfish or whatever, but if I look into my conscience, I know that I just can't do it, and anyone who truly could would be a genuinely good person, I'd admire them for it. (http://bbs.tiexue.net/post_5677348_1.html)

These and other examples of discrimination and public panic over HIV transmission have led to the diagnosis of the specific AIDS-related phobia or psychological condition which has been dubbed "AIDS panic" (*aizibing kongjuzheng*), with those suffering from it being known as the *kong'ai zu* or the *kong'ai min,* as discussed at the outset of this chapter. The earliest instance of the condition is recorded in scientific literature as "the worried well of AIDS" 2004 (J. Wang et al. 2004) but recorded outpatient cases have increased exponentially thereafter (F. Wang, Li, and Yue 2006; J. Fu et al. 2008; C. Wu 2009, Y. Xiao 2009; Y. Liu and

Shao 2010). The Chinese equivalent of Wikipedia offers references to many recent incidences as well (Baidu Encyclopedia [百度百科] 2012).

Conclusion

In view of the recent and increasing diagnosis and prevalence of the *kong'ai zu* (AIDS panickers) and *kong'ai zheng* (AIDS phobia), it is important to look closely at HIV media and the role it plays in shaping public perceptions. In this chapter I have examined the trends in HIV media representations and the public health role this plays in China. As I have described, China's stories about HIV communicate the impacts of HIV infection using particular kinds of people who often lack access to treatment. Over time, HIV has been embodied first by gay EuroAmericans and Black Africans, and later, by disadvantaged rural Chinese, minority folk, and other 'undesirable' types of people. The outcome is that the media has created a class of sufferers who are marked for their low social standing, their low quality, and their terrifying lack of health and social exclusion. Chinese leaders now espouse a rhetoric of care and recognition of the HIV positive, which they demonstrate by, for example, shaking hands with the HIV positive on World AIDS Day, or spending time in AIDS villages over the Chinese Spring Festival. Despite this, the effects of the media I have explored are longstanding and detrimental to population health and well-being. This embodiment of HIV and the reporting on its geosocial prevalence have driven problematic and contradictory sentiments of fear of and distance from HIV among urban Chinese.

China's case shows the importance of placing popular understandings of HIV within local knowledge of health and illness, and also within local cultures of representation. The longstanding impact that representations of HIV have had on China's public health, and on the discriminatory attitudes toward HIV positive should be taken into account by anyone overseeing communication strategies in public media and health advertisement strategies. Although in China HIV/ AIDS already receives exceptionally—and disproportionately—large amounts of external funding and attention in comparison to diseases that pose greater public health challenges such as TB and hepatitis, the latest biomedical research on future HIV trends in China advises that further investment be made in prevention (Jinghua Li et al. 2012). Yet, as I have shown in this chapter, any attempt to improve prevention messages within the medical and social science communities must consider the negative public health outcomes that HIV representations over the past three decades have had in China. Well-grounded communication strategies that address the visual culture and communication history of the virus will be key to the efficacy of any continued investment in prevention.

Filmography

*AIDS: The Super Epidemic (*超级瘟疫: 艾滋病*)* (dir. Shanghai Population and Family Planning Center, 1990).

*AIDS: Threatening the Chinese (*威胁中国人的艾滋病*)* (dir. The City of Shanghai Birth Control Planning Propaganda and Education Center,1996).

HIV/AIDS Public Service Announcements. (dir. Ruby Yang, 2002-2012).

*Julia's Story (*朱利亚的故事*).* (dir. Ruby Yang, 2005).

Julia's Story Trailer. (dir. Ruby Yang, 2005).

Migrant Workers PSA (dir. Ruby Yang, 2006).

*Together (*在一起*)* (dir. Zhao Liang, 2010). Available at: http://www.youtube.com/watch?v=waYsH_wYpgs.

*The epic of central plains: A story about the central plains farmers and HIV/AIDS (*中原纪事:关于中原农民和艾滋病的故事*)* (dir. Ai Xiaomin, 2006).

Bibliography

99 Healthnet *(99* 健康网*).* 2010c. Suspecting AIDS: the symptoms of AIDS panic (怀疑染艾滋:恐艾症的表现). [Online, 24 November, AIDS section]. Available at: http://www.99.com.cn/azb/zzzd/77335.htm [accessed: 12 August 2012].

Anagnost, A. 2006. Strange circulations: the blood economy in rural China. *Economy and Society*, 35(4), 509–529.

Asia Catalyst, and Korekata AIDS Law Center. 2012. *China's Blood Disaster: The Way Forward* [Online: Asia Catalyst and Korekata AIDS Law]. Available at: http://asiacatalyst.org/blog/2012/03/china–compensate–hiv–blood–disaster–victims.html [accessed: 4 April 2012].

Bai, S. 1995. The tragedy of homosexuals (同性恋的悲剧). *Southern Weekend* (南方周末), May 19: 5.

Baidu Encyclopedia (百度百科). 2012h. *AIDS panic (*艾滋病恐惧症*)* [Online:]. Available at: http://baike.baidu.com/view/5493614.htm [accessed: 10 January 2013].

Ballentine, P., and Sofer, K. 2012. *China's 2012 Party Leadership Transition: Key Faces to Watch.* Washington, DC: Center for American Progress. [Online] Available at: http://www.americanprogress.org/wp–content/uploads/issues/2012/08/pdf/china_profiles.pdf [accessed: 4 September 2012].

Beijing Yirenping Center. 2008. *The First Case Against Hepatitis Discrimination Opens in Court for Second Time (*乙肝歧视反诉第一案第2次开庭通知*).* [Online: Yirenping Center (益仁平中心)]. Available at: http://www.yirenping.org/article.asp?id=177 [accessed: 30 September 2008].

Blum, S.D. 2001. *Portraits of "Primitives": Ordering Human Kinds in the Chinese Nation.* Lanham, Maryland: Rowman & Littlefield.

Cai, P. 2012. Time for China to bottle up its Gini. Sydney Morning Herald [Online, February 27, World Business section] Available at: http://www.smh.com.au/business/world–business/time–for–china–to–bottle–up–the–gini–20120227–1txxs.html [accessed: 3 March 2012].

Carter, M. 2012. Combination prevention approach could have a big impact on HIV epidemic in China. *Aidsmap HIV & AIDS – Sharing Knowledge, Changing Lives.* [Online] Available at: www.aidsmap.com/Combination–prevention–approach–could–have–a–big–impact–on–HIV–epidemic–in–China/page/2441682/ [accessed: 10 August 2012].

CCTV 13 News (CCTV 13 新闻). 2012d. Man takes taxi pricked by needle possibly containing HIV (男子打车被扎针头或含HIV病毒). [Online, 25 August, *24 Hours (24小时)* section, news report video]. Available at: http://video.sina.com.cn/p/news/s/v/2012–08–25/003561849279.html [accessed: 25 August 2012].

Central Intelligence Agency. 2012. *The World Factbook China.* Washington, DC: Central Intelligence Agency Press. [Online]. Available at: https://www.cia.gov/library/publications/the–world–factbook/geos/ch.html [accessed: 4 October 2012].

Chan, A., Madsen, R., and Unger, J. 1984. *Chen Village: The Recent History of a Peasant Community in Mao's China.* Berkeley and Los Angeles: University of California Press.

Chen, B. 2010. *Open Letter to the General Secretary of the Chinese Communist Party Hu Jintao (*致中共中央总书记国家主席胡锦涛的公开*)* [Online, Beijing Aizhixing Institute]. Available at: http://aidslaw2010.blogspot.com.au/2010_11_01_archive.html [accessed: 1 December 2010].

Chen, Guidi, and Chun, T. 2004. *An Investigative Report on the Chinese Peasantry (*中国农民调查*).* Beijing: Renmin wenxue chubanshe.

Chen, Lei, Jiang, H., Yi, L., and Zhao, J. 2004. China's AIDS heroes (中国抗艾英雄). *Southern People Weekly (*南方人物周刊*),* December 1, 18–39.

*China Daily (*中国日报网*).* 2012f. Examining the degree of our country's hepatitis–based discrimination (看看我国乙肝歧视有多严重). [Online, 31 October, Health (名医频道) section] Available at: http://www.chinadaily.com.cn/jiankang/yg/yiganqishi/84127.html [accessed: 10 November 2012].

*China Medical Tribune (*医学论坛网*).* 2012g. Social humanities and ethical issues of AIDS research (艾滋病的社会人文和道德问题研究). [Online, 21 November] Available at: http://www.cmt.com.cn/detail/99181.html [accessed: 7 January 2013].

China Ministry of Health, and Department of Hygiene and Infectious Disease Prevention. 1988. *Manual for AIDS Prevention.* Beijing: Chinese Science and Technology Press.

China Ministry of Health. 2010. *The work and progress of China's hepatitis B prevention and control strategies (*中国乙肝防控策略和工作进展*)* [Online, Beijing: Ministry of Health. Available at: http://www.moh.gov.cn/publicfiles/

business/htmlfiles/mohjbyfkzj/s3582/201004/46912.htm [accessed: 18 July 2011].

Chris. 2006. Lu Guang and AIDS Villages (卢广与艾滋病村). *Public Good China (*公益中国) [Online, 27 October, repost of HIV/AIDS images and text] Available at: http://www.pubchn.com/blog/pubchn/articles/28020.htm [accessed: 1 December 2006].

Couzin, O. 2007. 2006/2007 China HIV/AIDS Directory (2006/2007 中国艾滋病名录). Beijing: China AIDS Info, AIDS Care China, China HIV/AIDS Information Network, Pengyou Tongxin.

Cui, L. 1992. China, Tanzania co-operate in AIDS treatment. *Beijing Review* 35(5-6), 38–41.

Dong, Y. 2006. Captured petty thief uses 'AIDS syringe' to escape police squadron (小偷行窃失手被抓 狂舞'艾滋'针逃出重围). *Xinhua News Online (*新华网 *news* [Online, 12 September, photo news section]. Available at: http://www.cq.xinhuanet.com/photonews/2006–09/12/content_8015980.htm [accessed: 21 March 2007].

Erwin, K. 2006. The circulatory system: blood procurement, AIDS, and the social body in China. *Medical Anthropology Quarterly* [Online], 20(2), 139–159. doi:10.1525/maq.2006.20.2.139.

Fan, M. 2007. Among Chinese, fear and prejudice about hepatitis B: job discrimination is widespread in land with 120 million carriers. *Washington Post*, 12 February, A15.

Fang, X., and Yu, L. 2012. Government refuses to release gini coefficient. *CaixinOnline* [Online, 18 January, Top Stories Politics section] Available at: http://english.caixin.com/2012–01–18/100349814.html [accessed: 20 January 2012].

Farmer, P. 1996. On suffering and structural violence: a view from below. *Daedalus* 125(1), 261–283.

Floyd, K., Baddeley, A., Dias, H.M., Falzon, D., Fitzpatrick, D., Gilpin, C., Glaziou, P., et al. 2011. *Global Tuberculosis Control 2011*. [Online: World Health Organization]. Available at: http://www.who.int/tb/publications/global_report/2011/en/index.html [accessed: 9 August 2012].

Fu, J., Ma, Y., Song, Y., and Li, J. 2008. Analyzing cases of AIDS panic in STD outpatient clinics (性病门诊艾滋病恐惧症病例分析). China Healthcare Frontiers (中国医疗前沿), 3(22), 93.

Fu, Q. 2007. Fearful shock — patients with AIDS (恐怖震撼——发病的艾滋病人). *Pinghu Community Forum of the Three Gorges Media Net (*平湖社区三峡传媒网旗下论坛). [Online, 1 August, Repost of HIV/AIDS images and text]. Available at: http://bbs.sxcm.net/forum.php?mod=viewthread&tid=35535 [accessed: 1 September 2009].

Gao, Y. 2007. The mirror can't lie: the reality of AIDS villages part one (镜头不会撒谎: 艾滋病村的真相(一). QQ. *Gao Yaojie's Blog*. [Online] Available at: http://qz.qq.com/622006522/blog?uin=622006522&vin=0&blogid=0&page=3 [accessed: 2 April 2008].

Gao, Y., Shang, H. and Guo, M. eds. 2003. STDs, AIDS: Knowing Through Stories (鲜为人的故事 - 艾滋病,性病防治大众读本). Zhengzhou, Henan: Hongyuan Farmer's Press.

Guo, G. 1997. Taking on the bloodselling market (直击卖血市场). *Southern Weekend (南方周末)*, 21 March.

Heinrich, L. 2008. *The Afterlife of Images: Translating the Pathological Body Between China and the West.* Durham, NC and London: Duke University Press.

Hodgson, A. 2012. *Special Report: Income Inequality Rising Across the Globe.* London, UK: Euromonitor International. [Online]. Available at: http://blog. euromonitor.com/2012/03/special–report–income–inequality–rising–across– the–globe.html [accessed: 20 May 2012].

Hood, J. 2011. *HIV/AIDS, Health and the Media in China: Imagined Immunity through Racialized Disease.* London and New York: Routledge.

———. 2012. China's AIDS underclass (Aimin): preserving power and inequality through media portrayals of HIV/AIDS. PhD diss., University of Technology Sydney.

Hossain, S.I. 1998. *Tackling Health Transition in China.* Washington, DC: The World Bank.

Hou, Y. 2009. *The Price of Development: A Collection of Research Papers on the Harm of Illicit Drugs and HIV in Areas of Ethnic Minorities in Western China* (发展的代价西部少数民族毒宾的伤害和艾滋病问题). Beijing: Central University of Ethnic Nationalities Press.

Huan, J. 2010. Ethnicity and gender in social research on HIV in China, in *HIV in China: Understanding the Social Aspects of the Epidemic*, edited by J. Jing and H. Worth. Sydney, NSW: UNSW Press, 196–214.

Huang, Y. 2010. Female sex workers in China: their occupational concerns, in *HIV in China: Understanding the Social Aspects of the Epidemic*, edited by J. Jing and H. Worth. Sydney, NSW: UNSW Press, 43–66.

Hyde, S.T. 2007. *Eating Spring Rice: The Cultural Politics of AIDS in Southwest China.* Berkeley and Los Angeles: University of California Press.

International Public Relations Network. 2012b. *Blue Focus PR Consulting: Hepatitis B Awareness Campaign* [Online:]. Available at: http://www.iprn. com/members/bluefocus//profile [accessed: 10 July 2012].

Jacka, T. 2009. Cultivating citizens: *suzhi* (quality) discourse in the PRC. *Positions: East Asia Cultures Critique* 17(3), 523–535.

Jacobs, A. 2009. HIV tests turn blood into cash in China. *The New York Times* [Online, 3 December, Health/Health Care Policy section]. Available at: http:// www.nytimes.com/2009/12/03/health/policy/03china.html [accessed: 3 December 2012].

Jiang, X., and Wang, S. 2009. *Special Report: Hepatitis B Carriers Challenge Discrimination.* [Online: Global Times (环球时报), 10 September]. Available at: http://special.globaltimes.cn/2009–09/471637.html [accessed: 29 December 2009].

Jin, W. 2002. The AIDS Iceberg and This Century's 'Titanic' (艾滋病冰山和本世纪的'泰坦尼克号'). *Xinmin Weekly (*新民周刊), 22 July, 20-25.

Jing, J. 2006. The social origin of AIDS panics in China, in *AIDS and Social Policy in China*, edited by J. Kaufman, A. Kleinman, and A. Saich. Cambridge, MA: Harvard University Asia Center, 176–193.

———. 2007. AIDS and Chinese society (艾滋病与中国社会). Public lecture given at the Central University for Nationalities (民族大学) East Humanities Building, 28 March.

———. 2010. Drugs, HIV and Chinese youth, in *HIV in China: Understanding the Social Aspects of the Epidemic*, edited by J. Jing and H. Worth. Sydney, NSW: UNSW Press, 67–100.

Jing, J. and Worth, H. 2010. An overview of China's HIV epidemic, in *HIV in China: Understanding the Social Aspects of the Epidemic*, edited by J. Jing and H. Worth. Sydney, NSW: UNSW Press, 11–42.

*Jinling Hotline (*金陵热线). 2009. Drunken man [has unprotected sex] and falls into a cycle of AIDS panic: all 'AIDS–phobic citizens' are of high quality (酒后放纵他陷入恐艾怪圈: 恐艾族很多是高素质). [Online, 1 December] Available at: http://www.jlonline.com/news/nanjing/2009–12–01/25817.html [accessed: 15 December 2010].

Kleinman, A. 1999. Experience and Its Moral Modes: Culture, Human Conditions, and Disorder, presented at the Tanner Lectures on Human Values, April 13, Stanford University. Available at: http://tannerlectures.utah.edu/lectures/documents/Kleinman99.pdf [accessed, 12 October 2005].

Kleinman, A., Das, V., and Lock, M. 1996. Introduction. *Daedalus* 125(1), xi–xx.

Kleinman, A., Das, V., and Lock, M., eds. 1997. *Social Suffering*. Berkeley, CA: University of California Press.

Lai, W., Yu, H., Luo, Y., Li, T., Liu, L., Zhou, J., Qin, G. and Zhang, L. 2011. Survival Analysis for AIDS Patients in Sichuan Province After Antiretroviral Therapy (四川省艾滋病抗病毒治疗患者生存时间分析). *Chinese Journal of Public Health (*中国公共卫生) 27(12) (December): 1521–1522. Available at: http://en.cnki.com.cn/Article_en/CJFDTOTAL–XBYA201103009.htm [accessed: 25 March 2012].

lanbh21 2012. Lucky in love, [unlucky] in AIDS! (撞了桃花运,得了艾滋病!) tiexue community (铁血社区) [Online, post, 2012] Available at: http://bbs.tiexue.net/post_5677348_1.html [accessed: 17 September 2012].

lanbh21 2012. Lucky in love, [unlucky] in AIDS! (撞了桃花运,得了艾滋病!) *tiexue community (*铁血社区) [Online, post, 2012] Available at: http://bbs.tiexue.net/post_5677348_1.html [accessed: 17 September 2012].

Levine, R. 2007. Case 3: controlling tuberculosis in China, in *Case Studies in Global Health: Millions Saved*. Sudbury, MA: Jones & Bartlett and The Centre for Global Development, 1–8.

Li, J. 2002. *The Last Declaration of War (*最后的宣战). Tianjin: Tianjin People's Press.

Li, Jiarui. 2012. Beijing security investigate case of taxi passenger pricked by needle and suspected to be infected by HIV virus (北京警方调查出租车乘客被扎疑似感染艾滋事件). *Beijing Evening Post (*北京晚报*)* [Online, 25 August]. Available at: http://news.sina.com.cn/c/2012–08–25/133925035410.shtml [accessed: 25 August 2012].

Li, Jinghua., Gilmour, S., Zhang, H., Koyanagi, A. and Shibuya, K. 2012. The Epidemiological Impact and Cost–effectiveness of HIV Testing, Antiretroviral Treatment and Harm Reduction Programs in China. *Aids* (July), 1. doi:10.1097/QAD.0b013e3283574e54.

Li, Q. 2003. Yongcheng: blood debacle investigation (永城血祸调查). *Xinmin Weekly (*新民周刊*)*, 30 July, 15–21.

Li, X., and Zhou, M., eds. 2005. *HIV/AIDS Media Reader (*艾滋病媒体读本*)*. Beijing: Tsinghua University Press.

Li, Y. 2001. The Shocking 'Plasma Economy'—interviewing Henan's 'AIDS Villages' (骇人的'血浆经济'——走访河南'艾滋病村'). *Sanlian Lifestyle Weekly (*三联生活周刊*)* [Online, 5 September]. Available at: http://www.cctv.com/special/289/2/25967.html [accessed: 3 October 2002].

Lin, V. 2012. Transformations in the healthcare system in China. *Current Sociology* 60 (July 4), 427–440. doi:10.1177/0011392112438329.

Liu, S. 2011. *Passage to Manhood: Youth Migration, Heroin, and AIDS in Southwest China*. Stanford, CA: Stanford University Press.

Liu, Y. 2004. Henan: Provincial cadres come to AIDS villages (河南: 艾滋村里来了干部)." *Newsweek (*新闻周刊*)*, 1 March.

Liu, Y. 2010. The urgent need to control STDs and HIV/AIDS (控制性病艾滋病刻不容缓). *The Chinese Journal of Human Sexuality (*中国性科学*)*, 11, 3.

Liu, Y., and Shao, C. 2010. 'AIDS–phobic Citizens': How to Get over Feelings of 'AIDS Phobia' ('恐艾族'怎样克服恐艾心理). *Shenzhen Special Zone Daily (*深圳特区报*)* [Online, 2 December] Available at: http://www.chinadaily.com.cn/hqss/jiankang/2010–12–02/content_1322210_2.html [accessed: 8 December 2010].

Liu, Y., Rao, K., and Hsiao, W.C. 2003. Medical expenditure and rural impoverishment in China. *Journal of Health and Population Nutrition*, 21(3), 216–222.

Liu, Z. 2003. AIDS lawsuits and blood transfusion phobia (艾滋病官司与输血恐惧). *Newsweek (*新闻周刊*)*, 11 August.

Long, Q. 2005. Getting away from AIDS knowledge misunderstandings: problems of AIDS ≠ problems of morality (走出艾滋认识误区 艾滋病问题≠道德问题). *Southern Daily (*南方日报*)* [Online, 6 December]. Available at: http://health.sohu.com/20051206/n240885156.shtml [accessed: 7 December 2012].

Ma, X., Zhang, J., Meessen, B., Decoster, K., Tang, X., Yang Y., and Ren, X. 2011. Social health assistance schemes: the case of medical financial assistance for the rural poor in four counties of China. *International Journal for Equity in Health* 10(44), 1–13.

*Medical Doctor Net (*医药医生网*)*. 2011c. Misunderstandings cause AIDS panic (误导引起对艾滋病的恐慌). [Online, 9 September, Social Concern (社会关爱) section] Available at: http://www.yywsb.com/lx/lxlist,896079.html [accessed: 10 September 2011].

Ministry of Health. 2010a. *Fifth National Tuberculosis Epidemiological Survey.* Beijing.

*People's Daily (*人民日报*)* . 2001. How did 'AIDS watermelons' cause such a stir? ('艾滋西瓜'是如何成熟的?). [Online, 6 July, Friday edition] Available at: http://www.renminbao.com/rmb/articles/2001/7/6/14261p.html [accessed: 12 February 2004].

*People's Daily Online (*人民网*)*. 2011a. 500 million suspected to carry tuberculosis virus. [Online, 23 March, China Society section] Available at: http://english. peopledaily.com.cn/90001/90776/90882/7329035.html [accessed: 28 May 2011].

Qi, Y. 1997. Bloodstand (血站). *Southern Weekend (*南方周末*)*, 17 July.

*Qilu.net (*齐鲁网*)*. 2012c. Man uses bottle of blood [said to be] infected with HIV in attempt to extort millions of RMB from hotel (男子用瓶装艾滋病血液敲诈酒店百万元). [Online, 25 August, *Lifestyle (*生活*)* section, news report video] Available at: http://video.sina.com.cn/p/news/s/v/2012–08–25/003561849279. html#61796641 [accessed: 4 September 2012].

Schein, L. 2002. *Minority Rules: The Miao and the Feminine in China's Cultural Politics.* Durham, NC: Duke University Press.

*Science and Technology of Family (*家庭科技*)*. 2012a. How to get over AIDS phobia (如何克服恐艾症).

Serlin, D. 2012. Introduction, in *Imagining Illness: Public Health and Visual Culture*, edited by D. Serlin. Minneapolis, MN: University of Minnesota Press, xi–xxxvii.

Shan, J. 2012. HIV Rises Sharply Among Chinese 50 and Older. *China Daily (*中国日报网*)* [Online, 23 August]. Available at: http://www.chinadaily.com.cn/ china/2012–08/23/content_15699324.htm [accessed: 24 August 2012].

Shan, M., and Xu, Y. 2012. Bitter Grass: Investigating Yunnan's HIV Positive Sex Workers《苦草》 云南艾滋性工作者调查. *Tengxun net (*腾讯网*)* [Online, photojournalism section, *Life in the Underworld (*地下人生*)*]. Available at: http://news.qq.com/photon/huozhe/kucao1bf.htm [accessed: 1 September 2012].

Shao, J. 2006. Fluid labor and blood money: the economy of HIV/AIDS in rural central China. *Cultural Anthropology* 21(4), 535–569.

Shao, J., and Scoggin, M. 2009. Solidarity and distinction in blood: contamination, morality and variability. *Body and Society* 15(2), 29–49. doi:10.1177/1357034X09103436.

Shao, Y. 2001. AIDS in South and Southeast Asia. HIV/AIDS: Perspective on China. AIDS Patient Care and STDs 14(8), 431–2.

Shen, H. 1997. Undercover investigation to Dianxi AIDS village (秘访滇西艾滋病村). *Southern Weekend (*南方周末*)*, 3 October, 1–2.

Shi, J., Zhi, R., and Li, F. 1991. Yunnan HIV poster series: preventing AIDS: protecting your family's prosperity, guaranteeing your body's health (预防 艾滋病: 维护家庭幸福, 保障身体健康). Public Health Poster. Kunming: Yunnan People's Press.

Shi, M. 2012. Taxi passenger pricked by needle likely to contain HIV (针头扎 伤打车乘客或含HIV病毒). *The Beijing News (*新京报*)* [Online, 24 August, Beijing News (北京新闻) section]. Available http://epaper.bjnews.com.cn/html/2012-08/24/content_366901.htm?div=-1 [accessed: 27 August 2012].

Siu, H.F., and Faure, D. 1995. Introduction, in *Down to Earth: The Territorial Bond in South China*, edited by H. F. Siu and D. Faure. Stanford: Stanford University Press, 1–20.

Stan, A. 2012. What's causing the spike in HIV infection in old Chinese men? Comment on research results. *Business Insider Contributor*. [Online, 23 August] Available at: http://mobile.businessinsider.com/whats–causing–the–spike–in–hiv–infection–in–old–chinese–men–2012–8 [accessed: 24 August 2012].

Su, C. 2010. 'Red oil': blood and the role of a machine in the HIV outbreak in central China, in *HIV in China: Understanding the Social Aspects of the Epidemic*, edited by J. Jing and H. Worth. Sydney, NSW: UNSW Press, 101–116.

Sullivan, S.G., Xu, J., Feng, Y., Su, S., Chen, X., Ding, X., Gao, Y., Dou, Z., and Wu, Z. 2010. Stigmatizing attitudes and behaviors toward PLHA in rural China. *AIDS Care* 22(1), 104–111. doi:10.1080/09540120903012528.

Sun, W., and Guo, Y. 2012. Introduction. In *Unequal China: The Political Economy and Cultural Politics of Inequality*, edited by W. Sun and Y. Guo, 1–26. New York and London: Routledge.

The Economist. 2012. Bad blood: in central China AIDS activists step up pressure on the government. [Online, 8 September] Available at: http://www.economist.com/node/21562241 [accessed: 8 September 2012].

The World Bank News. 2010b. Feature story. China: tuberculosis control project. [Online, 24 September, News and Views section]. Available at: http://www.worldbank.org/en/news/2010/09/24/china–tuberculosis–control–project0 [accessed: 20 August 2012].

The World Bank. 2011d. *China – tuberculosis control project*. Implementation Completion and Results Report. Washington, DC: The World Bank.

UNAIDS, China AIDS Media Project, Ogilvy, and Global Business Council. 2008. *AIDS–Related Knowledge, Attitudes, Behavior, and Practices: A Survey of Six Chinese Cities*. KAPB. Beijing: UNAIDS China.

UNAIDS, Marie Stopes International China office, and Institute of Social Development Research of the China Central Party School. 2009. *The China Stigma Index Report*. Beijing: UNAIDS China.

UNAIDS. 2011. *Highly Vulnerable Transport Sector Needs Effective HIV Programmes*. [Online: UNAIDS, 11 July, Feature Stories section] Available at: http://www.unaids.org/en/resources/presscentre/featurestories/2011/july/20110711transporthiv/ [accessed: 1 December 2011].

Unger, J., and Him C. 2012. The Guangdong Model: Collective Village Land, Urbanization, and the Making of a New Middle Class. *The Urbanization of Rural China*. Available at: http://www.eastasiaforum.org/2012/05/18/guangdong–collective–land–ownership–and–the–making–of–a–new–middle–class/ [accessed: 8 September 2012].

United Nations Theme Group on HIV/AIDS. 2002. *China's Titanic Peril: 2001 Update of the AIDS Situation and Needs Assessment Report*. Beijing: Joint United Nations Programme on HIV/AIDS UNAIDS, UNICEF, UNDP, UNFPA, UNDCP, ILO, UNESCO, WHO, WORLD BANK.

Wan, Q. 2004. Wu Yi: the first vice-premier to enter epidemic area (吴仪: 第一位进入疫区的副总理). *Southern People Weekly (*南方人物周刊*)*, 1 December, 20-21.

Wan, Y., and Beijing Aizhixing Institute. 2011. *Review of China's Response to Recommendations Raised during the UPR of Feb 2009*. Vancouver: Beijing Aizhixing Institute.

Wan, Y., Hu, R., Guo R., and Arnade, L. 2009. Discrimination against people with HIV/AIDS in China. *The Equal Rights Review* 4, 1–25.

Wang, J., Wang, S., Lin, X., Su, W., Chen, H., and Wu, H. 2004. The first explorative study on the worried well of AIDS (艾滋病恐惧症的研究初探). *Advances in Psychological Science* （心理科学进展*)* 12(2), 435-439.

Wang, F., Li, Y., and Yue, J. 2006. Number of 'AIDS panickers' far exceeds that of HIV positive: fear practically causing collapse ('恐艾症'远多于艾滋病感染者:让人濒临崩溃). *Xiaoxiang Morning Post (*潇湘晨报*)* [Online, 28 November] Available at: http://hn.rednet.cn/c/2006/11/28/1042045.htm [accessed: 2 December 2006].

Wang, J. 2012. Going viral: hepatitis sufferers need to make their voices heard. *South China Morning Post*, 13 March, Health section, 5-8.

World Health Organization. 2011b. Public health round–up. *Bulletin of the World Health Organization* 89 (7) (July 1): 472–473.

Wu, C. 2001. Gao Yaojie: AIDS blankets Henan (高耀洁: 河南艾滋病已无空白点). *Newsweek (*新闻周刊*)*, 28 May, 30-34.

Wu, C. 2009. What symptoms does AIDS panic have? (恐艾症有什么症状?). *Aids.39.net* [Online, 7 October, chat room (社区) section]. Available at: http://aids.39.net/yf/cs/0910/7/1018769.html [accessed: 11 July 2011].

Xia, G., and Yang, X. 2005. HIV/AIDS-related knowledge, attitudes, and behaviors among commercial sex workers and their clients (商业性性小姐艾滋病认识态度与行为调查). *Society (*社会*)* 5, 167–187.

Xia, Z. 2012. AIDS rape crime causes alarm (艾滋病患者强奸恩人,另类犯罪理由令人警醒). *Women's Life (*妇女生活*)*, 6.

Xiao, M. 2007. The mirror can't lie: the reality of AIDS villages (part one) (镜头不会撒谎：艾滋病村的真相(一). *Hanjiang Community (*汉江社区*)*. [Online, repost of HIV/AIDS images and text] Available at: http://www.hjsq.cn/thread–25847–1–1.html [accessed: 1 December 2008].

Xiao, Y. 2009. 'AIDS panic' recently made me wish I was dead ('恐艾症'曾让我痛不欲生). *Healthy Lifestyle (*健康生活*)*.

Xu, Chi. 2012. Landlord forces volunteers to close free AIDS shelter. *Shanghai Daily*, [Online, 17 September, Nation section]. Available at: http://www.shanghaidaily.com/article/print.asp?id=511980 [accessed: 17 September 2012].

Xu, Ming. 2012. Taxi AIDS needle incident. Passenger encounters unfortunate AIDS needle surprise. Why rumors fly. (出租车艾滋针乘出租车遭艾滋针袭击谣言为何满天飞). *Jiangnan Capital Post (*江南都市报*)* [Online, 27 August] Available at: http://www.banzhu.com/article/1494736 [accessed: 28 August 2012].

Xu, Weiwei. 2012. HIV Infection in old Chinese men rises. *Morning Whistle* [Online. 23 August, Politics and Society section]. Available at: http://www.morningwhistle.com/html/2012/PoliticsSociety_0823/213649.html [accessed: 24 August 2008].

Yan, L. 2006. *Ding Village Dream (*丁庄梦*)*. Shanghai: Shanghai Literature and Arts Press.

Yang, G. 2012. How to dispel suspicions over HIV needle prickings? (驱散出租车上的艾滋疑云被'艾滋针'扎伤该怎么办?). *Familydoctor Online (*家庭医生在线*)* [Online, 3 September] Available at: http://jkkt.familydoctor.com.cn/a/201209/52713994817.html [accessed: 12 November 2012].

Yang, J., and Huang, J. 2004. Houyang, the silence of being just two kilometers away (后杨,两公里外的沉寂). *Xinmin Weekly (*新民周刊*)*, 7 June, 20-21.

Yang, M.M.H. 2002. Mass media and transnational subjectivity in Shanghai: notes on (re)cosmopolitanism in a Chinese metropolis, in *Media Worlds: Anthropology on New Terrain*, edited by F. Ginsburg, L. Abu-loghod, and B. Larkin. Berkeley and Los Angeles: University of California Press, 189–210.

Ye, X., and Chun, Y. 2012. Experts: chronic disease, a critical issue in China. *People's Daily Online (*人民网*)* [Online, 20 September, English edition, Life and Culture section]. Available: http://english.peopledaily.com.cn/90782/7954814.html# [accessed: 20 September 2012].

Yun, L., Trout, S., Lu, K., and Creswell, J.W. 2005. The needs of AIDS-infected individuals in rural China. *Qualitative Health Research* 15(9), 1149–1163. doi:10.1177/1049732305276690.

Zhang, K. 2005. *Five Year Survey on AIDS in Henan Province (*河南艾滋病五年调查报告*)*. Beijing: Beijing You'an Hospital, AFAO, UNICEF, China-UK AIDS Foundation.

Zhang, Xiuzhen. 2012. AIDS Panic: don't overlook this psychological disorder (恐艾症不可忽视心理疾病). *Health Guide (*健康向导*)*.

Zhang, Yuhui. 2012. The development of non-communicable disease accounts for China. Understanding how different diseases impact on health expenditure. Research presentation given at Seminar Room 2, Ann Harding Conference Centre, Building 24, University Drive South, Bruce, Australian Capital Territory, 3 July.

Zhao, X., Yao, N., and Kang, L. 2005. Ending 'the plasma economy' (终结'血浆经济'). *Cai Jing (财经)* [Online, 2 May] Available at: http://magazine.caijing.com.cn/2005-05-02/110064242.html [accessed: 8 May 2005].

Zhao, Y., Xu, S., Wang, L., Chin, D.P., Wang, S., Jiang, G., Xia, H. et al. 2012. National survey of drug-resistant tuberculosis in China. *New England Journal of Medicine* 366(23), 2161–2170. doi:10.1056/NEJMoa1108789.

Zheng, T. 2007. Aizhi Dajiangtang (爱知大讲堂). Public presentation and guest lecture presented at the Aizi Dajiangtang, Central University for Nationalities. Beijing, East Wenzou Bldg 0101, 7 June.

Zhou, S. 2007. *Crying Out for Sunshine: The AIDS Community You Don't Understand* (呼唤阳光一你不了解的艾滋病群落). Beijing: Ancient Chinese Medicinal Book Press.

Zhu, Y. 2001. Henan's Wenlou village unexpectedly has 241 people infected with AIDS! Blame solely on illegal blood collection (河南文楼村竟有241人染艾滋!都是非法采血惹的祸). *Sohu.com (搜狐)* [Online, 23 August] Available at: http://news.sohu.com/45/99/news146359945.shtml [accessed: 27 November 2008].

Zhuang, K. 2005. Revelation of the Tiger's Day initiative in the Yi ethnic region of Xiaoliangshan (小梁山彝族虎日民间戒毒行动和人类学的实践). *Journal of Guangxi University for Nationalities (广西民族学院学报)* 27(2), 38–47.

Zhuang, K., and Hua, W. 2002. *Tiger Day (虎日)*. Documentary. Beijing: Institute for Anthropology, Renmin University of China. [Online] Available at: http://v.youku.com/v_show/id_XNDc3NTU3NzY4.html [accessed: 27 February 2007].

Index

Page numbers in italics indicate figures.